Violence among the Mentally Ill

NATO Science Series

A Series presenting the results of activities sponsored by the NATO Science Committee. The Series is published by IOS Press and Kluwer Academic Publishers, in conjunction with the NATO Scientific Affairs Division.

A. Life Sciences	IOS Press
B. Physics	Kluwer Academic Publishers
C. Mathematical and Physical Sciences	Kluwer Academic Publishers
D. Behavioural and Social Sciences	Kluwer Academic Publishers
E. Applied Sciences	Kluwer Academic Publishers
F. Computer and Systems Sciences	IOS Press
1. Disarmament Technologies	Kluwer Academic Publishers
2. Environmental Security	Kluwer Academic Publishers
3. High Technology	Kluwer Academic Publishers
4. Science and Technology Policy	IOS Press
5. Computer Networking	IOS Press

NATO-PCO-DATA BASE

The NATO Science Series continues the series of books published formerly in the NATO ASI Series. An electronic index to the NATO ASI Series provides full bibliographical references (with keywords and/or abstracts) to more than 50000 contributions from international scientists published in all sections of the NATO ASI Series.
Access to the NATO-PCO-DATA BASE is possible via CD-ROM "NATO-PCO-DATA BASE" with user-friendly retrieval software in English, French and German (WTV GmbH and DATAWARE Technologies Inc. 1989).

The CD-ROM of the NATO ASI Series can be ordered from: PCO, Overijse, Belgium

Series D: Behavioural and Social Sciences – Vol. 90

Violence among the Mentally Ill
Effective Treatments and Management Strategies

edited by

Sheilagh Hodgins

Université de Montréal,
Montréal, Quebec, Canada
and
Karolinska Institute,
Stockholm, Sweden

Kluwer Academic Publishers

Dordrecht / Boston / London

Published in cooperation with NATO Scientific Affairs Division

Proceedings of the NATO Advanced Study Institute on
Effective Prevention of Crime and Violence among Persons with Major Mental Disorders
Il Ciocco, Italy
16-26 May 1999

A C.I.P. Catalogue record for this book is available from the Library of Congress.

ISBN 0-7923-6437-6 (HB)
ISBN 0-7923-6438-4 (PB)

Published by Kluwer Academic Publishers,
P.O. Box 17, 3300 AA Dordrecht, The Netherlands.

Sold and distributed in North, Central and South America
by Kluwer Academic Publishers,
101 Philip Drive, Norwell, MA 02061, U.S.A.

In all other countries, sold and distributed
by Kluwer Academic Publishers,
P.O. Box 322, 3300 AH Dordrecht, The Netherlands.

Printed on acid-free paper

Printed in the Netherlands.

This volume was produced with funds from the
Scientific Division of NATO
and a grant from the
Institut für forensische Psychiatrie Haina e.V.

TABLE OF CONTENTS

V. PREVENTING VIOLENCE IN THE COMMUNITY

INTRODUCTION

The NATO Advanced Study Institute on the Prevention of Crime and Violence Among the Mentally Ill was held in May 1999 in Tuscany, Italy. Participants from 15 countries attended. Since care for persons with mental illness (schizophrenia, major depression, bipolar disorder, delusional disorder, atypical psychoses) has been deinstitutionalized, some persons with these disorders are committing crimes and serious violence. Consequently, societies around the world are confronted with a new challenge: to provide mental health care and social services to mentally ill persons in a humane way that will prevent illegal behaviours. Research in this field has been dominated by investigations designed to improve clinicians' accuracy in predicting violent behaviours, with little attention focused on the organization and implementation of treatments.

The premise of the Advanced Study Institute was that treatments must have empirically proven efficacy. Both professional ethics and public accountability require empirical evidence that each treatment will alleviate the problem that it targets. However, despite the fact that Western industrial societies provide treatment for mentally ill persons who have offended, there is a very limited base of knowledge on what constitutes effective treatment and how such treatments should be organized and delivered. The Advanced Study Institute was an attempt to stimulate and encourage research that will extend this knowledge base. The goals were to review what is known about mentally ill offenders and about effective treatments for them, and to provide a framework for the orientation of future investigations designed to improve treatment efficacy.

The participants in the Advanced Study Institute included scientists conducting research on criminality and violence among persons with mental illness and clinicians responsible for the treatment and management of those persons. As expected, the two groups of participants were not always comfortable with each other. The clinicians complained that much of the research in the field does not provide information useful for resolving the problems that plague the organization and delivery of services. Further, they suggested that information resulting from scientific studies is often not applicable to clinical settings. In addition, they insisted that the scientists fail to measure the positive changes in patients that result from treatment. One participant summed up the debate well after the meeting: "We clinicians were however in the minority and initially were silenced by the overwhelming level of debate amongst our academic colleagues. It was with some trepidation that we quietly entered in to the area of debate only to realize that research is of limited value unless the findings can be implemented in clinical practice and we are gate keepers of this process. Researchers value our feedback on clinical matters."[1] The scientists, while sympathetic to the clinicians' responsibilities, lack of time, and lack of resources, argued that research has produced a wealth of information that could be used to improve the efficacy of treatment but instead is being ignored.

A more serious debate also emerged, one that saw clinicians and researchers on both sides of the issue. This debate focused on the criteria to be used in developing and implementing treatment and management services for the mentally ill who have a history of criminality and/or violence. One side, consisting mainly of participants from North America and the United Kingdom, argued that treatment policy and services should be based on empirical findings of efficacy. The other side, consisting mainly of participants from Europe and the Scandinavian countries, argued that other, non-empirical, factors should determine the organization and delivery of services. Notably, those arguing against the necessity of an empirical basis for treatment policy and practices were for the most part working in settings with adequate funding and resources, while the supporters of scientifically based practice came in large part from settings in which financial and human resources were lacking. Some argued that once there is evidence that a particular treatment is effective or ineffective with a specific group of patients, it is morally imperative to use that information to modify services. I personally found it difficult to understand the argument against basing treatment policy and practice on empirical findings. Such a perspective suggests that science does not contribute to improved treatment. This contradicts the premise of the Institute and much evidence. The chapters in this volume support, I think, the idea that research can contribute to improved treatment, and that questions concerning what treatment to provide and how to provide it are best answered by conducting scientific studies. Few governments and societies continue to accept the word of experts on what should be done if those experts cannot demonstrate that their opinions are supported by empirical data.

The Institute began with a series of lectures reviewing knowledge about mentally ill persons who commit crimes and/or behave violently. These lectures, revised and presented in Section I of this volume, demonstrate that research has provided useful information about who those persons are and what they do. The evidence is clear that the population of mentally ill offenders is heterogeneous, composed of subgroups with different needs with respect to treatments and services. The research reviewed in these initial chapters also demonstrates that mentally ill offenders present multiple problems, each of which needs to be addressed with a specific intervention. Encouragingly, the chapters in the subsequent sections present concrete information about interventions that are effective. As will be seen, there is a lot we do not know, but perhaps more important at this juncture is the point that there is a lot we do know. This is the base from which future studies designed to improve treatment efficacy can begin.

The heterogeneity of the population of mentally ill offenders and the multiple problems that each case presents necessitate diverse means of organizing and delivering treatment and management services. Many different components of treatment must be considered—for example, medications for the symptoms of the major mental disorder, programmes designed to eliminate substance abuse, life skills training, social skills training, programmes to change antisocial attitudes and values, and anger management training. In addition, different levels of supervision must be provided, to ensure compliance. Much discussion during the Advanced Study Institute focused on the need for research to more specifically describe mentally ill offenders and their behaviours in various situations. Precision in understanding these individuals, the problems that they present, and the contexts and immediate antecedents of their illegal behaviours will, it was suggested, greatly increase the likelihood that effective interventions will be developed.

In order to build on what has been shown to be effective with certain subgroups of this population, it is necessary to borrow from other fields. Both research and treatment for mentally ill offenders have been isolated, from research and treatment for mental illness, from studies of the rehabilitation of offenders, and from the development of effective treatments for substance abuse. Yet, as repeatedly demonstrated in many of the chapters in Sections II through V, some components of treatment shown to be effective with other populations are worth modifying and adapting for use with mentally ill offenders. Whether or not they will be effective will have to be determined empirically. The following strategy won consensus at the meeting: (1) identify the multiple specific problems presented by mentally ill offenders; (2) identify a treatment that has been shown to be effective in treating the problem in another population; (3) modify the treatment for use with persons with a specific mental illness; (4) evaluate the outcome; and (5) if the outcome is positive, refine it, try it again, and measure the outcome.

One of the distinctive features of treating mentally ill offenders is that the clinician usually does not control admission and discharge nor choose the setting in which the treatment will be provided. The additional challenges of providing treatments in specialized forensic hospitals, in correctional facilities, and in the community are discussed in Sections III, IV, and V. There is evidence that specialized community forensic treatment programmes are less expensive than institutional care. Further, there is some evidence, from small, experimental studies, that community programmes that are organized and delivered in specific ways can prevent criminality and violence even among high-risk cases. The chronicity of mental illness requires that treatment be planned over the long term, often over many decades. While stays in hospital will usually be necessary, either for legal or for clinical reasons, the goal is to identify programmes that will allow patients to spend most of their lives safely in the community. The organization of services and the collaboration of health, social service, and justice ministries are essential for such long-term treatment planning.

The Advanced Study Institute was a small step in encouraging scientists and clinicians to collaborate and in encouraging clinicians to apply the knowledge that scientists provide. Only through such collaboration will we develop the treatments and management services, and the means to organize and deliver them, that will effectively prevent criminality and violence among the mentally ill. The premise, of course, is that empirical findings are the rational basis for making decisions on policy, the organization of treatment, and the content of treatment.

One regret I do have is that so many interested persons from Eastern European countries could not attend for financial reasons. Thanks to the efforts of R. Müller-Isberner, we succeeded in contacting many clinicians and scientists in these countries who are engaged in work in the field. Neither they nor we, however, succeeded in finding the funds to allow them to travel to Italy and participate in the Advanced Study Institute.

The Advanced Study Institute was supported by a grant from the Scientific programme of NATO.

Many individuals contributed to making the Institute a success. Joëlle Chevrier did all of the secretarial work, Jason Schiffman and Jasmine Tehrani made sure the audiovisual equipment worked, and Bruno Giannassi attended to many small details at the hotel in order to ensure our comfort. I thank them sincerely.

Finally, I would like to thank Jane Broderick and Jonathan Paterson, who skilfully and with good humour did the editing and layout, respectively, of this volume.

Sheilagh Hodgins
February 2000

Note

1. A. Thomas. *Report of the Sir Kenneth Calman Bursary Awards 1999,* p. 3.

Section I

VIOLENCE BY THE MENTALLY ILL:

PREVALENCE, TRIGGERS, AND DETERMINANTS

MAJOR MENTAL DISORDERS AND CRIME IN THE COMMUNITY

A Focus on Patient Populations and Cohort Investigations

PATRICIA A. BRENNAN
EMILY R. GREKIN
ERIC J. VANMAN

The public has a fear of the mentally ill. It has long believed that mentally ill individuals are more prone to crime, especially violent crime, than other members of society (Gerbener, 1980; Monahan, 1992; Rabkin, 1979). The media perpetuates this view with news stories revealing the psychiatric history of gunmen involved in shooting sprees. In some cases, as in the recent shooting in a Colorado high school that left 14 children and a teacher dead, it seems as if the public desperately looks for evidence of mental disorder to explain criminal acts that seem otherwise unexplainable.

Public perception of the mentally ill as dangerous can lead to labelling and stereotyping of these individuals (Link, Cullen, Frank, & Wozniak, 1987). Patient advocacy groups have therefore spoken out against the perception of the mentally ill as criminals. Research studies completed before the 1980s did not appear to adequately test the relationship between crime and mental illness. Many of these studies did not use appropriate comparison groups, and the crucial question of whether there was a relationship between crime and mental illness within samples of similar age, gender, and socioeconomic levels remained unanswered.

The past 2 decades have seen an influx of studies on the relationship between violent crime and mental illness, particularly at the level of large-scale, epidemiological samples (e.g., Link, Andrews, & Cullen, 1992; Swanson, Holzer, Ganju, & Jono, 1990). Results from these recent studies have prompted Monahan (1992) to conclude that "there is a relationship between mental disorder and violent behavior, one that cannot be fobbed off as chance or explained away by third factors that caused them both...I now think the no-relationship [between violence and mental disorder] conclusion is at least premature and may well be wrong...new studies find a consistent, albeit modest relationship between mental disorder and violent behavior."

The above conclusion has policy implications for the treatment of the mentally ill and the prevention of criminal violence. In light of the research evidence, denying the existence of this relationship would do disservice to the public as well as to individuals with mental illness. On the other hand, more in-depth examinations of this

3

S. Hodgins (ed.), Violence among the Mentally Ill, 3–18.
© 2000 *Kluwer Academic Publishers. Printed in the Netherlands.*

relationship are necessary if meaningful and useful policy suggestions are to be made for the treatment of mentally ill populations. Questions that need to be addressed include the following: Does the relationship between crime and mental illness differ across diagnostic categories? Relative to crime in general, is violent crime particularly likely to be associated with mental illness? How much is the risk for criminal behaviour associated with the symptoms or the course of the disorder? What is the relative utility of diagnostic status, medication compliance, demographic factors, and associated substance abuse in the prediction of criminal behaviour?

The purpose of this chapter is to review and critically evaluate the literature on major mental disorders (i.e., psychotic disorders such as organic psychoses, affective psychoses, and schizophrenia) and crime in the community. The primary focus will be whether individuals with major mental disorders are more likely than controls to exhibit criminal behaviour in a community context. In addition, the above-stated questions about the relationship between crime and mental illness will be addressed in an attempt to suggest policy considerations and directions for future research.

Douglas and Hart (in press) have recently presented a general narrative and quantitative review of the relationship between psychosis and violence, which includes all types of populations and violence, in both community and inpatient settings. This chapter has a more specific focus. We will not address violent behaviour that occurs in inpatient settings, nor rates of major mental disorder in violent or offender populations (for a specific review of the latter, see Bonta, Law, & Hanson, 1998). In addition, as we are particularly focused on major mental disorders, this chapter will not review the literature comparing the criminal behaviour of all mentally ill individuals or all psychiatric patients (as one group) to controls. For more inclusive reviews of the crime and mental disorder relationship, see Hodgins (1993), Monahan (1992), and Rabkin (1979). It should be noted that most of the studies that have looked at individuals with major mental disorders as a separate group have been completed in the last 2 decades. Therefore, the literature we will review reflects the relationship between crime and major mental disorders during the current era of deinstitutionalization, and our conclusions may not generalize to other historical time periods.

As Johnson (1989) notes, "narrative reviews often lack methodological rigor and rely too heavily on the level of statistical significance of a given study finding, to the exclusion of a consideration of the magnitude of the finding" (p. 5). Meta-analyses can also help to explain inconsistent findings and identify outlier studies in the literature under examination. Therefore, rather than simply providing a narrative review, we will, throughout this chapter, present average effect sizes and other meta-analytic findings.

We used the method for calculating effect sizes recommended by Haddock, Rindskopf, and Shadish (1998). We calculated the log odds ratios for each study that provided categorical data, and we converted them to a standardized mean difference statistic (by dividing them by 1.81). We also calculated standardized mean difference statistics for studies that provided continuous outcome variables. All effect sizes were then weighted by sample size and combined to estimate the overall effect of the relationship between crime and major mental disorder. It should be cautioned, however, that there were a limited number of studies available from which to compute these effects, and that there is considerable heterogeneity in the effects for the studies reviewed. Meta-analyses presented here should be considered as suggestive, rather than conclusive, and attempts should be made to replicate and expand these findings as more studies are published in this area.

Crime and Major Mental Disorders

Large-scale birth-cohort investigations provide optimal opportunities for the examination of the relationship between crime and major mental disorder. In these investigations, the crime rates of individuals with major mental disorder can be compared to the crime rates of non-mentally ill controls born and raised in the same country during the same historical time period. In the first investigation of this type, Ortmann (1981) examined the psychiatric hospitalization and criminal records of 11,540 men born in Copenhagen in 1953. He found that males hospitalized with a diagnosis of major mental disorder were more likely than non-disordered males to be convicted of a criminal offence by the age of 23.

A second large-scale birth-cohort study in Sweden ($N = 15,117$) also found an increase in criminal convictions for individuals with diagnoses of major mental disorder (Hodgins, 1992). This study found that men with major mental disorders were 2.56 times more likely than men with no disorder to be registered for a criminal offence by age 30, and that women with major mental disorders were 5.02 times more likely than women with no disorder to be registered for a criminal offence by age 30. Odds ratios for violent crime (males = 4.16, females = 27.45) were higher than those for index crimes in general.

Hodgins, Mednick, Brennan, Schulsinger, and Engberg (1996) recently examined the relationship between crime and major mental disorder in a population birth cohort of all individuals born in Denmark between 1944 and 1947 ($N = 358,180$). This study examined psychiatric hospitalization and criminal conviction histories through age 44. Males with major mental disorders were more likely than non-mentally ill controls to have a record of criminal conviction for violence, theft, fraud, vandalism, traffic offences, and drug offences. Females with major mental disorders were more likely than non-mentally ill controls to have a record of criminal conviction in all offence categories with the exception of drug offences. The pattern noted in the Swedish cohort of higher odds ratios for violence compared to crime in general was repeated for the females in this Danish birth-cohort study.

A fourth large-scale birth-cohort study in Finland (Tiihonen, Isohanni, Raesaenen, Koiranen, & Moring, 1997) examined the official criminal records and psychiatric hospital records of 12,058 individuals through age 26. This study replicated the previous birth-cohort studies in its finding that individuals with psychotic disorders were more likely than non-mentally ill controls to have an official criminal record and a record of criminal violence. These relationships were significant after controlling for socioeconomic status of family of origin.

The findings of the Danish, Swedish, and Finnish birth-cohort studies were consistent concerning the relationship between major mental disorder and criminal outcome. These studies all took place in Scandinavian countries, and they all focused on official records of criminal behaviour. It has been argued that mentally ill individuals might be more likely to be arrested than non-mentally ill individuals (Teplin, 1984). On the other hand, conviction rates for the mentally ill might be an underestimate of actual offences committed, as many psychotic individuals are referred to hospitals rather than prosecuted for their offences, and others are not convicted due to a finding of Not Guilty by Reason of Insanity (Paull & Malek, 1974). There is a need for studies that examine the self-reports of criminal or violent behaviour, to rule out this potential methodological confound. In addition, studies in regions other than Scandinavia would help to determine whether the findings noted in these birth-cohort studies could be generalized to other parts of the world.

In the last decade, four large-scale community studies have compared the self-reported violent behaviour of psychotic individuals and non-mentally ill controls. In the first of these, Link et al. (1992) found that a scale of psychotic symptoms significantly predicted self-reports of violent and illegal behaviour in mental patients and community controls in New York. This result was noted even when sociodemographic variables including age, gender, education, and ethnicity were controlled. In a community-based epidemiological study of 2,678 individuals in Israel, Stueve and Link (1997) also noted a positive relationship between psychotic disorders and self-report of fighting and weapons use. This relationship remained significant when statistical controls were applied for demographic characteristics, substance abuse, and antisocial personality diagnosis.

The largest self-report study of major mental disorder and violence was completed in the context of the National Institute of Mental Health (NIMH) Epidemiologic Catchment Area (ECA) survey (Swanson et al., 1990). This study examined the self-reported commission of four types of violence (hitting a partner, hitting a child, physically fighting with others, and using a weapon during a fight) over the previous year in a pooled sample of approximately 10,000 respondents. Diagnoses were determined from psychiatric interviews rather than hospitalization records. In findings similar to those of other self-report studies, individuals with a diagnosis of major mental disorder were found to report higher rates of violence than individuals with no psychiatric disorder. In addition, it was noted that a secondary diagnosis of substance abuse substantially increased the risk for violence within the major mental disorder group.

The MacArthur Violence Risk Assessment Study more fully examined the role of substance abuse in the relationship between major mental disorders and violence (Steadman et al., 1998). In this study, 1,136 patients discharged from inpatient facilities were compared to controls living in the same neighbourhoods. Rates of violent behaviour were obtained from arrest records, collateral interviews, and interviews with the individuals themselves. Rates of violence were found to be higher in those with major mental disorders than in controls. However, this finding was significant only for individuals who also reported substance abuse. Individuals with major mental disorders and no substance abuse did not exhibit more violent behaviour than individuals with no mental disorder and no substance abuse. Repeated survey data also revealed that the greater the time lapse since discharge from the psychiatric facility, the smaller the association between major mental disorder and violence. However, the statistical analyses used to reach this conclusion have since been called into question (Volavka, 1999).

Overall, the results of the self-report community surveys are similar to the results of the birth-cohort studies that relied solely on official measures of criminal outcome. There does seem to be an association among violence, crime, and major mental disorder. This finding remains significant when statistical controls for demographic factors are applied. Substance abuse appears to play an important role in the relationship between psychosis and criminal outcomes, which suggests a need for further study of the relative effects of substance abuse within psychotic groups.

Individual study and overall effect sizes for the relationship between major mental disorder and crime, as well as major mental disorder and violence, are presented in Figures 1 and 2. Each bar in the figure represents the 95% confidence interval around the calculated effect size. Studies that did not provide the necessary statistical information to compute an effect size were excluded from this analysis. For those studies that included more than one measure of crime or violence (e.g., self-reports of fighting and self-reports of weapon use), we randomly chose one crime variable for inclusion.

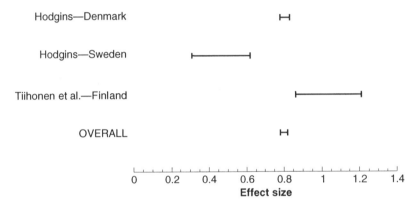

Figure 1. Crime and major mental disorder

According to Cohen (1992), effect sizes can be interpreted as follows: .20 is small; .50 is medium; .80 and above is large. The overall effect sizes for major mental disorder and crime and for major mental disorder and violence are significant and large. Although authors of several studies note that odds ratios for violence were found to be higher than those for crime, this effect-size analysis reveals that the psychotic-crime relationship is not stronger for violent crime than for overall crime.

A significant difference (QB(1) = 4.14, *p* <.05) was found between the effect sizes for those studies that examined violence as measured by official records and those studies that measured violence by self-report. When the studies are separated on the basis of this moderating variable, those that measure violence by self-report yield a larger positive effect size. This finding suggests that official statistics may be a biased underestimate of rates of violence in the mentally ill, or, alternatively, that individuals with major mental illness may be relatively more likely to commit minor forms of violence than major forms resulting in arrest or conviction.

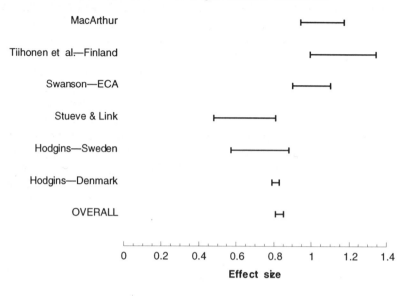

Figure 2. Violence and major mental disorder

The overall effect size of the relationship between crime and major mental disorder is similar for males and females (QB(1) = 1.15, p = ns). On examination of violent crime, however, females are found to have a higher effect size than males (QB(1) = 256.03, p <.001). Although studies often find higher odds ratios for criminal outcomes in mentally disordered females than males, our quantitative analysis suggests that this gender difference may be specific to violent crime.

Crime and Specific Psychotic Disorders

We have noted a relationship among psychotic disorders, crime, and violence. When considered as a group, major mental disorders are associated with crime and violence. But is the risk for crime and violence high for all types of psychoses, or is this overall relationship masking differential risk rates for specific psychotic disorders? In order to consider this question, we will examine the available research on rates of crime and violence for individuals with organic psychoses, affective psychoses, and schizophrenia in comparison to non-mentally ill controls.

ORGANIC PSYCHOSES

Organic psychosis has been associated with high rates of criminal violence. Organic psychosis is a persistent impairment of comprehension that may be caused by dementia, delirium, infection, injury, or substance abuse *(International Classification of Diseases, 8th ed)*. Tiihonen et al. (1997) noted a relationship between organic psychoses and violence in their Finnish cohort study. Brennan (1997) noted a similar relationship in the 1944–47 Danish population birth-cohort study. In that study, although males with organic psychosis but no substance-abuse diagnosis were found to be more violent than non-hospitalized males, the simultaneous control of demographic and diagnostic confounds rendered the organic psychosis-violence relationship non-significant. This suggests that the organic diagnosis might be a good risk indicator for violence because of its strong relationship with other demographic and diagnostic risks for violence. For example, organic psychosis may be the long-term outcome of substance abuse and may indicate a severe level of these problems, which in turn are directly linked to violence. Future analyses of the organic substance abuse-violence relationship across the lifetime might provide a better understanding of the proximal and distal factors for violence in these at-risk individuals.

AFFECTIVE PSYCHOSES

Few studies have examined the criminal behaviour or arrest of individuals with affective psychoses in comparison to the general population. The results of studies that have done so suggest that people with affective disorders are more prone to violence than those with no mental disorder. For example, the ECA study found higher rates of self-reported violence among people with depression and bipolar disorder than among those with no psychiatric disorder (Swanson et al., 1990). Data from the Finnish birth-cohort study also reveal higher rates of crime and violence among individuals with diagnoses of mood disorders with psychotic features than among those with no mental disorder (Tiihonen et al., 1997). Similarly, the 1944–47 Danish birth-cohort study found significant differences in violence between individuals with affective psychoses and individuals never hospitalized (Brennan, 1997). However, supplemental analyses revealed that affective psychoses in the absence of substance abuse or personality disorders did not result in an increased propensity for violence. Although a register linkage study in Australia noted a relationship between affective disorders and violence that remained significant when substance abuse was controlled (Wallace et al., 1998), most studies of the relationship between affective psychoses and violence have not looked at the potential mediating effects of substance abuse in the relationship.

One problem with most of the studies of affective psychoses and crime is a sole reliance on official crime records. Official arrest or conviction records do not include cases in which the affective disordered individuals kill themselves after committing a violent crime. Also, most of the studies in this area have examined hospitalized patients. Individuals who are hospitalized for affective psychoses may not be representative of people with these conditions. There is a need for studies that examine affective disorder in community populations, and that control for concomitant substance abuse, if we are to have a complete understanding of the affective disorder-substance abuse-violence connection.

SCHIZOPHRENIA

The psychotic disorder most frequently examined in terms of its relationship to criminal outcome is schizophrenia. Are there higher rates of crime for individuals with schizophrenia than for the general population? One method that has been used to address this research question is a comparison of the crime rates for schizophrenic inpatients and the general population. For example, a study with selected inpatients of a Veterans Administration hospital (95% diagnosed as schizophrenic) found that arrest rates of homicide, assault, and robbery were significantly higher for these patients than for the general population (Giovannoni & Gurel, 1967).

The past decade has seen a large increase in the number of studies directly comparing rates of violence for a schizophrenic population to non-mentally ill controls. Prior to 1988 there were only two studies of this type, and both used sampling methods that may have biased their results. In the first study, 42 schizophrenic patients were randomly selected from a psychiatric outpatient clinic and compared to 42 non-psychiatric medical patients drawn from the same Canadian hospital (Chuang, Williams, & Dalby, 1987). Self-reports of criminal involvement were compared for the samples and no differences were found in the rate of crimes committed against persons—three of the 42 individuals in each sample reported such behaviour. In the second study, psychiatric inpatients admitted to the only state mental hospital in the state of Wyoming during 1969 ($N = 461$) were compared to the general Wyoming population in terms of arrests for violence between 1964 and 1973 (Durbin, Pasewark, & Albers, 1977). No differences were found in the rate of offending for the two groups. Moreover, not one of the 40 schizophrenic males in the inpatient sample was arrested for a violent offence.

The low rates of violence found in these two samples of schizophrenics may reflect sampling biases rather than true rates of violent behaviour in schizophrenic populations. In the Chuang et al. (1987) study, the sample was drawn from a population of schizophrenics who were in compliance with an outpatient regimen. It is conceivable that such schizophrenics are a uniquely compliant, non-aggressive, less seriously ill subsample of the schizophrenic population. If that is the case, their rates of violence might be an underestimation of the rates of violence in the complete schizophrenic population. In the Durbin et al. (1977) study, individuals sent to the psychiatric hospital following arrest were excluded from the patient sample. Considering this sampling method, it seems plausible that the more violent schizophrenic patients may have been systematically selected out of the study. The remaining group of schizophrenic inpatients would be expected to display less violent behaviour than the general population, which indeed they did, according to their measure of violent arrests.

In the last decade, a series of studies has revealed a significant relationship between schizophrenia and criminal behaviour in the community. Lindqvist and Allebeck (1990b) carried out a longitudinal follow-up study of 644 schizophrenics in Stockholm. They compared the rates of violence and crime observed in their sample to the expected rates estimated from official statistics. Their results suggest an association between schizophrenia and an increased rate of violence for both males and females; however, an association between schizophrenia and crime in general was found only for the females in the sample. A patient-community study in Switzerland also noted an increased risk for violent convictions, but not general crime convictions, for male patients with schizophrenia compared to controls (Modestin & Ammann, 1996).

A comparison of White House case subjects in Washington, DC, to matched controls also revealed higher violent-crime arrest rates for the schizophrenics, but only when history of prior violent-crime arrests was statistically controlled (Shore, Filson, & Rae, 1990). In the ECA study as well, individuals diagnosed with schizophrenia self-reported more violent behaviour than individuals with no mental disorder (Swanson et al., 1990). In their Finnish birth-cohort study, Tiihonen et al. (1997) also compared rates of crime and violence for schizophrenics to those for individuals with no mental disorder. They found that male schizophrenics had a higher risk for violent crime, but not for other types of crime, compared to controls. These researchers noted that more than half of the schizophrenic offenders also had problems with alcohol, and that the rates of violence were especially high for schizophrenics with co-existing substance abuse.

Using data from the 1944–47 Danish birth-cohort study, Brennan (1997) examined the relationship between schizophrenia and violence. When demographic factors and secondary diagnoses of substance abuse and personality disorders were controlled together, schizophrenia was the only specific category of major mental disorder significantly related to arrest for criminal violence. Similar to Tiihonen et al. (1997), Brennan found that a secondary diagnosis of substance abuse substantially increased the risk for violence among the schizophrenic patients in the sample.

Effect sizes for individual studies and overall effect sizes for the relationship among schizophrenia, crime, and violence are presented in Figures 3 and 4. In contrast to the findings for psychotic disorders as a whole, individuals with a diagnosis of schizophrenia are relatively more likely to evidence higher rates of violent crime than of crime in general. The effect size for violence is large and significant. The effect size for crime, while significant, is quite small, and the confidence interval contains zero. This finding of a very small effect size for schizophrenia and crime, relative to that for major mental disorder and crime, suggests that future research should examine non-schizophrenic psychotic disorders in relation to crime.

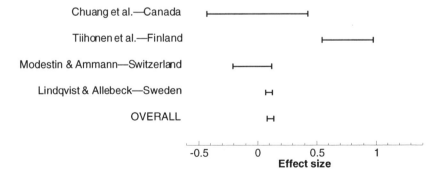

Figure 3. Crime and schizophrenia

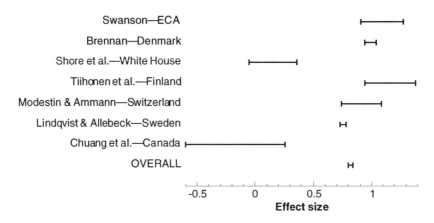

Figure 4. Violence and schizophrenia

The Nature of the Relationship Between Psychoses and Crime

SYMPTOMS

The above findings suggest a significant relationship between major mental disorders and crime, as well as between schizophrenia and violence. What is not clear, however, is the exact nature of these relationships. Schizophrenics may be more violent in response to, or as a result of, their psychotic symptoms. The acute phase of paranoid schizophrenia is often marked by delusions and hallucinations. In a study of 150 patients consecutively admitted to a state hospital and charged with murder, Lanzkron (1963) found that diagnosed paranoid schizophrenics were often living under a delusional system at the time of their crime. In their extensive study of mentally ill violent offenders in Germany, Hafner and Boker (1973) discovered that delusions, specifically those of love and jealousy, were more common among violent than among non-violent schizophrenics. These authors also found auditory and bodily hallucinations and paranoid feelings of malaise to be very common in their population of schizophrenic violent offenders. These results are consistent with those of Planansky and Johnston (1977), who found that a gross delusional hallucinatory disorganization, with prominent psychotic fears and loss of control, often accompanied the violent behaviour of schizophrenic inpatients. Taylor (1998) recently explored the relationship between delusions and crime in more detail. She noted that, although probably only 50–60% of psychotic individuals are suffering from delusions at any one time, 93% of the psychotic males in the sample reported having delusions when they committed their criminal offence. In addition, Taylor examined potential mediating and moderating factors in the relationship between psychotic symptoms and acting on such symptoms. She found that delusional beliefs resulting in depression, anxiety, or fear were more likely to be acted upon than delusional beliefs resulting in anger. This finding suggests that interesting work might be done in the future in terms of further examining the role of affective symptoms in the relationship between major mental disorder and crime.

A growing body of work on the role of psychotic symptoms in the relationship between mental disorder and violence suggests that a very particular symptom pattern may play a primary role in this process (Link et al., 1992; Link & Stueve, 1994; Swanson, Borum, Swartz, & Monahan, 1996; Wessely, Buchanen, Reed, & Cutting, 1993). In a hospital and community study of violence, active psychotic symptoms that reflected the perception of being out of control were found to fully explain the significant relationship between violence and psychiatric patient status (Link et al., 1992). In the same study, these particular psychotic symptoms also predicted the level of violence in the community control group. Link and Stueve later found that the psychotic symptoms related to feeling threatened or out of control ("threat-control override symptoms") were more predictive of violence in the community than other types of psychotic symptoms. Swanson et al. (1996) replicated this finding with the ECA data. The results of these studies imply that the relationship between major mental disorders and the potential for violence may be explained in part by psychotic symptoms. However, more recent results noting a curvilinear relationship between psychotic symptoms and violence (Swanson, Estroff, Swartz, & Borum, 1997) suggest that further work is needed to fully understand the predictive utility of psychotic symptoms for dangerousness risk assessment.

SUBSTANCE ABUSE

The large number of studies that have found a relationship among major mental disorder, crime, and violence after controlling for sociodemographic factors suggests that factors such as age or socioeconomic status do not fully explain the relationship. However, in addition to demographic factors, an increased rate of personality and social factors related to violence in the general population has been found in psychotic individuals presenting with violent behaviour. Alcohol- and drug-abuse rates of 27–55% have been found in violent, mentally ill populations (Lindqvist & Allebeck, 1990a). For example, Zitrin, Haradesty, Burdock, and Drossman (1976) found that, of the 42 schizophrenics arrested for violence in their sample, 20 also had a history of alcohol abuse and eight had a history of drug dependence. Substance abuse was also noted in the histories of most individuals in the 1944–47 Danish birth cohort who were diagnosed with organic brain disorders.

Steadman et al. (1998) suggest that substance abuse is a crucial factor in assessing the risk of violence among the mentally ill. They conclude, from their large-scale follow-up study, that co-occurring substance abuse accounts for increased violence in persons with major mental disorders such as schizophrenia. In a recent analysis of data from the Finnish birth cohort (Raesaenen et al., 1998), odds ratios for violent crime dropped from 25.2 for schizophrenics with comorbid alcoholism to 3.6 for schizophrenics without comorbid alcoholism. Drug abuse has also been found to play an important role in the commission of violence by individuals with affective disorders (Brennan, 1997; Hodgins, Lapalme, & Toupin, in press).

It appears that alcohol and drug abuse may play a substantial role in the overall findings of increased violence among individuals with major mental disorders. What is not clear from the research to date is the nature of the process by which substance abuse and major mental disorder may act together to produce an increased risk for violent outcomes. For example, is a person with schizophrenia more responsive to delusions while under the influence of alcohol, or is a schizophrenic who abuses alcohol less likely to be medication compliant and therefore more likely to experience symptoms that, in turn, lead to an increased risk for violence? Understanding this process should be a primary focus of research in this area, as it has implications both for the prediction of violence and for the treatment of individuals with major mental illness and comorbid substance abuse.

PERSONALITY DISORDERS

Personality disorders have long been associated with high rates of criminal violence, and antisocial personality disorder has been hypothesized to play a moderating role in the relationship between major mental disorder and crime (Hodgins, 1998). Specifically, it has been theorized that there are two types of violent individuals with major mental disorders. One type has comorbid antisocial personality disorder and is aggressive from a young age, whereas the other type becomes violent later in life, due to the symptoms of the major mental disorder. Support for this theory can be found in a study by Taylor (1998). She found that hallucinations and delusions were more related to violence in psychotic individuals who did not have a secondary diagnosis of personality disorder compared to those who did. Given this potential moderator relationship and the consistent finding of a relationship between personality disorder and violence, it seems appropriate to examine the role of personality disorders in the relationship between psychosis and violence. Examination of or control for personality disorders, however, is rarely carried out in studies of major mental disorder and criminal outcomes. It should also be noted that secondary diagnoses are less reliable and valid than primary diagnoses, and hospital-based diagnoses of personality disorder are underestimates of the true rate of these disorders in the population. Therefore, even those few hospital-based studies that have statistically controlled for this comorbid condition have not been able to fully assess its effect on the relationship between major mental disorder and crime. This is another area that needs to be addressed by future research.

Methodological Issues

The studies examined in this narrative and quantitative review used a variety of methods—community-based samples and birth cohorts, inpatient samples and outpatient samples, self-reports and official measures of crime. The weight of the evidence suggests a significant and large effect of major mental disorder on crime and violence. Is this likely an overestimate or underestimate of the true effect? It has been suggested that psychotic individuals who are identified for research studies as a result of being treated (particularly in inpatient samples) may be more criminal or violent than the overall population of psychotic individuals. Therefore the results of studies focused on treatment-based samples are presumed to overestimate the relationship between major mental disorder and crime. The community-based samples of Swanson et al. (1990) and Stueve and Link (1997), however, found effect sizes similar to those noted in treatment-identified samples. It has also been argued that the crime-mental disorder relationship may be overestimated if one relies on official measures of crime, in that individuals with mental disorders might be more likely to be caught or arrested for crimes (Teplin, 1984). Our effect-size analyses, however, reveal that the relationship between major mental disorder and violence is actually stronger in studies that utilize self-report than in official measures of violence. This suggests that the overall effect noted between major mental disorder and violence might be an underestimate of the true effect, as most of the studies reviewed used official measures of crime.

Several other methodological factors suggest that the studies reviewed here may have underestimated the true effect of the relationship among major mental disorder, crime, and violence. First, the relationship between major mental disorder and violence may be stronger with age, and most of the samples comprised primarily young adults. Second, most research studies have not been able to identify, or have excluded, individuals who died. In the 1944–47 Danish cohort, this exclusion resulted in an underestimate of the relationship between crime and mental disorder for females (Hodgins, 1998). Third, a psychotic individual's refusal to participate in a study or its follow-up interviews might be related to his or her propensity for violence. If so, the rates of violence for those included in the samples may be lower than the true rates for individuals with major mental disorder. Finally, most studies of crime and major mental illness do not control for the incapacitation effects of hospitalization, and most acts of violence in inpatient settings do not lead to arrest. Therefore, the true risk for violence in hospitalized, psychotic individuals may be underestimated in studies that rely only on official crime statistics.

Policy Issues

Our quantitative meta-analysis has noted large effect sizes for the crime-major mental disorder relationship. Moderator analyses also suggest that the effect size for major mental disorder and violence is higher for females than for males. The primary obstacle to applying this information on the level of individual prediction is the issue of base rates. Violence has a low base rate, particularly for females. A large effect size for major mental disorder and violence does not mean that psychotic females are likely to commit acts of violence. Most psychotic females, in fact, will not commit violence. Psychotic females are more likely than non-psychotic females to be violent; this is what the effect size tells us. However, unless we attend to base rates in risk assessments, our individual prediction equations will be fraught with false positive errors.

Overall, the findings of this review and meta-analysis suggest that different diagnoses are associated with different propensities for violence, as are contributing factors of gender, socioeconomic status, marital status, and drug/alcohol abuse. More specific questions as to the periods of highest risk and the symptoms associated with higher risk are currently being examined. Only when all of this information is used together, in association with information concerning dynamic risk predictors, do we see utility in predictions of individual risk.

Information on psychiatric conditions might be useful in risk assessment, when it is combined with demographic information and substance-abuse histories. For example, data from the Danish cohort study (Brennan, 1997) suggest that low SES males with a combination of organic psychosis and a substance-abuse diagnosis would be considered at much higher risk for violence than high SES males with no psychiatric or substance-abuse histories. The ultimate aim of such violence risk assessment would not be to stigmatize or to restrain all psychotic individuals in the community, but rather to prevent violence among mentally ill populations who are at particular risk. It is hoped that by preventing such violence, the community will be more likely to accept rather than reject the mentally ill.

References

Bonta, J., Law, M., & Hanson, K. (1998). The prediction of criminal and violent recidivism among mentally disordered offenders: A meta-analysis. *Psychological Bulletin, 123*(2), 123–142.

Brennan, P.A. (1997, June). Psychoses and violence in a total birth cohort. Symposium on mental disorder and violence, Leipzig.

Chuang, H.T., Williams, R., & Dalby, J.T. (1987). Criminal behaviour among schizophrenics. *Canadian Journal of Psychiatry, 32*(4), 255–258.

Cohen, J. (1992). A power primer. *Psychological Bulletin, 112,* 155–159.

Douglas, K.S., & Hart, S.D. (in press). Psychosis as a risk factor for violence: A quantitative review of the research. *Psychological Bulletin.*

Durbin, J.R., Pasewark, R.A., & Albers, D. (1977). Criminality and mental illness: A study of arrest rates in a rural state. *American Journal of Psychiatry, 134,* 80–83.

Gerbener, G. (1980). Stigma: Social functions of the portrayal of mental illness in the mass media. In J.G. Rabkin, L. Gelb, & J.B. Lazar (Eds.), *Attitudes toward the mentally ill: Research perspectives* (pp. 45–47). Washington: US Government Printing Office.

Giovannoni, J.M., & Gurel, L. (1967). Socially disruptive behavior of ex-mental patients. *Archives of General Psychiatry, 17,* 146–153.

Haddock, C.K., Rindskopf, D., & Shadish, W.R. (1998). Using odds ratios as effect sizes for meta-analysis of dichtomous data: A primer on methods and issues. *Psychological Methods, 3,* 339–353.

Hafner, H., & Boker, W. (1973). Mentally disordered violent offenders. *Social Psychiatry, 8,* 220–229.

Hodgins, S. (1992). Mental disorder, intellectual deficiency, and crime: Evidence from a birth cohort. *Archives of General Psychiatry, 49,* 476–483.

Hodgins, S. (1993). The criminality of mentally disordered persons. In S. Hodgins (Ed.), *Mental disorder and crime* (pp. 3–21). Newbury Park, CA: Sage.

Hodgins, S. (1998). Epidemiologic investigations of the associations between major mental disorders and crime: Methodological limitations and validity of the conclusions. *Social Psychiatry and Psychiatric Epidemiology, 33,* S29–S37.

Hodgins, S., Lapalme, M., & Toupin, J. (in press). Criminal activities and substance use of patients with major affective disorders and schizophrenia: A two-year follow-up. *Journal of Affective Disorders.*

Hodgins, S., Mednick, S.A., Brennan, P.A., Schulsinger, F., & Engberg, M. (1996). Mental disorder and crime: Evidence from a Danish birth cohort. *Archives of General Psychiatry, 53*(6), 489–496.

Johnson, B.T. (1989). *DSTAT: Software for the meta-analytic review of research literatures.* Hillsdale, NJ: Erlbaum.

Lanzkron, J. (1963). Murder and insanity: A survey. *American Journal of Psychiatry, 119,* 754–758.

Lindqvist, P., & Allebeck, P. (1990a). Schizophrenia and assaultive behaviour: The role of alcohol and drug abuse. *Acta Psychiatrica Scandinavica, 82,* 191–195.

Lindqvist, P., & Allebeck, P. (1990b). Schizophrenia and crime: A longitudinal follow-up of 644 schizophrenics in Stockholm. *British Journal of Psychiatry, 157,* 345–350.

Link, B., Andrews, H., & Cullen, F. (1992). The violent and illegal behavior of mental patients reconsidered. *American Sociological Review, 57,* 275–292.

Link, B.G., Cullen, F.T., Frank, J., & Wozniak, J.F. (1987). The social rejection of former mental patients: Understanding why labels matter. *American Journal of Sociology, 92,* 1461–1500.

Link, B.G., & Stueve, A. (1994). Psychotic symptoms and the violent/illegal behavior of mental patients compared to community controls. In J. Monahan & H.J. Steadman (Eds.), *Violence and mental disorder: Developments in risk assessment* (pp. 137–159). Chicago: University of Chicago Press.

Modestin, J., & Ammann, R. (1996). Mental disorder and criminality: Male schizophrenia. *Schizophrenia Bulletin, 22*(1), 69–82.

Monahan, J. (1992). Mental disorder and violent behavior: Perceptions and evidence. *American Psychologist, 47,* 511–521.

Ortmann, J. (1981). Psykisk afvigelse og kriminel adfaerd en undersogelse af 11533 maend fodt i 1953 i det metropolitane omrade kobenhavn *(Forksningsrapport, Vol. 17).* Copenhagen: Kommunehospitalet.

Planansky, K., & Johnston, R. (1977). Homicidal aggression in schizophrenic men. *Acta Psychiatrica Scandinavica, 55,* 65–73.

Rabkin, J.G. (1979). Criminal behavior of discharged mental patients: A critical appraisal of the research. *Psychological Bulletin, 86,* 1–27.

Raesaenen, P., Tiihonen, J., Isohanni, M., Rantakallio, P., Lehtonen, J., & Moring, J. (1998). Schizophrenia, alcohol abuse, and violent behavior: A 26-year followup study of an unselected birth cohort. *Schizophrenia Bulletin, 24*(3), 437–441.

Shore, D., Filson, C.R., & Rae, D.S. (1990). Violent crime arrest rates of White House case subjects and matched control subjects. *American Journal of Psychiatry, 147,* 746–750.

Steadman, H.J., Mulvey, E.P., Monahan, J., Robbins, P.C., Appelbaum, P.S., Grisso, T., Roth, L.H., & Silver, E. (1998). Violence by people discharged from acute psychiatric inpatient facilities and by others in the same neighborhoods. *Archives of General Psychiatry, 55*(5), 393–401.

Stueve, A., & Link, B.G. (1997). Violence and psychiatric disorders: Results from an epidemiological study of young adults in Israel. *Psychiatric Quarterly, 68*(4), 327–342.

Swanson, J., Estroff, S., Swartz, M., & Borum, R. (1997). Violence and severe mental disorder in clinical and community populations: The effects of psychotic symptoms, comorbidity, and lack of treatment. *Psychiatry: Interpersonal and Biological Processes, 60*(1), 1–22.

Swanson, J.W., Borum, R., Swartz, M.S., & Monahan, J. (1996). Psychotic symptoms and disorders and the risk of violent behaviour in the community. *Criminal Behaviour and Mental Health, 6,* 309–329.

Swanson, J.W., Holzer, C.E., Ganju, V.K., & Jono, R.T. (1990). Violence and psychiatric disorder in the community: Evidence from the Epidemiologic Catchment Area surveys. *Hospital and Community Psychiatry, 41,* 761–770.

Taylor, P.J. (1998). When symptoms of psychosis drive serious violence. *Social Psychiatry and Psychiatric Epidemiology, 33*(Suppl 1), S47–S54.

Teplin, L.A. (1984). Criminalizing mental disorder: The comparative arrest rate of the mentally ill. *American Psychologist, 39,* 794–803.

Tiihonen, J., Isohanni, M., Raesaenen, P., Koiranen, M., & Moring, J. (1997). Specific major mental disorders and criminality: A 26-year prospective study of the 1996 Northern Finland Birth Cohort. *American Journal of Psychiatry, 154*(6), 840–845.

Volavka, J. (submitted). Letter to the Editor. Submitted to *Archives of General Psychiatry.*

Wallace, C., Mullen, P., Burgess, P., Palmer, S., Ruschena, D., & Browne, C. (1998). Serious criminal offending and mental disorder. *British Journal of Psychiatry, 172*(6), 477–484.

Wessely, S., Buchanan, A., Reed, A., & Cutting, J. (1993). Acting on delusions: I. Prevalence. *British Journal of Psychiatry, 163,* 69–76.

Zitrin, A., Hardesty, A.S., Burdock, E.U., & Drossman, A.K. (1976). Crime and violence among mental patients. *American Journal of Psychiatry, 133,* 142–149.

Patricia A. Brennan, Emily R. Grekin, and Eric J. Vanman are associated with Emory University, Atlanta, Georgia, USA.

Authors' Note

Comments or queries may be directed to Patricia A. Brennan, PhD, Psychology Department, Emory University, Atlanta GA 30322 USA. Telephone: 404 727-7458. Fax: 404 727-0372. E-mail: <pbren01@emory.edu>.

REDUCING VIOLENCE RISK

Diagnostically Based Clues from the MacArthur Violence Risk Assessment Study

JOHN MONAHAN
PAUL S. APPELBAUM

A great deal of work in mental health law has been addressed to improving the assessment of violence risk among people with mental disorder (Borum, 1996; Monahan et al., in press; Steadman et al., in press). It is clear, however, as a number of researchers have recently emphasized, that risk assessment is only the first step in dealing with violence by people with mental disorder and must be followed by effective risk reduction (Carson, 1994; Heilbrun, 1997). The clinical and empirical literatures on risk reduction have been reviewed in a number of important sources (Eichelman & Hartwig, 1995; McNiel, 1998; Quinsey, Harris, Rice, & Cormier, 1998; Rice & Harris, 1997; Roth, 1987; Wettstein, 1998). A fair summary of that literature is that mental health professionals (particularly when assisted by actuarial instruments) appear to be better at estimating an individual's level of violence risk than lowering that estimated level of violence risk.

The purpose of this chapter is to identify "clues"—promising hypotheses—from the MacArthur Violence Risk Assessment Study for clinical intervention strategies to reduce violence risk among people hospitalized for mental disorder.

Terminology: The Various Types of "Risk Factor"

Clarity in terminology is crucial to progress in the fields of "risk assessment" and "risk reduction." Fortunately, a recent article, "Coming to terms with the terms of risk" (Kraemer et al., 1997), provides that clarity, as well as a useful framework for the present chapter. A "risk factor," according to Kraemer et al., is merely "a correlate that precedes the outcome" of interest (p. 340). To say that a variable is a risk factor for violence, in other words, is to say two things, and only two things: (a) the variable correlates significantly with the outcome of interest (violence in the community), and (b) the variable was measured prior to the time that the occurrence of the outcome was measured.

To be a target of clinical intervention, however, a risk factor must possess two characteristics in addition to statistical correlation and temporal precedence. First, it

19

S. Hodgins (ed.), Violence among the Mentally Ill, 19–34.
© 2000 *Kluwer Academic Publishers. Printed in the Netherlands.*

must be capable of change. According to Kraemer et al. (1997): "A risk factor that can be demonstrated to change spontaneously within a subject (e.g., age or weight) or to be changed within a subject by intervention (such as the administration of a drug or psychotherapy), we propose to call a *variable* risk factor." Second, changing the variable risk factor must result in a corresponding change in the criterion. According to Kraemer et al.: "A variable risk factor that can be shown to be manipulable and, when manipulated, can be shown to change the risk of the outcome we term a *causal* risk factor." As they state, "structuring effective treatment requires a focus on causal risk factors" (p. 343).

We modify the terminology of Kraemer et al. (1997) in one respect. Even if a measured risk factor is fixed (and therefore not a candidate for *direct* causal risk factor, since it is not variable), the measured risk factor can have an *indirect* relevance to treatment, in that it may suggest the existence of other, unmeasured, risk factors that may mediate the effect of the fixed risk factor on violence. These unmeasured risk factors may well be capable of change.

For example, being abused as a child has been found in several studies to be a risk factor for committing violence as an adult (Widom, 1989). While having been abused is an historical fact that cannot be changed, the abuse may still bear an important indirect causal relationship to violence, because, for example, sequelae of the abuse may include fear, anger, and inability to establish trusting relationships—all of which alone or in interaction may potentiate violent behaviour. These sequelae of trauma may indeed be changeable and may respond to treatment. In this illustration, we would say that fear, anger, and lack of trust mediate the causal relationship between abuse as a child and violence to others as an adult. Child abuse, then, would be a risk factor that could be *addressed* by clinical intervention, albeit by clinical intervention targeted at those (potentially changeable) factors that may be hypothesized to mediate the relationship between the abuse and violence.

Scope of the Current Analyses

We wish to be explicit at the outset about the exploratory and heuristic nature of the analyses we present in this chapter. In the preceding paragraph we refer to *potentially* changeable risk factors that may be *hypothesized* to mediate the relationship between a risk factor and violence. The subtitle of this chapter is *clues* for reduction of violence risk. We make no stronger empirical claim. Our research was designed for the purpose of improving assessment of violence risk. It did not extend to clinical trials attempting to change any risk factor we identified, or to studies attempting to test whether a change in a risk factor resulted in a corresponding change in the likelihood of violence.

Although definitive answers to questions about reduction of violence risk will have to await studies with experimental or quasi-experimental research designs, heuristic analyses such as the ones we present here may be valuable in suggesting which risk factors might most profitably be the targets of clinical risk-reduction research.

Disaggregation of Bivariate Relationships by Diagnosis

The "first step" in formulating "an adequate treatment plan," states the introduction to DSM-IV (American Psychiatric Association, 1994, p. xxv), is obtaining a diagnosis. Indeed, one of the primary purposes of DSM-IV "is to provide clear descriptions of diagnostic categories in order to enable clinicians [to] treat people with various mental disorders" (p. xxvii). Although disaggregating patients by specific diagnosis may not be the most productive strategy for assessing violence risk (Steadman et al., 2000), it may well be a productive approach to the reduction of violence risk (cf. Rice & Harris, 1997). Risk factors may differ for patients in different diagnostic categories, and clinical interventions, even for the same problem (such as substance abuse or anger), may vary according to the diagnosis of the patient. In this regard, "rapid differential diagnosis" has recently been recommended by McNiel (1998, p. 107) as the first step in formulating a violence risk management plan. Indeed, Mulvey and Lidz (1988) have demonstrated empirically that clinicians confronted with violent patients in the emergency room rapidly shift from dealing with the violent behaviour to treating the specific diagnostically defined disorder they hypothesize to underlie the violence.

In this chapter we search for clues to risk reduction among a set of bivariate risk factors for violence within a sample of acute civil patients disaggregated into four primary diagnostic groups: schizophrenia, major depression, bipolar disorder, and substance abuse.

Methodology of the MacArthur Violence Risk Assessment Study

SUBJECT ENROLMENT

Admissions were sampled from acute psychiatric inpatient facilities at three sites: Western Psychiatric Institute and Clinic (Pittsburgh, PA), Western Missouri Mental Health Center (Kansas City, MO), and Worcester State Hospital and the University of Massachusetts Medical Center (Worcester, MA). Selection criteria for research subjects were: (a) civil admissions, (b) between the ages of 18 and 40, (c) English-speaking, (d) white or African-American ethnicity (or Hispanic in Worcester only), and (e) a chart diagnosis of schizophrenia, schizophreniform, schizoaffective, depression, dysthymia, mania, brief reactive psychosis, delusional disorder, alcohol or drug abuse or dependence, or a personality disorder. The study was completely described to the subjects and written informed consent obtained.

SAMPLE DESCRIPTION

We approached a quota sample (to ensure representativeness across sites on gender, race, and age) of 1,695 potential participants. The refusal rate was 29.0% ($n = 492$). The final sample given a hospital interview was 1,136. Differences between the eligible admissions and the follow-up sample ($n = 939$) are discussed in detail elsewhere (Steadman et al., 1998). Males formed 57.3% of the sample. Ethnically,

68.7% of the sample was white, 29.1% African American, and 2.2% Hispanic. The mean age was 29.9 (*SD* = 6.2) years. Depression was the most frequent primary research diagnosis established using the DSM-III-R Checklist (Janca & Helzer, 1990) (41.9%), followed by Alcohol/Drug Abuse/Dependance (21.8%), Schizophrenia (17.0%), Bipolar Disorder (14.1%), Personality Disorder Only (2.1%), and Other (3.1%). The proportion of all cases with a primary research diagnosis of major mental disorder that had a co-occurring diagnosis of substance abuse or dependence was as follows: Depression, 49.6%; Schizophrenia, 41.0%; Bipolar Disorder, 37.7%; and Other Psychotic Disorder, 45.0%.

DATA COLLECTION

Hospital data collection was conducted in two parts: an interview by a research interviewer to obtain data on risk factors and violence, and an interview by a research clinician (PhD or MA/MSW in psychology or social work) to confirm the chart diagnosis using the DSM-III-R Checklist and to administer several clinical instruments.

The hospital data-set consisted of 134 risk factors from four conceptual domains: dispositional or personal factors (e.g., age), historical or developmental factors (e.g., child abuse), contextual or situational factors (e.g., social networks), and clinical or symptom factors (e.g., delusions) (Steadman et al., 1994).

The first 20 weeks after hospital discharge was chosen as the time frame for the analysis, because this was the period during which violence by patients in the community was most prevalent (Steadman et al., 1998). Research interviewers attempted two follow-up interviews with enrolled patients in the community during this period, approximately 10 weeks apart. A collateral informant who knew of the patient's behaviour in the community was interviewed using the same schedule. Arrest and rehospitalization records were the third source of information about the patient's behaviour in the community.

Patients and collaterals were asked independently whether the patient had been involved in any of several categories of violent behaviour in the previous 10 weeks. Answers were probed to ascertain the number of discrete incidents, and only the most serious act for each incident was coded. Violence to others was defined to include the following: acts of battery that resulted in physical injury; sexual assaults; assaultive acts that involved the use of a weapon; and threats made with a weapon in hand. Violence reported by any of the three data sources—subject self-report, collateral report, or official records—was reviewed by a team of trained coders to obtain a single reconciled report of violent behaviour.

Results of the MacArthur Violence Risk Assessment Study

Overall, 18.7% of all patients committed at least one violent act during the first 20 weeks following discharge from hospital. The prevalence of violence by primary research diagnosis, overall and as a function of a co-occurring diagnosis of substance abuse or dependence, is presented in Table 1. (For other studies that have found rates of violence to be lower among patients with schizophrenia than among patients with other, non-psychotic diagnoses, see Gardner, Lidz, Mulvey, & Shaw, 1996; Harris, Rice, & Quinsey, 1993; Wallace et al., 1998.)

Table 1. Percentage violent in follow-ups 1 or 2, by primary research diagnosis and co-occurrence of substance abuse/dependence diagnosis

Diagnosis	N	% of sample	% with substance Dx	Total % violent	% violent without substance Dx	% violent with substance Dx
Depression	393	41.9	49.6	18.8	10.3	27.9
Schizophrenia	160	17.0	41.0	8.1	5.4	11.8
Bipolar	132	14.1	37.7	15.2	14.3	16.7
Other psychotic	29	3.1	45.0	17.2	12.5	23.1
Alcohol/drug	205	21.8	100.0	28.8	NA	28.8
Personality only	20	2.1	0.0	25.0	25.0	NA

The bivariate correlations (Pearson's *r*) between each of the variables measured in the hospital and the occurrence of violence in the community, disaggregated by the patients' primary research diagnosis—for those four primary research diagnoses where the sample size was greater than 100 patients—is presented in Table 2. (The listed variables are more fully described in Steadman et al., 1994, and are available from the authors.)

Table 2. Bivariate correlations between variables measured in the hospital and violence during the first 20 weeks after discharge, by primary research diagnosis

	Schizophrenia	Depression	Bipolar	Substance abuse
Personal domain				
Sex—male	.126	.096	.144	.010
Age	.059	−.032	−.186*	−.138*
Race—white	−.153	−.107*	−.048	−.183**
Race—Hispanic	−.053	−.065	NA	.179*
Verbal IQ	−.049	−.155**	−.086	−.096
Ever married	.073	.044	.068	−.180**
Hare PCL:SV > 12	.229**	.346***	.123	.191**
Novaco anger—behaviour	.082	.249***	.071	.090
Novaco anger—cognitive	.044	.107*	−.030	.106
Novaco anger—arousal	.074	.127*	.013	.030
Novaco anger—intensity	.091	.119*	.032	.031
Barrett impulsivity, motor	−.014	.139**	−.074	.036
Barrett impulsivity, non-planning	.024	.082	−.026	−.047
Barrett impulsivity, cognitive	.072	.054	−.047	−.009
Historical domain				
Years of education	.050	−.131**	−.241**	−.062
Socioeconomic status	.002	.006	.265**	.078
Employed	−.148	−.063	−.088	−.036
Age at first hospitalization	−.029	−.003	−.236**	−.131
# prior hospitalizations	.041	−.074	.054	.015
Involuntary legal status	.030	.135**	.112	.036

	Schizophrenia	Depression	Bipolar	Substance abuse
Recent violent behaviour	.155*	.144**	.078	.089
Adult arrest—seriousness	.200*	.329***	.187	.162*
Adult arrests—frequency	.184*	.333***	.208*	.167*
Any arrest person crime (official report)	.309***	.048	.075	.133
Any arrest other crime (official report)	.199*	.106*	.113	.020
Sexually abused before age 20	−.073	−.062	.026	−.003
Seriousness of abuse as child	.067	.160**	.125	.204**
Frequency of abuse as child	.086	.163**	.086	.117
Father ever used drugs	.053	.091	.290**	.218**
Father ever arrested	.226**	.167**	.091	.155*
Father ever excess drinking	.027	.129*	.223*	.031
Father ever admitted to psychiatric hospital	.048	.035	.054	.013
Lived with father to age 15	−.058	−.100*	−.094	−.069
Mother ever used drugs	.058	−.018	−.126	.226**
Mother ever arrested	.389***	−.051	−.009	.128
Mother ever excess drinking	.136	.077	−.015	.081
Mother ever admitted to psychiatric hospital	−.014	−.002	−.142	.037
Lived with mother to age 15	−.033	.025	−.163	−.117
Parents ever fought with each other	.085	.046	.027	.114
Parents ever fought with others	.131	.007	.119	.081
Any head injury—loss of consciousness	.068	.100*	.140	.017
Any head injury—no loss of consciousness	.067	.061	.036	.016
Self-harm thoughts	.078	−.008	.036	−.048
Self-harm attempt	−.041	−.063	−.030	.020
Suicide attempt	−.081	.053	−.027	−.075
Contextual domain				
Living in private residence	−.018	−.077	−.140	−.020
Homeless	.048	.134**	.111	−.087
Living alone	−.063	−.063	−.140	−.091
Perceived stress	.081	.085	.060	−.012
Social networks				
# people in social network	−.008	−.028	−.150	.043
% mental health professionals in social network	−.026	−.100*	−.006	−.095
% family in social network	−.027	.011	.004	.028
# negative persons in social network	.077	.108*	.101	.015
# positive and material supporters	−.019	−.146**	−.155	.013
Average # mentions per negative person	.119	.003	.074	.078
Average # mentions per pos/mat person	.078	−.094	−.017	−.030
Frequency of social network contact	−.091	.001	.114	−.053
Duration of social network contact	.069	.023	.157	−.054
Clinical domain				
Chart antisocial personality disorder	.103	.226***	.119	.114
DSM-III-R checklist				
Major disorder, no substance	−.115	−.224***	−.032	NA

	Schizophrenia	Depression	Bipolar	Substance abuse
Major disorder + substance	.115	.224***	.032	−.121
Substance, no major disorder	NA	NA	NA	.121
Drug or alcohol	.115	.224***	.032	NA
Drug	.170*	.180***	.056	.088
Alcohol	.136	.184***	.058	−.040
Schizophrenia	NA	.105*	−.041	−.012
Mania	.046	NA	NA	−.063
Depression	.003	NA	.082	−.125
Other psychosis	−.024	NA	NA	.047
Personality disorder only	NA	NA	NA	NA
Brief Psychiatric Rating Scale (BPRS)				
Total score	−.046	.060	−.010	.061
Activation subscale	−.111	.024	−.054	−.050
Hostility subscale	.042	.169**	.004	.173*
Anergia subscale	−.035	−.053	.154	−.044
Thought disturbance subscale	.015	.087	.022	−.035
Anxiety/depression subscale	−.061	−.025	−.103	.036
Global assessment of functioning	−.071	−.056	−.119	−.084
Activities of daily living	.008	.010	−.062	−.031
Delusions				
Any delusions	.105	.011	−.085	.013
Persecutory	−.014	−.028	−.126	.016
Grandiose	.087	.116*	.043	.017
Body/mind control	.012	.013	−.042	−.136
Thought broadcasting	.118	−.007	−.060	−.077
Religious	−.102	−.055	.020	−.012
Jealousy	−.024	−.024	NA	NA
Guilt	.010	.107*	−.084	−.077
Somatic	.002	.105*	−.019	NA
Influence on others	−.033	−.024	NA	NA
Threat/control-override	−.067	−.012	−.009	−.121
Other	.210**	−.030	−.018	−.110
Violent fantasies				
Any	.162*	.051	.152	.207**
Frequent	.024	.105*	.260**	.115
Recent onset	.017	.048	−.038	.177*
Same type of harm	.162*	−.012	−.029	.100
Focus same person	.039	.058	.080	.212**
Escalating harm	.099	.037	.347***	.144*
While with target	.178*	.087	.055	.185**
Frequent, not escalating, not with target	.061	−.062	.053	.012
Frequent, escalating, not with target	NA	−.007	.372***	.102
Frequent, not escalating, with target	.−.012	−.126*	.031	..070
Frequent, escalating, with target	NA	.098	.082	.047
Not frequent, not escalating, not with target	−.187*	−.041	−.208*	−.198**

	Schizophrenia	Depression	Bipolar	Substance abuse
Any hallucinations	.106	.070	.053	.009
Command hallucinations	.064	.034	.064	.118
Present at time of admission				
Substance abuse	.135	.162**	−.035	.016
Paranoia	−.026	−.038	−.132	−.060
Delusions	.018	−.022	−.069	−.030
Decompensation	−.037	−.120*	.015	−.005
Violence	−.103	.058	.090	.212**
Hallucinations	.034	.017	−.239**	−.048
Bizarre behaviour	−.012	−.065	−.132	.040
Medication non-adherence	−.096	.000	−.071	−.094
Aggressive (non-violent)	.022	.047	.165	.089
Anxiety	.003	−.054	.017	−.192**
Suicide attempt	−.081	.065	.119	−.007
Mania	.027	−.034	−.062	.013
Personal problems	−.061	−.011	−.094	.076
Evaluation	.046	.034	.073	−.063
Other	−.059	−.016	.049	−.060
Medication change	−.073	−.016	.070	−.044
Unable to care for self	−.068	.046	−.064	.194**
Suicide threat	−.030	−.068	.055	−.106
Property damage	.099	−.030	−.041	.067
Court order	.053	.107*	−.084	−.095
Depression	.018	−.044	−.137	−.047
Drug use				
Any drug	−.006	.133**	−.085	.140*
Cocaine	.045	.067	.088	.068
Alcohol	.176*	.149**	−.075	−.069
Other	−.034	.152**	−.052	.109
Marijuana	.019	.129*	−.126	−.055
Stimulants	−.034	−.035	NA	.056
Sedatives	−.054	.007	.026	.082
Opiates	−.041	.027	.049	.006
Mini mental status	.006	.105*	.075	−.055
Perceived coercion at admission	.082	.034	−.115	.059

* $p < .05$ ** $p < .01$ *** $p < .001$

Three of these findings bear comment. First, one might expect the correlation between antisocial personality disorder and violence during the first 20 weeks post-discharge to be higher than the .103–.226 reported here. Note, however, that the variable being measured was *chart* antisocial personality disorder. It is common—in the United States, at least—for clinicians not to record an Axis II diagnosis of antisocial personality disorder in a patient's chart, particularly if the patient has an Axis I diagnosis of a major mental disorder.

Second, grandiose delusions correlated positively with violence in the group of patients whose primary research diagnosis was depression. This does indeed appear anomalous: Can patients correctly diagnosed with major depression also have grandiose delusions? Further examination of the data reveals that a grandiose delusion was reported on the delusions screening questions of the Diagnostic Interview Schedule for only 11 of the 393 patients with a primary research diagnosis of depression (2.8% of the depressed patients). Whether these 11 patients were misdiagnosed as depressed, or were misassessed as having a grandiose delusion—or whether it is indeed possible (albeit rare) for a person correctly diagnosed as depressed to experience a co-occurring grandiose delusion—is not known.

Finally, one variable found to correlate significantly with violence in some recent retrospective self-report research, "threat/control-override symptoms" (Link, Monahan, Stueve, & Cullen, 1999; Link & Stueve, 1994), did not correlate with violence in any diagnostic in this prospective clinical study. The reasons for this failure to replicate are considered in detail in Appelbaum, Robbins, and Monahan (in press).

Which of the variables from Table 2 can be designated as risk factors for violence within a diagnostic group? All of the variables were measured in the hospital, before the occurrence or non-occurrence of violence during the outcome period, so all fulfil one of Kraemer et al.'s (1997) two criteria for designation as risk factor: temporal precedence. The other criterion is a statistically significant correlation with the outcome. Given the number of multiple comparisons being made here, we chose a high alpha level ($p <.01$) for considering a correlation to be "significant." Variables in Table 2 accompanied by at least two asterisks, therefore, may be considered to fulfil both of Kraemer et al.'s criteria for designation as risk factors for violence within a given diagnostic group. These risk factors are listed in Table 3. To simplify this exploratory analysis, Table 3 aggregates the separate subscales or dimensions of a given risk factor. Thus, a significant correlation between any subscale of the Novaco (1994) anger scale and violence is referred to as the risk factor of "anger," and a significant correlation between any subscale of the Grisso, Davis, Vesselinov, Appelbaum, and Monahan (in press) violent fantasy measure is referred to as "violent fantasies."

Which of the diagnostically based risk factors listed in Table 3 are "addressable" by clinical intervention? That is, which of the listed risk factors are changeable—either directly or indirectly—*and*, when changed, can be expected to result in a correspondingly changed (i.e., lowered) rate of violence? Again, our research design did not extend to clinical trials attempting to change risk factors or to studies testing whether changes in risk factors resulted in changes in the likelihood of violence. Therefore, in identifying "clues" to risk reduction, we limit ourselves here to those risk factors listed in Table 3 for which there is other, independent, empirical evidence regarding changeability and, in some instances, the effects of change on violence. We address several of these clues to violence risk reduction in the following section.

Table 3. Bivariate correlations (*p* < .01) with violence in follow-ups 1 or 2, by diagnosis

Schizophrenia (*n* = 160)	Depression (*n* = 393)	Bipolar (*n* = 132)	Substance abuse (*n* = 205)
Psychopathy	Verbal IQ (-)	Years of education (-)	White (-)
Violent arrest record	Psychopathy	SES	Ever married (-)
Father arrested	Anger	Age at 1st hospital (-)	Psychopathy
Mother arrested	Impulsiveness	Father used drugs	Serious child abuse
Other delusions	Years of education (-)	Violent fantasies	Father used drugs
	Involuntary status	Admission: hallucinations (-)	Mother used drugs
	Recent violence		Violent fantasies
	Arrest seriousness		Admission: violence
	Arrest frequency		Admission: anxiety (-)
	Serious child abuse		Admission: unable to care for self
	Frequent child abuse		
	Father arrested		
	Homeless		
	Social support (-)		
	Chart ASPD		
	Alcohol Dx		
	Drug Dx		
	BPRS hostility		
	Admission: substance abuse		
	Alcohol use		
	Drug use		

Clues to Violence Risk Reduction

SUBSTANCE ABUSE

Substance abuse was a strong risk factor for violence, particularly in patients with a primary research diagnosis of depression, whether it was measured by the patient having a co-occurring DSM-III-R diagnosis of alcohol or drug abuse, by the patient's reporting problematic alcohol or drug use prior to being hospitalized, or by substance abuse being recorded in the patient's chart as one of the reasons for admission. Is substance abuse in people with a mental disorder such as depression "addressable" by existing treatment methods? A growing body of research recently reviewed by Drake, Mercer-McFadden, Mueser, McHugo, and Bond (1998) indicates that it is.

Drake et al. (1998) conclude that 10 recent studies of integrated outpatient treatment programmes "provide encouraging evidence of the programs' potential to engage dually diagnosed patients in services and to help them reduce substance abuse and attain remission" (p. 589). The key features of the integrated programmes that Drake et al. consider successful are: one programme treats both disorders, the same clinician treats both disorders, and clinicians are well trained to treat both disorders. The treatments themselves are tailored to the dually diagnosed population, and focus on:

- preventing anxiety rather than breaking through denial
- building trust rather than expecting confrontation
- reducing harm rather than concentrating on immediate abstinence
- the long-term perspective rather than short-term treatment
- stage-wise motivational counselling rather than front-loaded counselling
- clinicians being readily available rather than holding only office hours
- 12-step groups being available rather than mandated
- psychiatric medication when indicated, rather than contraindicated for all.

It should be emphasized that to date none of the studies of integrated mental disorder/substance abuse treatment have focused on violence reduction as an outcome measure. Rather, existing studies have focused on reduced substance use and attenuated psychiatric symptoms (e.g., McHugo, Drake, Teague, & Xie, 1999). Research explicitly addressing the violence-reduction effects of integrated treatment would seem a clear priority in the field.

ANGER CONTROL

Anger (as measured by the Novaco Anger Scale [Novaco, 1994]) and hostility (as measured by the BPRS) were strong risk factors for violence, primarily in patients diagnosed with depression. Is there independent evidence that anger can be successfully treated, and that treatment will result in lowered violence risk? The recent work of Raymond Novaco (1997) suggests that there is. He has developed a cognitive-behavioural anger treatment programme, the components of which are:

- self-monitoring of the frequency, intensity, and situational triggers of anger
- constructing a personal anger provocation hierarchy, for use in practising coping skills
- training in the arousal-reduction techniques of relaxation and guided imagery
- cognitive restructuring by altering attentional focus, modifying appraisals, and using self-instruction
- training in behavioural coping, communication, and assertiveness through role play
- practising new anger coping skills while visualizing and role playing progressively more intense anger-arousing scenes.

Evaluations of cognitive-behavioural treatment to improve anger management (e.g., Chemtob, Novaco, Hamada, & Gross, 1997; Renwick, Black, Ramm, & Novaco, 1997) have shown very promising results in both civil and forensic patient populations.

Self-report of having been seriously or frequently abused as a child is a significant risk factor for committing violence as an adult (Table 3), particularly for patients with a primary research diagnosis of depression or substance abuse. As stated above, while child abuse is a fixed, historical risk factor that cannot be changed, the sequelae of the trauma of having been abused may indeed be changeable and may respond to treatment. In a chapter titled "Anger and Trauma," for example, Novaco and Chemtob (1998) write that "the activation of anger has long been recognized as a feature of clinical disorders that result from trauma" (p. 162). Thus, to the extent that the causal path runs from abuse to anger and from anger to violence, anger control programmes such as Novaco's (1997) cognitive-behavioural intervention may be effective in reducing violence risk.

It is important to note that an adult's self-report of having been abused as a child must be distinguished from actual child abuse (as measured, for example, from school or hospital records [e.g., Widom, 1989]). Reports of having been abused as a child are known to be common among offenders. Recent surveys by the U.S. Bureau of Justice Statistics indicate that "19% of State prison inmates, 10% of federal inmates, and 16% of those in local jails or on active probation told interviewers they had been physically or sexually abused before their current offense. Just under half of the women in correctional populations and a tenth of the men indicated past abuse" (Harlow, 1999, p. 1). The extent to which these self-reports of childhood abuse indicate actual abuse or are offered by patients to explain or excuse their past violent behaviour cannot be determined. Note that while the distinction between actual and reported abuse is important for risk-reduction purposes—if the patient was not actually abused it would be counterproductive to attempt to treat the "trauma" that was hypothesized to mediate the relationship between abuse and violence—it is not relevant to risk assessment. The self-report of having been abused—*whether or not it is true*—is a significant risk factor for violence (Table 3). For example, psychopaths are more likely than non-psychopaths to report having been abused as a child (Coid, 1998). Even if one took the view that these self-reports are often merely a reflection of a psychopathic lack of responsibility-taking, the predictive fact would remain that a self-report of having been abused was significantly and prospectively correlated with violence.

LACK OF SOCIAL SUPPORT

For patients with a diagnosis of depression or substance abuse, a lack of social support—as indicated by the Estroff social support inventory (Estroff & Zimmer, 1994), or by being homeless at the time of hospitalization, or by being "unable to care for self" as noted in the hospital chart—was a significant risk factor for violence.

Many methodologies have been developed to provide social support to people with mental disorder in the community. The literature on this topic is voluminous, and is ably reviewed by Høyer in this volume. We refer the reader to that chapter for an analysis of the provision of social support in the community as a strategy for risk reduction.

Conclusions

In this chapter we have sought to identify "clues"—promising hypotheses—from the MacArthur Violence Risk Assessment Study for clinical intervention strategies to reduce violence risk among people hospitalized for mental disorder. Since most clinicians approach clinical intervention in terms of diagnosis, we have disaggregated patients into one of four groups based on their primary research diagnosis—schizophrenia, depression, bipolar disorder, or substance abuse. Within each of the groups, we have identified those variables measured in hospital that correlated significantly ($p < .01$) with violence during the first 20 weeks after discharge to the community. Finally, we have searched for independent evidence as to whether these variables—which qualify as "risk factors" for violence (Kraemer et al., 1997)—are capable of being therapeutically addressed by existing treatment interventions.

One puzzle left by the current analyses has to do with reduction of violence risk in persons diagnosed with schizophrenia. Of 134 variables measured in the hospital, only five significantly correlated ($p < .01$) with violence during the first 20 weeks after discharge, and only one of these five ("other delusions," which refers to a diverse category of delusions defined by the fact that they were *not* persecutory, grandiose, etc.; see Table 3) appears even arguably addressable by clinical intervention. Part of this finding may be due to the relatively small sample size ($n = 160$; 17% of the total sample) of the schizophrenic group, especially as compared to the depressed group ($n = 393$; 41.9% of the total sample). However, if, in response to the small size of the schizophrenic group, the p value for considering a correlation to be "significant" were to be lowered from .01 to .05, there would still not be many "significant" correlations, certainly not many—apart from drug and alcohol abuse—that would be easily interpretable in terms of risk reduction (Table 2).

In addition to the issue of sample size, the baserate of violence during the first 20 weeks after discharge was only 8.7% for persons with schizophrenia, the lowest of any diagnostic group (see Table 1). This is less than half the baserate of the sample as a whole (18.7% violent) and less than one third the baserate of the most violent group, those with a primary research diagnosis of substance abuse (28.8% violent). It should be noted that patients who refused to participate in the study were significantly more likely to have a medical chart diagnosis of schizophrenia (43.7%) than patients who consented to be part of the hospital sample (20.0% of whom had a chart diagnosis of schizophrenia). It is impossible to determine whether the patients with schizophrenia who refused to participate were more violence-prone than the patients with schizophrenia who consented to participate. One methodological difficulty in uncovering risk factors for violence among people with schizophrenia appears to be that the baserate of community violence among persons in that diagnostic group—at least among the consenting acute civil psychiatric patients whom we studied—is so comparatively low.

We conclude that treatment of several of the risk factors for given diagnostic groups may have promise for reducing violence risk. Although definitive answers to questions about violence risk reduction must await studies with experimental or quasi-experimental research designs, heuristic analyses such as the ones we present here may be useful in suggesting which risk factors might most profitably be the targets of further clinical risk-reduction research.

References

American Psychiatric Association. (1994). *Diagnostic and statistical manual of mental disorders (4th ed.)*. Washington: American Psychiatric Press.

Appelbaum, P., Robbins, P., & Monahan, J. (in press). Violence and delusions: Data from the MacArthur Violence Risk Assessment Study. *American Journal of Psychiatry*.

Borum, R. (1996). Improving the clinical practice of violence risk assessment: Technology, guidelines, and training. *American Psychologist, 51,* 945–956.

Carson, D. (1994). Dangerous people: Through a broader conception of "risk" and "danger" to better decisions. *Expert Evidence, 3,* 51–69.

Chemtob, C., Novaco, R., Hamada, R., & Gross, D. (1997). Cognitive-behavioral treatment for severe anger in posttraumatic stress disorder. *Journal of Consulting and Clinical Psychology, 65,* 184–189.

Coid, J. (1998). The management of dangerous psychopaths in prison. In T. Millon, E. Simonsen, M. Birket-Smith, & R. Davis (Eds.), *Psychopathy: Antisocial, criminal, and violent behavior* (pp. 431–457). New York: Guilford.

Drake, R., Mercer-McFadden, C., Mueser, K., McHugo, G., & Bond, G. (1998). Review of integrated mental health and substance abuse treatment for patients with dual disorders. *Schizophrenia Bulletin, 24,* 589–608.

Eichelman, B., & Hartwig, A. (Eds.). (1995). *Patient violence and the clinician*. Washington: American Psychiatric Press.

Estroff, S., & Zimmer, C. (1994) Social networks, social support, and violence among persons with severe, persistent mental illness. In J. Monahan & H. Steadman (Eds.), *Violence and mental disorder: Developments in risk assessment* (pp. 259–295). Chicago: University of Chicago Press.

Gardner, W., Lidz, C., Mulvey, E., & Shaw, E. (1996). A comparison of actuarial methods for identifying repetitively violent patients with mental illness. *Law and Human Behavior, 20,* 35–48.

Grisso, T., Davis, J., Vesselinov, R., Appelbaum, P., & Monahan, J. (in press). Violent thoughts and violent behavior following hospitalization for mental disorder. *Journal of Consulting and Clinical Psychology*.

Harlow, C. (1999). *Prior abuse reported by inmates and probationers*. Washington: Bureau of Justice Statistics Selected Findings (NCJ 172879).

Harris, G., Rice, M., & Quinsey, V. (1993) Violent recidivism of mentally disordered offenders: The development of a statistical prediction instrument. *Criminal Justice and Behavior, 20,* 315–335.

Heilbrun, K. (1997). Prediction versus management models relevant to risk assessment: The importance of legal decision-making context. *Law and Human Behavior, 21,* 347–359.

Janca, A., & Helzer, J. (1990). DSM-III-R criteria checklist. *DIS Newsletter, 7,* 17.

Kraemer, H., Kazdin, A., Offord, D., Kessler, R., Jensen, P., & Kupfer, D. (1997). Coming to terms with the terms of risk. *Archives of General Psychiatry, 54,* 337–343.

Link, B., Monahan, J., Stueve, A., & Cullen, F.(1999). Real in their consequences: A sociological approach to understanding the association between psychotic symptoms and violence. *American Sociological Review. 64,* 316–332.

Link, B., & Stueve, A. (1994). Psychotic symptoms and the violent/illegal behavior of mental patients compared to community controls. In J. Monahan & H. Steadman (Eds.), *Violence and mental disorder: Developments in risk assessment* (pp. 137–159). Chicago: University of Chicago Press.

McHugo, G., Drake, R., Teague, G., & Xie, H. (1999). Fidelity to assertive community treatment and client outcomes in the New Hampshire dual disorders study. *Psychiatric Services, 50,* 818–824.

McNiel, D. (1998). Empirically based clinical evaluation and management of the potentially violent individual. In P. Kleespies (Ed.), *Emergencies in mental health practice: Evaluation and management* (pp. 95–116). New York: Guilford.

Monahan, J., Steadman, H., Appelbaum, P., Robbins, P., Mulvey, E., Silver, E., Roth, L., & Grisso, T. (in press). Developing a clinically useful actuarial tool for assessing violence risk. *British Journal of Psychiatry.*

Mulvey, E., & Lidz, C. (1988). *What clinicians talk about when assessing dangerousness.* Paper presented at the biennial meeting of the American Psychology-Law Society, Miami, FL.

Novaco, R. (1997). Remediating anger and aggression with violent offenders. *Legal and Criminological Psychology, 2,* 77–88.

Novaco, R., & Chemtob, C. (1998). Anger and trauma: Conceptualization, assessment, and treatment. In V. Follette, J. Ruzek, & F. Abueg (Eds.), *Cognitive-behavioral therapies for trauma.* New York: Guilford.

Novaco, R.W. (1994). Anger as a risk factor for violence among the mentally disordered. In J. Monahan & H. Steadman (Eds.), *Violence and mental disorder: Developments in risk assessment* (pp. 21–59). Chicago: University of Chicago Press.

Quinsey, V., Harris, G., Rice, M., & Cormier, C. (1998). *Violent offenders: Appraising and managing risk.* Washington: American Psychological Association.

Renwick, S., Black, L., Ramm, M., & Novaco, R. (1997). Anger treatment with forensic hospital patients. *Legal and Criminological Psychology, 2,* 103–116.

Rice, M., & Harris, G. (1997). The treatment of mentally disordered offenders. *Psychology, Public Policy, and Law, 3,* 126–183.

Roth, L. (Ed.) (1987). *Clinical treatment of the violent person.* New York: Guilford.

Silver, E., Mulvey, E., & Monahan, J. (1999). Assessing violence risk among discharged psychiatric patients: Toward an ecological approach. *Law and Human Behavior, 23,* 235–253.

Steadman, H., Monahan, J., Appelbaum, P., Grisso, T., Mulvey, E., Roth, L., Robbins, P., & Klassen, D. (1994). Designing a new generation of risk assessment research. In J. Monahan & H. Steadman (Eds.), *Violence and mental disorder: Developments in risk assessment* (pp. 297–318). Chicago: University of Chicago Press.

Steadman, H., Mulvey, E., Monahan, J., Robbins, P., Appelbaum, P., Grisso, T., Roth, L., & Silver, E. (1998). Violence by people discharged from acute psychiatric inpatient facilities and by others in the same neighborhoods. *Archives of General Psychiatry, 55,* 1–9.

Steadman, H., Silver, E., Monahan, J., Appelbaum, P., Robbins, P., Mulvey, E., Grisso, T., Roth, L., & Banks, S. (2000). A classification tree approach to the development of actuarial violence risk assessment tools. *Law and Human Behavior, 24,* 83–100.

Wallace, C., Mullen, P., Burgess, P., Palmer, S., Ruschena, D., & Browne, C. (1998). Serious criminal offending and mental disorder: Case linkage study. *British Journal of Psychiatry, 172,* 477–484.

Wettstein, R. (Ed). (1998). *Treatment of offenders with mental disorders.* New York: Guilford.

Widom, C. (1989). The cycle of violence. *Science, 244,* 160–166.

John Monahan is associated with the University of Virginia School of Law, Charlottesville, Virginia, USA. Paul S. Appelbaum is associated with the University of Massachusetts Medical Center, Worcester, Massachusetts, USA.

Authors' Note

Comments or queries may be directed to John Monahan, School of Law, University of Virginia, 580 Massie Road, Charlottesville VA 22903-1789 USA. Telephone: 804 924-3632. Fax: 804 982-2845. E-mail: < jmonahan@law5.law.virginia.edu>.

IMMEDIATE PRECURSORS OF VIOLENCE AMONG PERSONS WITH MENTAL ILLNESS

A Return to a Situational Perspective

HENRY J. STEADMAN
ERIC SILVER

After a lull of nearly a decade, the field of violence research has once again turned its attention to the importance of situational factors as precipitants of violent behaviour. This movement is clearly reflected in a comprehensive review of the criminological literature recently conducted by Sampson and Lauritsen (1994). While their thoughtful integration focuses primarily on criminal violence in communities, it also provides very important insights for questions of immediate precursors of violence for persons with serious mental illnesses. Sampson and Lauritsen's focus on situational factors is presented within the context of a "multilevel perspective" that demands that individual-, situational-, and community-level data be combined for optimal explanatory power. In an observation that applies very directly to research on violence and mental disorder, Sampson and Lauritsen note:

> An equally important limitation of prior individual-level analyses of both violent offending and victimization is that they generally have not considered the possible effects that situational- or community-level factors might have on an individual's experience with violence. (p. 29)

The notion that community-level risk factors are important for understanding the violent behaviour of persons with mental illnesses was recently examined by Silver, Mulvey, and Monahan (1999). Combining individual-level data on discharged psychiatric patients with data on neighbourhood poverty rates drawn from the 1990 United States Census, these researchers found that psychiatric patients residing in high-poverty neighbourhoods (i.e., neighbourhoods with a greater than 30% rate of poverty) were significantly more likely to engage in violence compared to similar patients residing in neighbourhoods with less poverty. This finding emphasizes the importance of assessing community contextual factors, in conjunction with individual-level characteristics, when assessing risk for violence among persons with mental illnesses, and suggests that the situational determinants of such violence may vary across community contexts. Although supportive of the multilevel approach,

35

S. Hodgins (ed.), Violence among the Mentally Ill, 35–48.
© 2000 *Kluwer Academic Publishers. Printed in the Netherlands.*

however, this finding says little about the unique situational antecedents of violent events.

Sampson and Lauritsen's (1994) integration of the criminological literature and the recent study by Silver et al. (1999) directly link to some earlier work of ours (Felson & Steadman, 1984; Steadman, 1982) on persons discharged from state psychiatric centres. That work suggested that a situational/interactional perspective could inform our understanding of the types of interaction sequences that culminate in violence in comparison with those that truncate at some point prior to violence. We relied heavily on a sociopsychological approach emphasizing situational identities or self-images (Felson, 1978; Luckenbill, 1977). Also, we tried to distinguish between contextual factors (e.g., location, time of day, number of people present and their size, strength, and relationship to the subject) and situational factors (e.g., threats, initial insults, immediate dispute context and mediations) (Steadman, 1982).

Two major conclusions emerged from our prior work: (1) interactional sequences were very similar across discharged psychiatric patients, released offenders, and the general population; and (2) discharged psychiatric patients tended to use fewer instances of account-giving, a type of behaviour found to be associated with interaction sequences that truncated prior to physical violence. Thus, although Monahan's (1975) suggestion that "rather than attempting to identify and modify violence-prone persons, energy could be expended in the attempt to identify and modify situations conducive to violence" (p. 27) was made in 1975, it still has not been heeded by the research community.

Our goal in this chapter is to take data from the MacArthur Violence Risk Assessment Study, the most comprehensive data-set available on community violence by recently hospitalized mentally ill persons, to promote interest in the situational perspective as a way of approaching the study of violence. However, we noted early on in our project that a research design developed to carefully look at situational and contextual factors related to violence was quite different from the design needed to achieve our core goals of assessing the importance of the clinical, historical, and personal risk factors that the field was suggesting were the factors most likely to be associated with community violence by persons with mental disorders.

In this chapter, we are thus limited to a small set of situational factors that are primarily descriptive of 608 violent incidents committed in the community over a 1-year period by people recently discharged from acute inpatient psychiatric facilities in the United States. Our main purpose is to describe the types, locations, and targets of violence committed by discharged psychiatric patients and to present data pertaining to the immediate contexts of those violent events. These data are presented for the sample of incidents as a whole and in terms of several diagnostic categories, including the presence of co-occurring alcohol- and substance-abuse disorders. These data can help to frame the research design that ultimately will be needed to thoroughly test the situational approach to understanding the relationship between serious mental disorder and violent behaviour.

Methods

PATIENT SAMPLE

Psychiatric admissions were sampled from acute inpatient facilities at three sites: Western Psychiatric Institute and Clinic (a university-based specialty hospital) (Pittsburgh, PA); Western Missouri Mental Health Center (a public mental-health centre) (Kansas City, MO); and Worcester State Hospital (a state psychiatric hospital) and University of Massachusetts Medical Center (a university-based general hospital) (Worcester, MA). Patients included in the study met the following eligibility criteria: (1) civil admissions, (2) between the ages of 18 and 40, (3) English-speaking, (4) white or African-American ethnicity (or Hispanic in Worcester only), and (5) a chart diagnosis of schizophrenia, schizophreniform, schizoaffective, depression, dysthymia, mania, brief reactive psychosis, delusional disorder, alcohol or drug abuse or dependence, or a personality disorder.

Eligible patients were sampled according to age, gender, and race to maintain a consistent distribution of these characteristics across sites. The mean time between hospital admission and approach by a research interviewer to obtain informed consent was 4.5 days. As the object was a sample of acute rather than chronic patients, otherwise eligible subjects who had been hospitalized for 21 days or more prior to being approached for enrolment were not interviewed. All subjects were asked for written informed consent to participate in the study. Data collection began in mid-1992 and ended in late 1995.

HOSPITAL DATA COLLECTION

In-hospital interviews were conducted in two parts: (1) an interview by the research interviewer to obtain data on demographic and historical factors, and (2) an interview by a research clinician (PhD or MA/MSW) to confirm the chart diagnosis using the DSM-III-R Checklist (Janca & Helzer, 1990) or, when no eligible Axis I diagnosis was present, to confirm a personality disorder using the Structured Interview for DSM-III-R Personality (Pfohl, Blum, Zimmerman, & Stangl, 1989). DSM-III-R Checklist diagnoses corresponded to a chart diagnosis in 85.7% of the cases. Discrepant diagnoses were resolved by a consultant psychiatrist at each site.

POST-DISCHARGE DATA COLLECTION

Five attempts were made to recontact and interview enrolled patients in the community (approximately every 10 weeks) over 1 year from the date of discharge from the target hospitalization. A collateral informant was also interviewed using the same interview schedule. A collateral was the person who was most familiar with the patient's behaviour and functioning in the community through direct contact with the patient, usually at least weekly. Collateral informants were nominated by patients during each follow-up interview. If the collateral nominee did not have at least weekly contact with the subject, the interviewer suggested a more appropriate person based on a review of the subject's social-network data. Collaterals were most often family members (47.1%), but were also friends (23.9%), professionals (13.9%), significant others (12.4%), or others (e.g., co-workers) (2.7%). Patients and collaterals were paid for their participation.

Official records provided a third source of information about patients' behaviour in the community. During the follow-up interviews, patients were asked whether they had been re-admitted to a psychiatric facility. If a patient reported being re-admitted and gave approval for release of information, the hospital was contacted to obtain information regarding the rehospitalization, including dates of hospitalization, diagnosis, and reasons for admission. Arrest records for all patients were obtained at the end of the 1-year follow-up.

ENROLMENT AND RETENTION

A complete description of recruitment and enrolment procedures is provided by Steadman et al. (1998). In brief, we approached a quota sample of 1,695 to partici-pate. The refusal rate was 29.0% (n = 492). The final sample given a hospital inter-view was 1,136. The median length of hospitalization for enrolled patients at the three sites was 9.0 days. We obtained at least one follow-up interview for 83.7% of the patients. Three or more follow-up interviews were obtained for 72.0% of the patients and 77.3% of the collaterals, and all five follow-up interviews were ob-tained for 49.6% of the patients and 44.7% of the collaterals.

VIOLENCE CODING AND RECONCILIATION

Questions about violence were adapted from the Conflict Tactics Scale as modified by Lidz, Mulvey, and Gardner (1993). Subjects and collaterals were asked whether the subject had committed each of eight categories of violent behaviour in the pre-ceding 10 weeks, including: (1) pushing, grabbing, or shoving; (2) kicking, biting, or choking; (3) slapping; (4) throwing an object; (5) hitting with a fist or an object; (6) sexual assault; (7) threatening with a weapon in hand; and (8) using a weapon. If a positive response was given, the subject or collateral was asked to list the number of times the behaviour occurred and to provide details about the incidents (e.g., place, other participants, level of injury). Incidents of child discipline without injury were excluded.

Acts were categorized as *violence* if they included battery resulting in physical injury, sexual assault, assault involving the use of a weapon, or threat made with a weapon in hand. Physical injury varied from bruises to death. Violent acts reported by any of the three data sources—subject self-report, collateral report, or official records—were reviewed by a team of trained coders to obtain a single "reconciled" report of violence. This triangulation of information sources was achieved by having two coders independently review each case in which a violent act was reported by any of the information sources in any of the follow-ups.

Results

Of the 951 subjects who completed at least one of the five community follow-up interviews, 262 (27.5%) committed at least one act of violence while in the community. Across the 951 subjects, the average time covered by community interviews was approximately 41 weeks. Of the 262 subjects with community violence, three quarters (75.1%) had completed at least four of the five community follow-up interviews. Table 1 shows the frequency distribution of violent acts for these 262 subjects. Of the subjects for whom a violent act was recorded during the follow-up period, 145 (55.3%) committed a single violent act and 224 (85.5%) committed three or fewer violent acts. Five subjects, however, were found to have committed 10 or more violent acts each. From the point of view of characterizing the situations surrounding violent incidents, these five subjects pose a substantial difficulty, as their presence was found to distort the overall patterns observed. Thus, for the purpose of these analyses, a smaller representative group of incidents from among the many committed by these five subjects was included to form a total sample of 522 violent incidents.

Table 1. Numbers of incidents committed by discharged patients
during 1-year follow-up period

Number of violent incidents	Number of discharged patients
1	145
2	50
3	29
4	17
5	8
6	4
7	2
8	1
9	1
10	1
16	1
21	1
25	1
41	1
Total = 608	Total = 262

We begin by examining the types of violent acts committed by discharged patients and the resulting levels of injury incurred by the target. Of the 522 incidents, 271 (51.9%) involved kicking, biting, choking, hitting, or beating up a target. Of these incidents, 212 (78.2%) resulted in bruises or cuts to the target. In addition, 135 incidents (25.9%) involved the use of a weapon or the imminent threat of weapon use (i.e., a threat made with the weapon in the subject's hand). The majority of these incidents (67.4%) did not result in injury. Eighteen of the 522 incidents (3.4%) involved forced sex, and a total of six incidents (1.0%) resulted in death to the target. After we complete our statistical analyses of all violent incidents, we will return to these six incidents because of the intense interest such incidents tend to generate.

As stated above, a primary purpose of this chapter is to examine violent incidents by subject's primary diagnosis to assess whether diagnosis-specific patterns emerge. Table 2 presents the distribution of diagnoses for the full follow-up sample (*n* = 951) and the full sample of violent incidents (*n* = 522). These data show that although 17.0% of the follow-up sample were diagnosed with a schizophrenia-related disorder, only 7.7% of all the violent acts were committed by persons with such diagnoses (Test of Proportions, *p* < .001). Conversely, although 22.5% of the follow-up sample were diagnosed with a primary alcohol- or substance-abuse-related disorder, 30.7% of the violent acts were committed by persons with such diagnoses (Test of Proportions, *p* < .001). In the remaining analyses, the two smallest diagnostic groupings, *Other major disorders* (2.9%) and *Non-major disorders only* (1.9%), were omitted because their small numbers produced unreliable estimates of the situational characteristics surrounding the violent acts committed by these subjects. The final sample for the remaining analyses consists of 497 violent acts.

Table 2. Primary diagnosis

Primary diagnosis (%)	Follow-up sample *n* = 951	All violent incidents *n* = 522
Depression/dysthymia	41.7	44.6
Schizophrenia/schizoaffective*	17.0	9.0
Mania/bipolar	13.9	10.9
Alcohol or drug abuse*	22.5	30.7
Other major mental disorder	3.0	2.9
Non-major mental disorder only	2.1	1.9

Test of Proportions
* *p* < .001

Table 3 displays the types of violent acts that were committed in terms of the subject's primary diagnosis. These data show that, compared to the total sample of violent acts, those committed by persons with schizophrenia-related diagnoses were less likely to involve weapons (19.1% versus 28.6%) and more likely to involve forced sex (14.9% versus 3.6%).

Although violent acts committed by persons with schizophrenia-related diagnoses were less likely to be targeted at strangers (7.0% versus 15.8% for the total sample), and violent acts committed by persons with mania/bipolar disorders and alcohol- or drug-abuse disorders were somewhat more likely to be targeted at strangers (23.6% and 18.4%, respectively), these differences were not statistically significant. In addition, although violent acts committed by persons with schizophrenia-related diagnoses were more likely to occur in the subject's home (65.1% versus 47.1% for the total sample), again this difference was not statistically significant.

For each violent incident reported, the subject was asked what had brought him or her into contact with the target. Table 4 shows that violent acts committed by persons with schizophrenia-related diagnoses were more likely to begin with a chance meeting between subject and target (40.6% versus 25.4% for the total sample).

Table 3. Types of violence, by primary diagnosis [a]

Type of violence [b]	Primary diagnosis				
	Depression/ dysthymia $n = 233$	Schizophrenia/ schizoaffective $n = 47$	Mania/ bipolar $n = 57$	Alcohol or drug abuse $n = 160$	Total sample $n = 497$
Throw object, push, grab, shove, slap	36 (15.5)	1 (2.1)	11 (19.3)	19 (11.9)	67 (13.5)
Kick, bite, choke, hit, beat up	124 (53.2)	26 (55.3)	28 (49.1)	85 (53.1)	263 (52.9)
Forced sex	7 (3.0)	7 (14.9)	2 (3.5)	2 (1.3)	18 (3.6)
Weapon use or threat with weapon in hand	57 (24.5)	9 (19.1)	15 (26.3)	43 (26.9)	124 (24.9)
Other, type unknown	9 (3.9)	4 (8.5)	1 (1.8)	11 (6.9)	25 (5.0)

[a] Column percentages shown in parentheses
[b] Pearson χ^2 ($df = 12$), $p < .01$

Table 4. Reason for contact between subject and target, by primary diagnosis [a]

Reason for contact [b]	Primary diagnosis				
	Depression/ dysthymia $n = 196$	Schizophrenia/ schizoaffective $n = 32$	Mania/ bipolar $n = 44$	Alcohol or drug abuse $n = 138$	Total sample $n = 410$
Chance meeting	38 (19.4)	13 (40.6)	17 (38.6)	36 (26.1)	104 (25.4)
Regularly scheduled activity	75 (38.3)	9 (28.1)	12 (27.3)	31 (22.5)	127 (31.0)
Irregularly scheduled activity	37 (18.9)	3 (9.4)	8 (18.2)	40 (29.0)	88 (21.5)
Subject sought out target	23 (11.7)	3 (9.4)	2 (4.5)	15 (10.9)	43 (10.5)
Target sought out target	16 (8.2)	2 (6.3)	5 (11.4)	13 (9.4)	36 (8.8)
Other	7 (3.6)	2 (6.3)		3 (2.2)	12 (2.9)

[a] Column percentages shown in parentheses
[b] Pearson χ^2 ($df = 15$), $p < .05$

In addition, each violent act reported in this study was categorized in terms of the level of "provocation" leading to the violence. Although violent acts committed by persons with schizophrenia-related diagnoses were somewhat more likely to be categorized as unprovoked (35.3% compared to 23.7% for all incidents), the differences in these data did not attain statistical significance.

For each act of violence, subjects were asked whether they had been drinking alcohol, using street drugs, or taking prescribed medications prior to the act. Table 5 shows that, not surprisingly, violent acts committed by subjects with alcohol- or drug-abuse primary diagnoses were more likely to have been preceded by alcohol consumption (60.3%, compared to 31.6% for subjects with schizophrenia and 29.5% for subjects with mania). As shown in Table 6, a similar pattern was not found in drug consumption, where no significant differences were found across the primary diagnostic groups.

Table 5. Alcohol consumption prior to incident, by primary diagnosis [a]

Alcohol consumption [b]	Primary diagnosis				
	Depression/ dysthymia $n = 198$	Schizophrenia/ schizoaffective $n = 38$	Mania/ bipolar $n = 44$	Alcohol or drug abuse $n = 136$	Total sample $n = 416$
No	102 (51.5)	26 (68.4)	31 (70.5)	54 (39.7)	213 (51.2)
Yes	96 (48.5)	12 (31.6)	13 (29.5)	82 (60.3)	203 (48.8)

[a] Column percentages shown in parentheses
[b] Pearson χ^2 $(df = 3)$, $p < .001$

Table 6. Street-drug consumption prior to incident, by primary diagnosis [a]

Street-drug consumption [b]	Primary diagnosis				
	Depression/ dysthymia $n = 196$	Schizophrenia/ schizoaffective $n = 38$	Mania/ bipolar $n = 42$	Alcohol or drug abuse $n = 130$	Total sample $n = 406$
No	161 (82.1)	27 (71.1)	36 (85.7)	94 (72.3)	318 (78.3)
Yes	35 (17.9)	11 (28.9)	6 (14.3)	36 (27.7)	88 (21.7)

[a] Column percentages shown in parentheses
[b] Pearson χ^2 $(df = 3)$, n.s.

Subjects who committed violent acts were asked whether they had been taking prescribed psychiatric medications at the time of the act. As shown in Table 7, violent acts committed by persons with alcohol- or substance-abuse diagnoses were less likely to have been committed while the subject was taking prescribed medications (33.3% versus 48.7% for all violent acts); however, this result was not statistically significant. By contrast, violent acts committed by persons with mania/bipolar disorders and with schizophrenia-related diagnoses were more likely to have been committed while the subjects were taking prescribed medications (57.6% and 60.0%, respectively).

Table 7. Taking prescribed medications, by primary diagnosis [a]

Taking prescribed medications—self-report[b]	Primary diagnosis				
	Depression/ dysthymia $n = 103$	Schizophrenia/ schizoaffective $n = 20$	Mania/ bipolar $n = 33$	Alcohol or drug abuse $n = 33$	Total sample $n = 189$
No	53 (51.5)	8 (40.0)	14 (42.4)	22 (66.7)	97 (51.3)
Yes	50 (48.5)	12 (60.0)	19 (57.6)	11 (33.3)	92 (48.7)

[a] Column percentages shown in parentheses
[b] Pearson χ^2 ($df = 3$), n.s.

So far, we have described violent acts in terms of subjects' primary psychiatric diagnoses. Next, we turn our attention to co-occurring alcohol- and substance-abuse disorders. Following procedures we developed in an earlier report (Steadman et al., 1998), we placed violent acts in three diagnostic categories involving the subject's primary diagnosis as well as the presence of co-occurring alcohol- or substance-abuse disorders. The first group ($n = 121$ violent acts) were committed by patients with a diagnosis of major mental disorder—schizophrenia, schizophreniform, schizoaffective, depression, dysthymia, mania, cyclothymia, or other psychotic disorder (including delusional disorder, atypical psychosis, and brief reactive psychosis)—who did not also have a diagnosis of alcohol or drug abuse or dependence (the MMD/NSA group). The second group ($n = 255$ violent acts) were committed by patients with a diagnosis of major mental disorder and a co-occurring diagnosis of substance abuse/dependence (the MMD/SA group). The third group ($n = 121$ violent acts) were committed by patients with a diagnosis of "other" mental disorder (i.e., a personality or an adjustment disorder, and several cases of "suicidality") and a co-occurring diagnosis of substance abuse/dependence (the OMD/SA group).

Table 8. Targets of violence, by diagnostic category [a]

Target of violence[b]	Diagnostic category			
	Major mental disorder, no sub-stance abuse $n = 114$	Major mental disorder, substance abuse $n = 239$	Other mental disorder, substance abuse $n = 114$	Total sample $n = 467$
Family member	61 (53.5)	106 (44.4)	45 (39.5)	212 (45.4)
Friend, acquaintance	36 (31.6)	103 (43.1)	42 (36.8)	181 (38.8)
Stranger	17 (14.9)	30 (12.6)	27 (23.7)	74 (15.8)

[a] Column percentages shown in parentheses
[b] Pearson χ^2 ($df = 4$), $p < .05$

Table 8 displays the targets of the violent acts committed by persons with these diagnostic characteristics. As shown, violent acts committed by the MMD/NSA group were more likely to be targeted at family members (53.5%) and less likely to be targeted at strangers (14.9%) compared to acts committed by the OMD/SA group, 39.5% of which were targeted at family members and 23.7% at strangers. In terms of the reason for contact between subject and target, Table 9 shows that violent acts committed by the MMD/NSA group were more likely to occur during the course of regularly scheduled activities (48.5%), compared to violent acts committed by the MMD/SA group (26.5%) and the OMD/SA group (22.3%). In terms of provocation (data not shown), violent acts committed by persons in the MMD/NSA group were less likely to have been unprovoked (15.1%), compared to violent acts committed by the MMD/SA group (25.2%) and the OMD/SA group (28.3%); however, this result was not statistically significant.

Table 9. Reason for contact between subject and target, by diagnostic category [a]

| Reason for contact [b] | Diagnostic category | | | |
	Major mental disorder, no substance abuse $n = 103$	Major mental disorder, substance abuse $n = 204$	Other mental disorder, substance abuse $n = 103$	Total sample $n = 410$
Chance meeting	24 (23.3)	51 (25.0)	29 (28.2)	104 (25.4)
Regularly scheduled activity	50 (48.5)	54 (26.5)	23 (22.3)	127 (31.0)
Irregularly scheduled activity	11 (10.7)	47 (23.0)	30 (29.1)	88 (21.5)
Subject sought out target	10 (9.7)	25 (12.3)	8 (7.8)	43 (10.5)
Target sought out target	7 (6.8)	18 (8.8)	11 (10.7)	36 (8.8)
Other	1 (1.0)	9 (4.4)	2 (1.9)	12 (2.9)

[a] Column percentages shown in parentheses
[b] Pearson χ^2 ($df = 10$), $p < .05$

Table 10 shows that, not surprisingly, violent acts committed by the MMD/NSA group were far less likely to be preceded by consumption of street drugs (5.0%) compared to violent acts committed by the MMD/SA group (28.8%) and the OMD/SA group (23.7%). There were no differences between the groups in terms of alcohol consumption (data not shown).

Finally, Table 11 indicates that violent acts committed by persons in the MMD/NSA group were more likely to have occurred while the subject was taking prescribed psychotropic medications (73.0%), compared to the OMD/SA group (47.6%) and the MMD/SA group (34.3%).

Table 10. Street-drug consumption prior to incident, by diagnostic category [a]

Street-drug consumption [b]	Diagnostic category			
	Major mental disorder, no substance abuse $n = 101$	Major mental disorder, substance abuse $n = 208$	Other mental disorder, substance abuse $n = 97$	Total sample $n = 406$
No	96 (95.0)	148 (71.2)	74 (76.3)	318 (78.3)
Yes	5 (5.0)	60 (28.8)	23 (23.7)	88 (21.7)

[a] Column percentages shown in parentheses
[b] Pearson χ^2 ($df = 3$), $p < .001$

Table 11. Taking prescribed medications, by diagnostic category [a]

Taking prescribed medications [b]	Diagnostic category			
	Major mental disorder, no substance abuse $n = 63$	Major mental disorder, substance abuse $n = 105$	Other mental disorder, substance abuse $n = 21$	Total sample $n = 189$
No	17 (27.0)	69 (65.7)	11 (52.4)	97 (51.3)
Yes	46 (73.0)	36 (34.3)	10 (47.6)	92 (48.7)

[a] Column percentages shown in parentheses
[b] Pearson χ^2 ($df = 3$), $p < .001$

SIX INCIDENTS OF MURDER

Clearly, murder is rarely perpetrated by discharged psychiatric patients. However, when it does occur, the particular cases are of extreme public and clinical interest. While such an analysis is not central to our discussion of immediate precursors of most community violence committed by discharged psychiatric patients, a brief description of the six incidents of murder is presented here to provide greater detail on these rare but extremely serious acts of violence.

To begin with, four of the six deaths were caused by a single subject and the remaining two deaths were caused by different subjects, for a total of three killers out the 951 subjects interviewed in our community sample (less than a third of a percentage point).

The first of these subjects was a 28-year-old African-American male with a Grade 10 education who was single (never married) and without children at the time of the incident. Upon voluntary admission to hospital, the subject was given a primary diagnosis of depression with severe psychoactive substance dependence and alcohol dependence. The subject reported suicidal thoughts and, for the preceding 2 years, hearing multiple male voices. He also believed that people wanted to harm him and had reported homicidal ideation directed towards his ex-girlfriend. The violent incident occurred approximately 4 months after discharge at his ex-girlfriend's apartment, where he fired shots at two males, killing one. The incident description states that the subject was jealous of the ex-girlfriend and may have been delusional at the time of the incident.

The second of these subjects was a 38-year-old African-American male with a Grade 9 education. The subject had been voluntarily admitted to hospital, prior to study enrolment, at his girlfriend's urging because he had apparently been talking to the television and had exhibited increasingly paranoid behaviour. During the target hospitalization, the subject was given a primary diagnosis of schizophrenia and had a history of psychoactive substance dependence and alcohol dependence. The subsequent violent incident involved an argument with the subject's girlfriend, which occurred in the subject's home about 5 weeks after discharge. During the argument, the subject struck his girlfriend on the head with an ashtray, resulting in her death. Believing the girlfriend was asleep, the subject proceeded to shave her head. The incident description indicates that the subject may have been delusional at the time of the incident and that he may not have intended to kill her.

The third of these subjects, a 21-year-old white male with a high-school education who had never been married and had no children, was responsible for four killings. The subject had lived with his parents until he was 9 years old, at which time he was placed in a "boys' home" for shooting his biological father. He lived in the home until age 16 and was in prison from age 17 to 21. Evidence of childhood physical abuse and parental alcohol and drug abuse was also reported. Both parents had been arrested many times—his mother for manslaughter. The incident descriptions indicate that all four victims were shot; two of the shootings occurred outdoors, one occurred in a residence, and one occurred in a fast-food restaurant. All four victims were strangers; two were male and two were female. The incidents were reported to have occurred while the subject was on an extended automobile trip. The motive for the killings is unclear. For his target hospitalization, the subject had been admitted voluntarily for evaluation for homicidal ideation after stabbing his male roommate. The subject denied hearing voices and was not delusional upon admission. The primary diagnosis given the subject was psychoactive substance abuse.

Discussion

Certainly, the descriptive analyses in this chapter do not do justice to a fully developed situational perspective. They do, however, help inform and frame the type of research design that would be needed to produce the data that would move us towards the integrated approach suggested by Sampson and Lauritsen (1994) with which we began this chapter (i.e., consisting of individual-, situational-, and community-level measures). The analyses presented here indicate that the characteristics and precursors of violent incidents among persons with serious mental illnesses are capable of being categorized by content, target, recent alcohol and drug use, and medication use. For example, these analyses suggest that violent acts committed by persons with major mental disorders without co-occurring substance-abuse disorders tended to be targeted at family members during the course of regularly scheduled activities and were less likely to occur while the subject was taking street drugs; and that those committed by persons with co-occurring alcohol- or substance-abuse disorders tended to have an opposite pattern.

Missing from these analyses, however, is a systematic look at the sequence of acts leading up to each violent event (what we have referred to elsewhere as the unit-act-sequence; Felson & Steadman, 1984). Also missing is a richer set of contextual measures within which to situate these interaction patterns. To further the situational perspective advanced here, future research will need to collect more detailed data on the sequence of behaviours leading up to violent events, including the behaviour of perpetrators and targets of violence, as well as involved third parties. In addition, data on interaction sequences in which violence could have occurred but did not occur would be of considerable value in helping to inform violence-reduction interventions. Although the prior methods used by Felson and Steadman seem to work, the coding processes are time-consuming, involving the detailed examination of audiotaped descriptions of violent events (or the transcriptions thereof). As we have found in this study, such data are difficult to collect in the context of otherwise lengthy interview protocols. In addition, the statistical analyses involved in discerning unique unit-act-sequences presents additional challenges. Finally, to advance our understanding of the role of macro-level factors in influencing these interaction patterns (what we have referred to elsewhere as an ecological approach; Silver et al., 1999), future research will need to begin collecting data on the communities in which violent events occur. Only then may differences across community contexts be examined.

Ultimately, we believe the integrated approach advocated here points to the need for interdisciplinary teams of researchers, much like the one used to conduct the MacArthur Violence Risk Assessment Study, because the types of issues raised at each of the relevant levels of analysis tend to map on to the substantive expertise of particular behavioural-science disciplines. It has been our experience that a diversity of perspectives is invaluable for executing a research agenda aimed at integrating these multiple perspectives.

References

Felson, R. (1978). Impression management and the escalation of aggression and violence. *Social Psychology Quarterly, 41,* 205–213.

Felson, R., & Steadman, H.J. (1984). Situational factors in disputes leading to criminal violence. *Criminology, 21,* 59–74.

Janca, A., & Helzer, J. (1990). DSM-III-R Criteria Checklist. *DIS Newsletter, 7,* 17.

Lidz, C.W., Mulvey, E.P., & Gardner, W. (1993). The accuracy of predictions of violence to others. *Journal of the American Medical Association, 24,* 1007–1011.

Luckenbill, D.F. (1977). Criminal homicide as a situational transaction. *Social Problems, 25,* 176–186.

Monahan, J. (1975). The prediction of violence. In D. Chappell & J. Monahan (Eds.), *Violence and criminal justice.* Lexington, MA: Lexington Books.

Pfohl, B., Blum, N., Zimmerman, M., & Stangl, D. (1989). *Structured interview for DSM-III-R personality.* Iowa City, IA: Department of Psychiatry, University of Iowa.

Sampson, R.J., & Lauritsen, J.L. (1994). Violent victimization and offending: Individual-, situational-, and community-level risk factors. In A.J. Reiss & J.A. Roth (Eds.), *Understanding and preventing violence, Vol. 3* (pp. 1–114). Washington: National Academy Press.

Silver, E., Mulvey, E.P., & Monahan, J. (1999). Assessing violence risk among discharged psychiatric patients: Toward an ecological approach. *Law and Human Behavior, 23*(2), 235–253.

Steadman, H.J. (1982). A situational approach to violence. *International Journal of Law and Psychiatry, 5,* 171–186.

Steadman, H., Mulvey, E., Monahan, J., Robbins, P., Appelbaum, P., Grisso, T., Roth, L., & Silver, E. (1998). Violence by people discharged from acute psychiatric inpatient facilities and by others in the same neighborhoods. *Archives of General Psychiatry, 55,* 393–401.

Henry J. Steadman is President of Policy Research Associates, Inc., Delmar, New York, USA. Eric Silver is Assistant Professor of Crime, Law and Justice at Pennsylvania State University, University Park, Pennsylvania, USA.

Authors' Note

This research was supported by the John D. and Catherine T. MacArthur Foundation Research Network on Mental Health and the Law and by the National Institute of Mental Health (NIMH Grant R01 49696).

Comments or queries may be directed to Henry J. Steadman, Policy Research Associates, Inc., 262 Delaware Avenue, Delmar NY 12054 USA. Telephone: 518 439-7415. Fax: 518 439-7612. E-mail: <hsteadman@prainc.com>.

COMMENTARY

Monahan and Appelbaum, "Reducing Violence Risk: Diagnostically Based Clues from the MacArthur Violence Risk Assessment Study"

Steadman and Silver, "Immediate Precursors of Violence Among Persons with Mental Illness: A Return to a Situational Perspective"

GILLES CÔTÉ

The work of Drs. Monahan and Steadman, presented here with, respectively, Dr. Appelbaum and Dr. Silver, has been widely and favourably received. Their research constitutes a benchmark for the scientific community interested in the study of risk factors of violent behaviour among the mentally ill. The results presented derive from the MacArthur Violence Risk Assessment Study, which, according to Borum (1996), marks a third generation of studies of dangerousness or, to use today's terminology, the risk factors of violent behaviour. This study by Drs. Steadman and Monahan stands out for a number of reasons: the range of risk factors considered; the large number of participants—more than a thousand; the pains taken to ensure that participants were drawn from various settings; and the sources of information used to index violent behaviour—official criminal records, self-reports, collateral reports. The purpose of the presentation by Drs. Monahan and Appelbaum is to "search for clues to risk reduction," whereas Drs. Steadman and Silver seek "to promote interest in the situational perspective." The ultimate goal of both presentations is to identify factors that can be modified by interventions in order to diminish the risk of violent behaviour. However, the heuristic value of their endeavours can be assessed and put into perspective only by discussing the MacArthur project as a whole.

Certain Principles Advanced Within the Context of the MacArthur Project

In several published articles, Drs. Steadman and Monahan (Monahan, 1997; Monahan & Steadman, 1994; Steadman et al., 1993, 1994) propose a number of principles to remedy the shortcomings of earlier studies and to orient research in this field. I will evaluate the results presented in these two papers and the methodology of the MacArthur project using these principles. This is an effort to provide an alternative to the approach employed by all the studies in the field. My goal is to raise a number

49

S. Hodgins (ed.), Violence among the Mentally Ill, 49–57.

of points that might enable us to put into perspective the type of research that has been favoured to date.

The researchers responsible for the MacArthur project advance five principles. First, violence risk assessment must have clinical relevance. In other words, although based largely on actuarial science, risk assessment cannot limit its focus to predictors but must seek to contribute to clinical practice. In my opinion, this means that consideration must be given to processes. Consequently, current risk assessment procedures are not limited to static variables, but also take account of dynamic variables. These latter variables are those that are likely to change as a result of intervention (a theme developed by Drs. Monahan and Appelbaum) such as the patient's evolution, and situational factors that play or may play a role in a given context (a theme developed by Drs. Steadman and Silver).

Second, Drs. Monahan and Steadman try to assess not only risk, but also risk management. This can only be done, in my opinion, by clearly identifying the processes involved. Not everyone agrees with me; Klassen and O'Connor (1994), for example, limit risk-management variables to those that are associated with an increased or decreased risk for violent behaviour and that can be targeted by intervention. Nevertheless, in their presentation Drs. Monahan and Appelbaum lay down the requirements of clinical interventions likely to diminish the risks of violent behaviour, citing Kraemer et al. (1997), who write that "structuring effective treatment requires a focus on causal risk factors." For their part, Drs. Steadman and Silver set as their ultimate goal "understanding the relationship between serious mental disorder and violent behaviour," recognizing that this requires a different research design from the one used in the MacArthur Violence Risk Assessment Study.

The third principle is not entirely independent of the first two, but it is set apart here in order for its importance to be stressed. On the basis of what Klassen and O'Connor (1994) state, Drs. Steadman and Monahan note the importance of having a theory of violent behaviour which informs the choice of predictor variables to be investigated (Monahan & Steadman, 1994). Steadman et al. (1994), however, point out that there exists no articulated and validated theory of violent behaviour or of mental disorder.

Fourth, drawing on the work of Dietz and colleagues, Drs. Steadman and Monahan state that "the predictors of one form of violence may be quite different than the predictors of another" (Monahan & Steadman, 1994, p. 10).

And finally, the fifth principle: The authors of the MacArthur project chose to explore a wide range of variables rather than focus intensely on a small number of specific variables, or, as they put it, "we have made a trade-off between *breadth* and *depth*" (Steadman et al., 1993, p. 47).

Operationalization of the Clinical Variables

The decision to examine a wide range of variables seems to have been made to the detriment of precision concerning the diagnoses, especially given what is known about the clinical specificity of violent patients with major mental disorders. It appears difficult to classify dysthymia as a major mental disorder given that this disorder, as defined in the DSM, is more a problem of chronicity than of severity. Indeed, the impairment of functioning in dysthymia is described as mild or moderate. The same is true for brief reactive psychosis, a disorder that can last for only a few hours, after which time the individual returns to premorbid levels of functioning. Also, the classification of so-called "schizophrenia-related diagnoses" directly affects the accuracy of the analyses, but in a more subtle way. Delusional disorder and psychotic disorder not otherwise specified (NOS) cannot be grouped together with schizophrenia. Finally, it is somewhat surprising to note a significant positive correlation between grandiose delusions and depression, as presented in Table 2 of the text of Drs. Monahan and Appelbaum.

Our own research has shown that violent behaviour is much more common among patients with delusional disorder and with a psychotic disorder NOS than among those with schizophrenia and schizoaffective disorder (Côté, Lesage, Chawky, & Loyer, 1997). What is more, those with delusional disorder and psychoses NOS tend to manifest behavioural problems at a much younger age than those with schizophrenia and schizoaffective disorder (Côté & Lesage, 1995). This finding supports an etiological hypothesis proposed by my colleague Sheilagh Hodgins, who distinguishes between "early starters"—persons with a severe mental disorder who display a pattern of antisocial behaviour beginning at a very young age and persisting through adulthood—and "late starters"—persons with a severe mental disorder whose antisocial behaviour onsets simultaneous with the mental disorder. Paranoia symptoms and intoxication have been reported to play a major role in the antisocial behaviour of late starters (Hodgins, Côté, & Toupin, 1998). There is no way of knowing how many participants in the MacArthur study met the criteria for delusional disorder and psychotic disorder NOS, but grouping them with schizophrenic participants weakens the measure,[1] as these participants may present distinct problems. This, together with the fact that the diagnoses were made shortly after admission, raises questions regarding the appropriateness of the classification of diagnoses. As well as being questionable at the theoretical level, the classification includes diagnoses that were made after a relatively short time in hospital. In such a short time, it is difficult, if not impossible, to distinguish symptoms attributable to the effects of substance abuse from symptoms of genuine psychogenic origin.

Representativeness of the Sample

If there were in fact few individuals with delusional disorder and psychotic disorder NOS recruited for the study, then we must wonder about the representativeness of the sample. The participants were recruited at three sites in different parts of the United States. These included a university-based specialty hospital, a state psychiatric hospital, and a university-based general hospital. If the authors wanted the results of their study to be generalizable to severely mentally ill patients who behave violently, should they not have included a subsample recruited in forensic hospitals or correctional facilities? One of our studies found that persons with mental illness in prison settings were clinically distinct from patients recruited in psychiatric hospitals (Côté et al., 1997). This clinical specificity characterized not only those with psychotic disorders, but also those with major mood disorders. Our study found that the most prevalent psychotic disorders in correctional facilities were delusional disorder and psychoses NOS and the most prevalent affective disorder was major depression. By contrast, the psychotic subjects recruited in psychiatric hospitals more often met criteria for schizophrenia or schizoaffective disorder. Furthermore, 91.3% of the subjects with a severe mental disorder who were recruited in correctional facilities had been convicted at one time or another for a violent offence, compared with only 18.3% of the subjects recruited in psychiatric hospitals. To conclude, it would appear questionable to undertake a study of factors associated with violent behaviour in persons with mental illness without including in the sample participants from judicial and prison settings.

In addition, Steadman et al. (1998) maintain that certain patients in the present study are at lower risk of committing violent acts "owing to more time spent in hospitals or jails in the later follow-up periods" (p. 397). We also have reason to believe that those persons who refused to take part in or who dropped out of the MacArthur study during the follow-up were more violent, given that, and I quote, "followed-up patients were less likely to have a documented history of violence than patients lost to follow-up" (p. 401). It should be noted in this regard that, based on the data provided in the presentation, the final sample represented 49.6% of the 1,136 patients who were interviewed in the hospitals, but only 33.2% of the initial population—that is, 563 of the 1,695 patients who were recruited. Consequently, if indeed violent patients are clinically distinct from non-violent patients, especially those in prison settings, then the representativeness of the MacArthur sample would appear to be skewed.

What is more, given the differing rates of violence that have been identified for the various diagnostic categories, and the associations identified with certain situational factors, the statistical analyses presented in the study by Drs. Steadman and Silver raise a number of questions. First, the number of violent incidents does not take into account the period in which subjects were at risk. Second, the frequency of violent incidents shows exponential growth, as 55.3% of the participants who engaged in violent behaviour did so only once (this percentage is inconsistent with the data presented in Table 1, as the cumulative percentage of incidents must also take into account those persons who committed no violent acts), while five patients registered a frequency of violent incidents that deviates considerably from that observed among the others. In order to sidestep this problem, the authors focus their attention on "a smaller representative group of incidents from among the many committed" by these subjects without giving any indication of the weighting procedure used. However, as the analyses are based on the number of incidents, any artificial reduction of this number for the purpose of weighting skews the results.

The Importance of Distinguishing Among Forms of Violence

Violent behaviours are not homogeneous. Monahan and Steadman (1994), drawing on the work of Dietz and colleagues, state that "the predictors of one form of violence may be quite different than the predictors of another" (p. 10). Consequently, it seems difficult to consider homicide with other forms of violence such as sexual assaults, threats made with a weapon, pushing, or batting with a fist. We, and others, have shown that the prevalence of major mental disorders is higher among homicide than non-homicide offenders (Côté & Hodgins, 1992). While the score on the Hare Psychopathy Checklist (Hare, 1991) is associated with violent behaviours (Hare & McPherson, 1984; Williamson, Hare, & Wong, 1987; see also the meta-analyses of Gendreau, Little, & Goggin, 1996), homicide is rare among psychopaths (Hare, 1981; Hare & Jutai, 1983). In fact, more homicides are observed among non-psychopaths than among psychopaths (Hare & McPherson; Williamson et al.). In samples of offenders recruited in psychiatric settings, PCL-R scores are not associated with homicide (Pham, Remy, Dailliet, & Lienard, 1997). The PCL-SV score was one of the most powerful predictors of violent behaviour identified in the MacArthur project (Monahan, 1998). Placing all violent behaviours on an equal footing increases the inaccuracy of the criterion variable, as the factors associated with one type of violent behaviour are not the same as those associated with another. Only six subjects in the MacArthur project committed a homicide. Consequently, homicides were included as violent events simply for practical reasons. However, the point made here should at least force us to think about the problem at the theoretical level in order to qualify the scope and generalization of the conclusions. It must be admitted, however, that this is not a serious problem for the MacArthur study.

Limitations of the Research Design Relative to the Implicit Theoretical Framework

It is important to situate the MacArthur study within a wider context, in order to identify alternatives to the current way of doing things. However, it is much harder to propose new ideas than to criticize established ones. Although Dr. Monahan recognizes the importance of having a theoretical framework to inform the choice of variables to be investigated, and although Dr. Steadman asserts that there exists no genuine theory of violence or mental illness, the fact remains that all ideas and all research designs are based on a theoretical framework that is implicit if not explicit. The implicit theoretical framework of the MacArthur project is essentially associationist. Drs. Steadman and Silver have as their objective to "thoroughly test the situational/interactional approach to understanding the relationship between serious mental disorder and violent behaviour." They recognize that a different research design is needed to allow us to obtain a real "understanding" of the relationship between mental disorder and violent behaviour. Understanding refers to processes, cause-and-effect relationships. The MacArthur study used a quasi-experimental design of the correlational type. This experimental design is essentially linear and based on comparisons. It cannot lead to an understanding of processes, as a correlation is not necessarily indicative of a causal relationship.

In order to deal with the problem of causality, the linear approach favours longitudinal studies, simply because cause precedes effect. The problem, however, is much more complex than it seems. There are so many intervening factors that it is difficult to control their effects. An exhaustive control of all variables would require samples of unthinkable sizes. As a case in point, allow me to use the data from the Stockholm Metropolitan Project presented by Hodgins (in press). Based on a birth cohort comprising 15,117 persons, she observed that only 82 men and 79 women developed a major mental disorder over a 30-year follow-up period. Of these, 41 men and 15 women committed crimes. If, in addition, we wished to take into account, for example, age at first offence, the subgroups become even smaller. Consequently, given the small number of subjects and the great number of intervening variables, possible interactions are impossible to measure.

Beyond these practical considerations, the linear approach has limitations at the theoretical level. Linear analysis supposes that a variable can be considered by itself and that it has the same influence on all individuals. Thus, differences observed among individuals are differences not in nature but in intensity. Indeed, variables are approached from a quantitative rather than qualitative angle. However, does a problem not take on meaning through an integrated pattern of variables or indices? An alternative to the correlational approach is the holistic or systems approach. According to this approach, the contribution of a variable cannot be gauged without taking into account the relationship of this variable with other variables. The pattern observed is no longer quantitatively different from the pattern presented by another individual or another group of individuals, but it may be qualitatively different. In sum, the meaning that a given variable takes on depends on the system of variables of which it is part. At the methodological level, this entails a shift from linear to typological analysis, or from a linear to a taxonomic approach. At the epistemological level, it entails a shift from linear causality to circular causality (Von Bertalanffy, 1967, p. 67).

The idea of a holistic approach has inspired, among others, Bergman and Magnusson (1997). Drawing on the general systems theory of Von Bertalanffy (1968), and underscoring the contribution of this approach in the field of the pure sciences (physics, chemistry, biology), Bergman and Magnusson propose that we shift from analyses centred on variables to analyses centred on persons. Von Bertalanffy (1968) defines systems as "complexes of elements standing in interaction" (p. 33). Thus, an element (a variable) can be studied only as a function of its relationships with other elements. Cluster analysis can be used to identify typologies that already take into account a multitude of interactions, some of which are clearly identified while others are identified only through their effects. Cluster analysis thus makes it possible to take into account the system as a whole.

The linear approach also influences the definition of clinical variables. In this regard, Drs. Monahan and Appelbaum define psychopathy according to the score on the PCL-SV. Their operationalization of psychopathy thus measures the intensity of a variable. Scores on the PCL-SV can also be used to make a diagnosis which allows for the study of psychopathy as a taxon. The score then reflects a difference in nature rather than intensity—that is, a qualitative difference. The linear conception of psychopathy is promoted by Widiger (1998). An alternative position is based on a holistic conception of psychopathy. It is the approach adopted by Hare (1991). Empirical data have confirmed that psychopathy is a distinct syndrome which does not overlap with other disorder syndromes (Hart & Hare, 1989; Hodgins et al., 1998).

Harris, Rice, and Quinsey (1994) demonstrate empirically that psychopathy is a taxon. It is entirely possible that no psychopaths were included in the MacArthur project, despite the fact that the PCL-SV score was found to be significantly associated with violence in all diagnostic groups other than bipolar disorder.

Conclusion

It is never easy to find the right tone and the appropriate level of analysis for a discussion of someone else's research. The task is even more difficult when it comes to a project on the scale of the MacArthur study. I could have made specific technical points, such as by questioning the decision to draw a comprehensive profile based on three distinct crossed tables without ensuring that the violent acts committed were the same in all three cases: (1) targeted family members, (2) occurred "during the courses of regularly scheduled activities," and (3) "were less likely to occur while the subject was taking street drugs." However, it seemed more constructive to focus on certain aspects of the investigation that force us to think about fundamental research questions. This is why, for example, I described an alternative approach to data analysis even though I did not have the space to elaborate on its strengths and limitations. However, the very idea of more closely examining the implicit theoretical framework of studies militates in favour of an epistemological re-assessment. We must ask ourselves whether giving more in-depth thought to the framework and methods of research would not allow us to ensure that ongoing projects are well grounded and to question our ways of doing things. More time spent thinking about epistemology would surely lead to better research and would help us to avoid being guided only by pragmatism.

Note

1 . It is less clear how the delusional disorder and psychotic disorder NOS are classified in the study by Drs. Monahan and Appelbaum, but it would be surprising to find them categorized under "other psychotics."

References

Bergman, L.R., & Magnusson, D. (1997). A person-oriented approach in research on developmental psychopathology. *Development and Psychopathology, 9,* 291–319.

Borum, R. (1996). Improving the clinical practice of violence risk assessment: Technology, guidelines, and training. *American Psychologist, 51,* 945–956.

Côté, G., & Hodgins, S. (1992). The prevalence of major mental disorders among homicide offenders. *International Journal of Law and Psychiatry, 15*(1), 89–99.

Côté, G., & Lesage, A. (1995). *Diagnostics complémentaires et adaptation sociale chez des détenus schizophrènes ou dépressifs.* Montreal: Centre de recherche de l'Institut Philippe Pinel de Montréal.

Côté, G., Lesage, A., Chawky, N., & Loyer, M. (1997). Clinical specificity of prison inmates with severe mental disorders: A case-control study. *British Journal of Psychiatry, 170,* 571–577.

Gendreau, P., Little, T., & Goggin, C. (1996). A meta-analysis of the predictors of adult offender recidivism: What works? *Criminology, 34,* 575–607.

Hare, R.D. (1981). Psychopathy and violence. In J.R. Hays, T.K. Roberts, & K.S. Soloways (Eds.), *Violence and the violent individual* (pp. 53–74). Jamaica, NY: Spectrum.

Hare, R.D. (1991). *The Hare Psychopathy Checklist: Revised.* Toronto: Multi-Health Systems, Inc.

Hare, R.D., & Jutai, J.W. (1983). Criminal history of the male psychopath: Some preliminary data. In K.T. Van Dusen & S.A. Mednick (Eds.), *Studies of crime and delinquency* (pp. 225–236). Boston: Kluwer Nijhoff.

Hare, R.D., & McPherson, L.M. (1984). Violent and aggressive behavior by criminal psychopaths. *International Journal of Law and Psychiatry, 7,* 35–50.

Harris, G.T., Rice, M.E., & Quinsey, N. (1994). Psychopathy as a taxon: Evidence that psychopaths are a discrete class. *Journal of Consulting and Clinical Psychology, 62,* 387–397.

Hart, S.D., & Hare, R.D. (1989). Discriminant validity of the Psychopathy Checklist in a forensic psychiatric population. *Psychological Assessment: Journal of Consulting and Clinical Psychology, 1,* 211–218.

Hodgins, S. (in press). Studying the etiology of crime and violence among persons with major mental disorders: Challenges in the definition and measurement of interactions. In L. Bergman & B. Cairns (Eds.), *Developmental science and the holistic approach.* Mahwah, NJ: Erlbaum.

Hodgins, S., Côté, G., & Toupin, J. (1998). Major mental disorders and crime: An etiological hypothesis. In D. Cooke, A. Forth, & R.D. Hare (Eds.), *Psychopathy: Theory, research and implications for society* (pp. 231–256). Dordrecht: Kluwer.

Klassen, D., & O'Connor, W.A. (1994). Demographic and case history variables in risk assessment. In J. Monahan & H.J. Steadman (Eds.), *Violence and mental disorder developments in risk assessment* (pp. 229–258). Chicago: University of Chicago Press.

Kraemer, H., Kazdin, A., Offord, D., Kessler, R., Jensen, P., & Kupfer, D. (1997). Coming to terms with the terms of risk. *Archives of General Psychiatry, 54,* 337–343.

Monahan, J. (1997). Clinical and actuarial predictions of violence. In D. Faigman, D. Kaye, M. Saks, & J. Sanders (Eds.), *Modern scientific evidence: The law of science and expert testimony, Vol. 1* (pp. 300–318). St. Paul, MN: West Publishing.

Monahan, J. (1998, June). *Violence and mental health.* Paper presented at the 23rd International Congress of Law and Mental Health, Paris.

Monahan, J., & Steadman, H.J. (1994). Toward a rejuvenation of risk assessment research. In J. Monahan & H.J. Steadman (Eds.), *Violence and mental disorder developments in risk assessment* (pp. 1–18). Chicago: University of Chicago Press.

Pham, T.H., Remy, S., Dailliet, A., & Lienard, L. (1997, June). *Psychopathy and prediction of violent behaviors: An assessment in security hospital.* Poster session presented at the 5th International Congress on the Disorders of Personality, Vancouver.

Steadman, H.J., Monahan, J., Appelbaum, P.S., Grisso, T., Mulvey, E.P., Roth, L.H., Clark Robbins, P., & Klassen, D. (1994). Designing a new generation of risk assessment research. In J. Monahan & H.J. Steadman (Eds.), *Violence and mental disorder developments in risk assessment* (pp. 297–318). Chicago: University of Chicago Press.

Steadman, H.J., Monahan, J., Robbins, P.C., Appelbaum, P., Grisso, T., Klassen, D., Mulvey, E.P., & Roth, L. (1993). From dangerousness to risk assessment: Implications for appropriate research strategies. In S. Hodgins (Ed.), *Mental disorder and crime* (pp. 39–62). Newbury Park, CA: Sage.

Steadman, H.J., Mulvey, E.P., Monahan, J., Robbins, P.C., Appelbaum, P.S., Grisso, T., & Roth, L.H. (1998). Violence by people discharged from acute psychiatric inpatient facilities and by others in the same neighborhoods. *Archives of General Psychiatry, 55,* 393–401.

Von Bertalanffy, L. (1967). *Robots, men and minds: Psychology in the modern world.* New York: Braziller.

Von Bertalanffy, L. (1968). *General system theory: Foundations, development, applications.* New York: Braziller.

Widiger, T.A. (1998). Psychopathy and normal personality. In D.J. Cooke, A. Forth, & R.D. Hare (Eds.), *Psychopathy: Theory, research and implications for society* (pp. 47–68). Dordrecht: Kluwer.

Williamson, S., Hare, R.D., & Wong, S. (1987). Violence: Criminal psychopaths and their victims. *Canada Journal of Behavioral Science, 19,* 454–462.

Gilles Côté is a professor at the Université du Québec à Trois-Rivières, Trois-Rivières, Quebec, Canada, and is Head, Centre de recherche de l'Institut Philippe Pinel de Montréal, Montreal, Quebec, Canada.

Author's Note

Comments or queries may be directed to Gilles Côté, PhD, Centre de recherche de l'Institut Philippe Pinel de Montréal, 10 905 boulevard Henri-Bourassa est, Montréal QC H1C 1H1 Canada. Telephone: 819 376-5085. Fax: 819 376-5195. E-mail: <gilles_cote@uqtr.uquebec.ca>.

ETIOLOGICAL FACTORS LINKED TO CRIMINAL VIOLENCE AND ADULT MENTAL ILLNESS

JASMINE A. TEHRANI
SARNOFF A. MEDNICK

Introduction

Criminal violence is of great concern to our society. Although we are unable to consistently predict which individuals will become violent, research and official crime statistics have suggested that certain individuals may be more prone to engage in criminal offending than others.

One group which has been found to be over-represented in our correctional facilities are mentally ill persons. Although some initially believed the association between mental illness and criminal offending to be spurious or non-existent (Monahan & Steadman, 1983), an impressive body of evidence, based on official crime statistics and self-reported data, has accumulated to suggest that mentally disordered individuals are at greater risk of criminal offending, and violent offending in particular, than non-mentally disordered individuals. This is not to say that all mentally ill persons do or will evidence violent tendencies. In fact, the majority of mentally ill persons remain law-abiding. Yet this particular population may be at increased risk of engaging in criminal violence. In this chapter, we will highlight some of our work addressing violent offending among the mentally ill. For the past 2 decades our research group has focused on identifying potential explanations for the comorbidity between criminal violence and mental illness. Two such candidate explanations are genetic factors and disruptions in foetal neural development. We are claiming not that these are the only explanations or that these two factors explain all of the comorbidity, but that these factors may provide a promising new direction in investigating the link between mental illness and criminal violence.

Violence Among the Mentally Ill

Mentally ill persons commit more than their share of criminal acts. This interpretation has been bolstered by large-scale epidemiological studies, most of which have been summarized by Brennan in this volume. For example, in a Swedish birth cohort, Hodgins (1992) noted that men hospitalized with major mental disorders, a

59

S. Hodgins (ed.), Violence among the Mentally Ill, 59–75.
© 2000 *Kluwer Academic Publishers. Printed in the Netherlands.*

category of mental disorders including mood disorders and schizophrenia, were four times more likely to be registered for a violent offence than non-hospitalized men. Mentally ill women, however, were 27 times more likely to be registered for a violent offence than non-mentally ill women. This finding tends to imply an association between violence and mental illness and to suggest that the presence of mental illness may pose a greater risk for violent offending among females than among males.

Some argue that the relationship between mental illness and criminal violence may be spurious. This interpretation is grounded in the observation that mentally disordered persons may be highly visible, attracting the attention of law-enforcement personnel and subsequently being targeted for arrest more than non-mentally ill persons (Teplin, 1984). Data collected from countries where police practise little discretion and must arrest any individual who displays antisocial behaviour does not support this contention. In Denmark, for example, police exercise little to no discretion (Mednick, personal communication).

In order to complete a rather definitive study of the relationship between mental illness and criminal violence, we assembled a complete national birth cohort in Denmark consisting of 358,180 individuals born in Denmark from 1944 to 1947 (Hodgins, Mednick, Brennan, Schulsinger, & Engberg, 1996). For each of these individuals, we compiled their lifetime psychiatric hospitalization and arrest records from 44 to 48 years of age. These data came from two national registers, the Danish psychiatric register and the Danish criminal register, both of which have been described as the most complete and accurate in the world (Wolfgang, 1977). These data permitted us to examine a totally unselected and exhaustive population of men and women who had reached an age at which further violent acts and initial psychiatric hospitalizations were unlikely.

Of non-hospitalized men of the cohort, 2% were registered for violent criminal acts. Of the males who had at least one psychiatric hospitalization, however, 14% had committed violent acts. For males, there is a seven-fold increase in the risk for violent offences associated with having been admitted to a psychiatric hospital, supporting the claim that mentally disordered persons are more likely to engage in violent acts. For females, the results are even more disturbing. The findings indicate that 1.6% of mentally ill females are registered for violent offences, compared to .1% of non-mentally ill females being registered for violent offences. Mentally ill females were 16 times more likely to commit violent crimes than non-mentally ill females. Consistent with the Hodgins (1992) study using a Swedish birth cohort, these findings suggest a co-occurrence, which may be greater in females than males, of mental illness and criminal violence.

RECIDIVISTIC VIOLENT OFFENDING AMONG THE MENTALLY ILL

Mentally ill persons, however, represent only a small segment of our society. How much of a societal problem does their violence constitute? The answer to this question lies in the fact that the mentally ill are recidivistically violent. It has been demonstrated that the small number of recidivistic offenders commit a disproportionately large number of crimes (Wolfgang, Figlio, & Sellin, 1972). Although the males admitted to psychiatric hospitals represented only 5% of the total population of males, they were responsible for 29% of all violent crimes committed by the 173,559 men in the cohort. Female mental patients formed slightly over 5% of the 162,312 females in the population. However, they were responsible for 50% of the violent offences committed by females in the cohort (Hodgins et al., 1996). Given the nature of the cohort, it is perhaps justified to generalize and say that 29% of all the violent crime perpetrated in the community by males is committed by mentally ill men and 50% of all the violent crime perpetrated by females is committed by mentally ill women. The violent offences committed by the mentally ill are a significant social problem. These estimates hold for Denmark and perhaps can be generalized to most Western nations.

These findings led us to search for clues as to why the mentally ill are excessively violent. There are many different types of explanations. Are there factors which are etiologically significant in mental illness that might also be relevant to violence? We know that mental illnesses have important genetic influences. We have demonstrated that criminal behaviour has important genetic influences.

Genetic Influences in Criminal Behaviour

We carried out a study of the genetic influence on criminal behaviour using an extensive data-set consisting of 14,427 Danish adoptees (ranging in age from 29 to 52 years) and both sets of biological and adoptive parents (Mednick, Gabrielli, & Hutchins, 1984). We found that adopted-away sons had an elevated risk of having a court conviction if their biological parent, rather than their adoptive parent, had one or more court convictions. If neither the biological nor adoptive parents were convicted, 13.5% of the sons were convicted. If the adoptive parents were convicted and the biological parents were not, this figure increased only to 14.7%. An examination of sons whose biological parents were convicted and whose adoptive parents remained law-abiding, however, revealed that 20% of the adoptees had one or more criminal convictions. Moreover, as the number of biological parental convictions increased, the rate of adoptees with court convictions increased.

Having demonstrated a genetic effect for criminal behaviour, we then turned our attention towards examining the types of offences committed by the male adoptees. Specifically, we hypothesized that an elevated proportion of adopted-away males whose biological parents had a criminal conviction would evidence increased rates of violent offences. An unexpected finding emerged in this adoption context.

Genetic factors played a significant role in property offending but not in violent offending (see Figure 1). This finding does not appear to be an anomaly, as it is congruent with the findings from a Swedish adoption cohort (Bohman, Cloninger, Sigvardsson, & von Knorring, 1982). (It should be noted, however, that some twin studies have suggested that violence is heritable [Cloninger & Gottesman, 1987].)

Perhaps the heritability of violence is mediated through a third, unidentified, factor. With this in mind, we combed the literature for clues which might help us to better understand our finding. A study carried out in Oregon suggested a new hypothesis. In this classic study, Heston (1966) followed up a sample of 47 offspring born to schizophrenic mothers. These offspring were separated from their mothers shortly after birth and placed in foster care or an orphanage. Heston was primarily interested in determining if adopted-away offspring were at increased risk of becoming schizophrenic themselves. The findings support the original hypothesis, as five of the 47 offspring became schizophrenic. An interesting finding is that an even greater number of the adopted-away offspring of schizophrenic biological mothers actually had been incarcerated for violent offences. Eleven (23.4%) of the adoptees had been incarcerated for violent offences. Since these offspring were not raised by their schizophrenic mothers, this suggested to us that mental illness and criminal violence may have a common genetic basis.

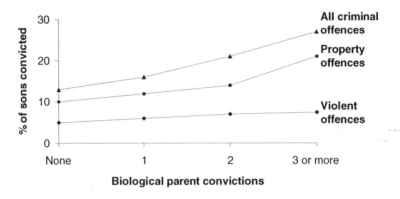

Figure 1. Adoptee criminal offenders, violent offenders, and property offenders, by biological parent convictions

With the Heston (1966) study in mind, Moffit (1987) took another look at our original adoption study findings and investigated the role of parental mental illness in the emergence of violent offending among adopted-away sons. When only the criminal behaviour of the biological parents was considered, she found no increase in violent offending in the adoptees. Violent offending in the offspring was predicted by the combined effect of psychiatric hospitalization and recidivistic criminal offending in the biological parents.

As seen in Figure 2, a significant increase in the rate of violent offending was noted only among offspring whose biological parents were severely criminal (typically the biological father) and had been hospitalized one or more times for a psychiatric condition (typically the biological mother). This study, along with the Heston (1966) study, provides convincing evidence that mentally ill parents transmit to their children a biological predisposition to commit violent acts. This transmission appears to be genetic and not social in nature.

What mechanisms underlie this genetic relationship between violent behaviour and mental illness? The comorbidity of mental illness and violence may depend on a third factor. This third factor may be a condition which shares genes with both violence and mental illness. An example of a third factor may be a genetic predisposition to alcohol abuse. Alcohol abuse is known to be very common in violent offenders, and alcohol intoxication is regularly associated with violent offending.

Alcohol abuse is also common among the mentally ill (Lindquist & Allebeck, 1989; Virkkunen, 1974).

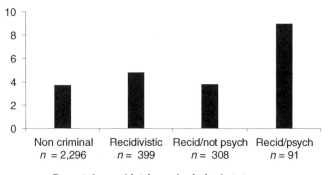

Parents' recidivism and psychopathology predict offspring violent crime in adoption cohort

Figure 2. Parents' recidivism and psychopathology predict offspring violent crime in adoption cohort

THE GENETIC LINK BETWEEN VIOLENCE AND ALCOHOLISM

There are reasons to suspect that violence and alcoholism may be genetically linked. Recent molecular genetics studies report that a gene related to the serotonin system may be associated with increased risk for the co-occurrence of violence and alcoholism (Hallikainen, Saito, Lachman, & Volavka, in press; Lappalainen et al., 1998). These efforts have been fuelled by the well-replicated finding that alcoholism and violence, in humans and in non-human primates, may be related to serotonergic dysregulation (Fils-Aime et al., 1996; Hibbeln et al., 1998; Higley et al., 1993; Higley, Suomi, & Linnoila, 1992; Linnoila, DeJong, & Virkkunen, 1989; Virkkunen et al., 1994; Virkkunen, Eggert, Rawlings, & Linnoila, 1996; Virkkunen, Nuutila, Goodwin, & Linnoila, 1987). This finding tends to suggest that violence and alcoholism may have a common genetic background. Family, twin, and adoption studies, which have partially supported the contention that criminality and alcoholism share a genetic basis, have generally focused on criminality per se and have neglected to differentiate between violent and non-violent types of offending. Epidemiological studies, therefore, are comparatively undeveloped in evaluating the familial association between alcoholism and violence. In a re-analysis of data from the Swedish Adoption Study, Carey (1993) found that paternal violence was linked to alcoholism in adopted-away males. Among biological fathers who had a conviction for violent offending, 24.7% of the adopted-away sons evidenced alcoholism, whereas 16.6% of adopted-away sons of non-violent biological fathers evidenced alcohol problems (chi-square (1) = 4.145, $p < .05$).

We are currently investigating the possible genetic link between violence and alcoholism (Tehrani & Mednick, 1999). Within the context of the Danish Adoption Cohort, we examined whether having an alcoholic biological parent placed the adopted-away sons at risk for violent offending. It should be noted that the criteria we have used to classify subjects as violent or alcoholic are strict, as this information was ascertained from the criminal register and psychiatric records. Subjects were classified as property offenders if they had committed property offences only. Violent offenders consisted of a group of individuals who had committed violent offences but possibly also some property offences.

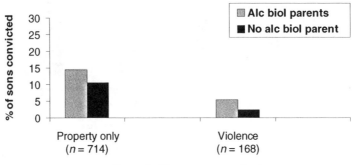

Figure 3. Alcohol problems in biological parents predicting type of offence in male adoptees

Our findings indicate a significant relationship between severe alcohol-related problems in the biological parents and violent offending in the adopted-away males (see Figure 3). Alcoholic biological parents were twice as likely as non-alcoholic biological parents to have a violent adopted-away son. This difference was significant. In contrast, the risk for property offences in adopted-away sons of biological parents with alcohol problems was not significantly elevated. The significant genetic effect was specific to violent offenders.

Moreover, violent offending, but not property offending, among the biological parents was related to severe alcohol-related problems in the adopted-away males. As demonstrated in Figure 4, there were no differences in the rate of alcohol-related problems between sons of biological parents with convictions for property offences and sons of non-criminal biological parents (about 2% in both groups of sons). The risk of alcohol-related problems in the males doubled to 4.1% when the biological parents evidenced violent offending.

These findings from our adoption cohort are in agreement with data from the Swedish Adoption Study. Moreover, evidence from epidemiological studies, particularly from adoption studies which are able to parcel out most environmental sources of influence, support the overall interpretations of recent molecular genetic studies.

We have presented data which indicate that the link between mental illness and criminal behaviour may be genetically mediated. By what mechanism might genetic predisposition increase the risk for mental illness and violence? We have suggested that genetically programmed disruptions during critical periods of foetal neural development may be an important predisposing factor in certain mental illnesses such as schizophrenia and affective disorders. We will argue that this may also be true for violence. We have also hypothesized that neural developmental disruption might result from non-genetic teratogens at critical developmental periods. One type of teratogen which may disrupt foetal neural development is prenatal exposure to the influenza virus. This hypothesis was first tested in a Helsinki birth cohort whose foetal developmental period overlapped the major influenza epidemic of 1957. In this population, we examined the risk for schizophrenia, major affective disorder, and criminal violence.

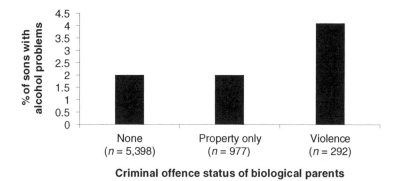

Figure 4. Type of offending in biological parents predicting alcohol problems in male adoptees

HELSINKI INFLUENZA PROJECT

Schizophrenia

In Helsinki, we reported that second-trimester maternal influenza significantly increased the risk for adult schizophrenia in the exposed foetuses (Mednick, Machon, Huttunen, & Bonnet, 1988). Specifically, the sixth month of gestation appeared to be the period of highest risk for the development of adult schizophrenia. This finding has been replicated in numerous epidemiological studies using independent samples as well as by numerous neuropathology studies (Adams, Kendell, Hare, & Munk-Jorgensen, 1993; Fahy, Jones, Sham, Takei, & Murray 1993; Kendell & Kemp, 1989; Kunugi, Takei, & Nanko, 1994; Machon & Mednick, 1994; Mednick, Machon, Huttunen, & Barr, 1990; O'Callaghan, Sham, Takei, Glover, & Murray, 1991; Waddington, 1992; Welham, McGrath, & Pemberton, 1993). It should be noted that four studies have failed to replicate our findings (Bowler & Torrey, 1990; Crow, Done, & Johnstone, 1991; Selton & Slaets, 1994; Susser, Lin, Brown, Lumey, & Erlenmeyer-Kimling, 1994). These studies, however, did not rely on official sources of data to corroborate the presence of a maternal influenza virus during pregnancy.

If exposure to the influenza virus during the second trimester of gestation is associated with elevated risk for schizophrenia, we may hypothesize that a significant proportion of schizophrenic patients in our sample suffered a maternal second-trimester infection. A review of clinical records revealed that among the schizophrenic patients whose second trimester of gestation coincided with the height of the 1957 influenza epidemic, 86.7% were exposed in utero to the influenza virus. In contrast, only 20% of those exposed in the first or third trimester had documented cases of maternal influenza exposure (Machon & Mednick, 1994).

We also hypothesized that differences could emerge in the symptom profiles of these second-trimester schizophrenics. Schizophrenia associated with a teratogenic-related disturbance, such as the influenza virus, may present with a distinctive symptomatology pattern. To test this hypothesis, we coded schizophrenia-related symptoms based on hospital records and personal interviews with the patients. Compared to the control groups (i.e., schizophrenics who were prenatally exposed to the influenza virus during trimesters one or three or not at all), the second-trimester schizophrenics displayed a predominance of symptoms associated with paranoia, such as suspiciousness, delusions of reference, and delusions of jealousy (Machon & Mednick, 1994).

Major affective disorder

More recently, we demonstrated that second-trimester exposure to the influenza virus may also be associated with other forms of mental illness, such as affective disorder (Machon, Mednick, & Huttenen, 1997). We reported that within the context of the Helsinki Influenza Project, subjects exposed to the influenza virus during the second trimester of gestation were at elevated risk for affective disorders later in life, as measured by psychiatric records. We noted that this effect was stronger in males than in females, as well as for unipolar versus bipolar forms of depression.

Our findings suggest that exposure to the influenza virus during the second trimester of gestation may be related to schizophrenia and affective disorder later in life. In any second-trimester-exposed individual, what determines whether schizophrenia or affective disorder will be manifested? To examine this question, we distributed the cases of schizophrenia and affective disorder according to their dates of exposure to the maternal influenza infection. We found that half of the second-trimester schizophrenics, as opposed to only 10% of the affective disorder cases, sustained a maternal infection in the sixth month of gestation. On the other hand, the majority of those with affective disorder suffered a maternal infection in the fifth month of gestation. This suggests more precise temporal specificity of the effects of the influenza teratogen.

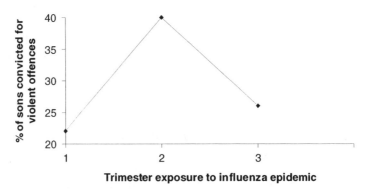

Figure 5. Violence in Helsinki cohort born after 1957 influenza epidemic

Violent offending

Within the context of the Helsinki Influenza Project, we investigated the relationship between type of offending and gestational period of exposure (Tehrani, Brennan, Hodgins, & Mednick, 1998). We hypothesized that maternal influenza during the second trimester was associated with an increased risk, among exposed foetuses, for violent offending but not property offending. To test this hypothesis, we searched the Finnish criminal register for all Helsinki residents born in the 9 months after the 1957 influenza epidemic.

We noted no relationship between property crime and period of exposure to the maternal influenza infections. Convictions for violent crimes, however, were significantly associated with second-trimester maternal infection. Individuals who had been exposed to the influenza virus during the second trimester of gestation were significantly more likely to have a criminal conviction for a violent offence than individuals who were exposed to the influenza virus during the first or third trimesters or not exposed to the virus at all. Moreover, violent offenders tended to have been exposed at the cusp of the sixth and seventh months.

Thus, we found that within the context of the Helsinki Influenza Project: (1) maternal infection in the fifth month of gestation is associated with major affective disorder; (2) maternal infection in the sixth month of gestation is associated with schizophrenia; and (3) maternal infection in the sixth and seventh months of gestation is associated with violent criminal offending. We might speculate that the fact that violence and schizophrenia share the sixth month of gestation as a vulnerable period helps to explain their frequent comorbidity. The gestational period of vulnerability for affective disorder, on the other hand, is almost restricted to the fifth month. It may be speculated that this separation of vulnerability periods for violence and affective disorder helps to explain the low levels of violent offending reported in affective disorder patients.

DISTURBANCE IN FOETAL NEURAL DEVELOPMENT

How might exposure to the influenza virus during the second trimester of gestation be associated with mental illness and criminal outcomes 15, 20, or even 30 years later? The maternal influenza virus acts as a teratogen, disrupting the normal development of the foetal brain. However, to increase the risk for criminal violence, for example, this neural disruption must satisfy two conditions. First, it must have occurred during a period or periods of rapid development of specific brain regions. Second, a deficit in these specific brain regions must play a significant role in increasing risk for criminal violence.

We are proposing that there exists one or more periods of foetal brain development during which a disturbance may increase the risk for certain negative outcomes, such as criminal violence. We hypothesize that if the genetic or teratogenic developmental disruption is introduced in a gestational period different from the identified "critical period," the risk for criminal violence will not be increased. Perhaps the teratogen introduced in a different gestational period will increase risk for another behavioural disorder, such as affective disorder. One hypothesis is that some of the great diversity seen in behavioural and mental disorders may be related to the consequences of teratogens encountered at different times during gestation. This does not mean that all mental disorders function according to this principle, but we offer it as one possible explanation for the etiology of certain mental disorders and criminal violence.

Drosophila larva development

The development of the Drosophila provides an instructive model for this hypothesis. The effect of teratogen on Drosophila development has been a subject of intense study since Gloor (1947). The most commonly studied teratogen has been heat shock; one example of heat shock is exposure of a Drosophila larva to a temperature of 40.8° Celsius for 35 minutes (Schlesinger, Ashburner, & Tissieres, 1982). Heat shock has been tested systematically with the Drosophila. Different structural abnormalities (e.g., missing wings, legs) have been observed with heat-shock exposure at different stages of larval development.

When the heat-shock teratogen is presented, cell activity is dominated by heat-shock proteins; normal gene expression is put on hold. When the danger to the cell has passed, the genes begin to express normally again. There is, however, an internal timing process that informs the cell which part of the Drosophila is scheduled for rapid development. Thus, 37 hours into the pupal stage the wings are scheduled for development. This wing development must be completed in the next 4 hours, because at 41 hours the head will begin rapid development and wing development will cease or be severely diminished. The genes express on schedule and will not return to an organ to remedy developmental errors. If the heat-shock teratogen is presented between 37 and 41 hours, the development of the wings will be disturbed and the wings will develop abnormally or not at all. Whatever element of the Drosophila (e.g., wings, legs) should have undergone rapid development during the heat-shock-induced interruption will suffer incomplete or abnormal development.

The relevance of this model to the human brain is clear. In response to a teratogen (such as maternal influenza infection or severe stress), the cells will assume a defensive stance. Heat-shock proteins will dominate cell behaviour; normal gene expression will be put on hold. If an element of the prefrontal cortex or thalamus is scheduled for rapid development at the time that the teratogen strikes, that development will suffer a deficit. When the influence of the teratogen dissipates, gene expression will once again dominate development. The gene expression, however, will skip the development of the element interrupted by the teratogen (in our example, the specific element of the prefrontal cortex or thalamus) and move on to the next brain area scheduled for rapid development. If we simply substitute a list of brain areas for the different elements of the Drosophila, and change the time scale from hours to days of gestation, we can see the relevance of the Drosophila model for human brain development.

TERATOGENIC DISTURBANCE AND HUMAN BRAIN DEVELOPMENT

In humans, several areas of the foetal brain may undergo rapid development at the same time. A period of rapid development is a period of special vulnerability for a brain region. During a vulnerable period of development, a teratogen will have exaggerated effects on the specific brain regions undergoing rapid growth at that time. The period or periods of vulnerability of specific brain regions must span some days in the second trimester of gestation. For example, if a failure of development of a sub-area of the prefrontal cortex or thalamus is a risk factor for criminal violence, then one period of vulnerability might comprise those days of gestation that the pre-frontal cortex and/or thalamus is most rapidly developing.

We hypothesize that normal mental functioning is dependent on a brain which has developed during gestation without serious disturbance. Deficits in specific brain areas, systems, and circuits may be associated with specific mental, behavioural, and cognitive disorders. Each of these areas, systems, and circuits has its appointed time during gestation to flourish. If this assigned developmental period is disturbed (by genetic or teratogenic influence), that area, system, or circuit will suffer a develop-mental deficit. If this specific brain deficit is a part of the etiology of a specific mental disorder, the risk for that disorder will be elevated.

It is well known that there is a specific sequence of organ development for the foetus. In the first trimester, the effect of a teratogen is dependent upon its timing. In a well-known example, thalidomide is effective as a teratogen only during 1 week in the first trimester. Taken in another period, it has no known teratogenic effect. The timing of a teratogen may determine which brain areas will fail to develop fully; the functional characteristics of these flawed brain areas may play a predispositional role in a variety of human outcomes. In concert with other teratogenic events, such as genetic factors and postnatal environmental events, these teratogenic disturbances can predispose an individual to a major mental or behavioural disorder; or the tera-togen may play a predispositional role in shaping the specific characteristics of the cognitive ability, the personality, and/or the temperament of the adult.

The impact of a teratogen on foetal neural development, either negative or neu-tral, appears contingent upon the timing of the virus. The effects of other types of teratogens on human development, however, may not function based on the "timing of exposure" hypothesis. It is also possible that the timing of exposure will be diffi-cult to determine. For example, it may be difficult to identify a specific month or trimester associated with the highest risk of negative outcome in cases where the teratogen is present throughout development, or when the long-term effects of the teratogen linger and have residual effects throughout the period of gestation. Intro-duction of some types of teratogens, such as illegal drugs, alcohol, and nicotine, may represent substances which, regardless of when they are introduced, are potentially harmful to the exposed foetus.

Much attention has recently been paid to the association between maternal smoking during pregnancy and negative behavioural outcomes among exposed foe-tuses. These negative outcomes include impulsivity and attentional problems (Fergusson, Woodward, & Horwood, 1998; Milberger, Biederman, Faraone, Chen, & Jones, 1996). Prenatal nicotine exposure has also been associated with criminal offending.

Maternal Prenatal Smoking and Criminal Violence

An investigation conducted in Finland by Rantakallio, Laara, Isohanni, and Moilanen (1992) examined the criminal records of 5,966 members of a birth cohort and found that prenatal maternal smoking predicted criminal offending at age 22. These findings persisted after controlling for the effects of social variables such as socioeconomic status. Most subjects, however, had not passed through most of the age of risk for criminal behaviour. Therefore, it is unclear whether maternal smoking during pregnancy may serve as a salient predictor of more serious or persistent types of criminal offending, such as recidivistic violent offending.

With these recent findings in mind, we investigated the association between maternal smoking and criminal violence using a Danish birth cohort of 4,129 males between the ages of 31 and 34 years (Brennan, Grekin, & Mednick, 1999). Accordingly, most of the males in our sample had passed through the age of risk for serious criminal offending. We hypothesized that maternal smoking would be related to an increased risk of violent offending among males and may be specific to certain types of offending patterns.

One of the major strengths of the study was that maternal prenatal smoking was assessed through interviews during the pregnancy as opposed to retrospectively. Moreover, we relied on the Danish criminal register to identify cases where the individuals were arrested for property or violent offences.

Maternal prenatal smoking was assessed during the third trimester of pregnancy. In addition, maternal drug use, pregnancy and delivery complications, parental psychiatric and criminal history, and maternal rejection were also assessed. The longitudinal nature of this project allowed for differentiation between less serious types of offending (as defined by criminal offending prior to age 18, or "adolescent-limited offending") and life-course-persistent offending (as defined by criminal offending prior to and after the age of 18) (Moffit, 1993). The second category represents a more serious form of antisocial behaviour.

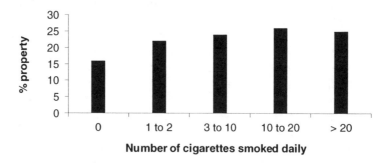

Figure 6. Maternal smoking and property offending in males

The data suggest that maternal smoking is related to life-course-persistent offending (p <.00001) and not to adolescent-limited offending (p = ns). This linear relationship persists despite accounting for potential confounds, such as: parent psychiatric hospitalization, pregnancy complications, delivery complications, maternal use of drugs during pregnancy, paternal criminal history, and socioeconomic status.

A relationship was observed between amount of maternal prenatal smoking and violent (chi-square (1) = 39.77, $p < .001$) and non-violent (chi-square (1) = 34.58, $p < .001$) offending (see figures 6 and 7). Potential confounds did not account for this relationship. These results indicate a dose-response relationship between amount of maternal prenatal smoking and arrests for persistent criminal behaviour and violent offending in nicotine-exposed male offspring.

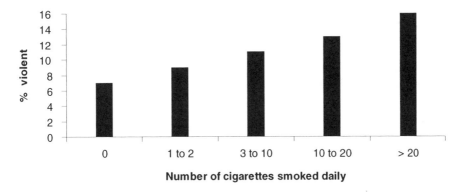

Figure 7. Maternal smoking and violent offending in males

Conclusions

The data summarized suggest that genetic and non-genetic teratogenic factors may increase the risk of violent offending. Genetic factors which we have targeted are related to parental mental illness and alcoholism. We have reported that mental illness in the biological parents is associated with an increase in a child's risk for violent offending. This is true even when the child is adopted away from his biological family and raised separately. This tends to suggest that biological parents may transmit some type of characteristic(s) predisposing their offspring to criminal violence. Secondly, we have recently found that alcohol problems and violence, two outcomes which are found to aggregate within families and within individuals, may have common genetic factors. This finding supports recent molecular genetic studies which have identified a gene common to alcoholism and violence.

We propose that disruptions to foetal neural development, through the introduction of some type of teratogen, may be associated with an increased risk for certain mental and behavioural disorders. This is not to say that all forms of criminal behaviour and mental illness are attributable to a teratogenic disturbance. Our finding that schizophrenia marked by paranoid features is associated with exposure to the second-trimester maternal influenza virus supports our contention that certain mental illnesses or subtypes of mental illnesses (but not all) may operate according to the timing-of-exposure hypothesis. We also found criminal violence to be elevated among offspring prenatally exposed to the influenza virus and among offspring whose mothers smoked cigarettes during pregnancy.

Taken together, these studies provide clues to the potential etiological factors linked to violence and mental illness and may help to elucidate the nature of their co-occurrence. Moreover, research into etiological factors may translate into useful intervention strategies for reducing the incidence of criminal violence and mental illness. Identification of children at genetic risk for mental illness or criminal violence (e.g., through the mental or criminal status of the biological parents) may facilitate the implementation of early intervention programmes to reduce the child's risk of negative outcomes later in life. Moreover, prenatal health care aimed at reducing or eliminating maternal smoking during pregnancy, for example, may in turn decrease the likelihood that a child will later engage in acts of criminal violence. Such possibilities illustrate the utility of etiological research to treatment issues, and may help to bridge the gap between research and the development and implementation of intervention and treatment strategies.

References

Adams, W., Kendell, R.E., Hare, E.H., & Munk-Jorgensen, P. (1993). Epidemiological evidence that maternal influenza contributes to the etiology of schizophrenia: An analysis of Scottish, English, and Danish data. *British Journal of Psychiatry, 163,* 522–534.

Bohman M., Cloninger, C.R., Sigvardsson, S., & von Knorring A.L. (1982). Predisposition to petty criminality in Swedish adoptees. *Archives of General Psychiatry, 39,* 1233–1241.

Bowler, A.E., & Torrey, E.F. (1990). Influenza and schizophrenia: Helsinki and Edinburgh. *Archives of General Psychiatry, 47,* 876–877.

Brennan, P.A, Grekin, E.R., & Mednick, S.A. (1999). Maternal smoking during pregnancy and adult male criminal outcomes. *Archives of General Psychiatry, 56,* 215–219.

Carey, G. (1993). Genetics and violence. In A.J. Reiss, K.A. Miczek, & J.A. Roth (Eds.), *Understanding and preventing violence. Vol. 2: Biobehavioral influences* (pp. 21–58). Washington: National Academy Press.

Cloninger, C.R., & Gottesman, I.I. (1987). Genetic and environmental factors in antisocial behavior disorders. In S.A. Mednick, T.E. Moffitt, & S.A. Stack (Eds.), *The causes of crime: New biological approaches* (pp. 92–109). New York: Cambridge University Press.

Crow, T.J., Done, D.J., & Johnstone, E.C. (1991). Schizophrenia and influenza. *Lancet, 338,* 116–117.

Fahy, T.A., Jones, P.B., Sham, P.C., Takei, N., & Murray, R.M. (1993). Schizophrenia in Afro-Caribbeans in the UK following prenatal exposure to the 1957 A2 influenza pandemic. *Schizophrenia Research, 9,* 132.

Fergusson, D.M., Woodward, L.J., & Horwood, J. (1998). Maternal smoking during pregnancy and psychiatric adjustment in late adolescence. *Archives of General Psychiatry, 55,* 721–727.

Fils-Aime, M.L., Eckardt, D., George, D.T., Brown, G.L., Mefford, I., & Linnoila, M. (1996). Early-onset alcoholics have lower cerebrospinal fluid 5-hydroxyindoleacetic acid levels than late-onset alcoholics. *Archives of General Psychiatry, 53,* 211–216.

Gloor, H. (1947). Versuche mit aether an drosophilia. *Revue Suisse Zoologique, 54,* 637–712.

Hallikainen, T., Saito, T., Lachman, H.M., & Volavka, J. (in press). Association between low activity serotonin transporter promoter genotype with habitual impulsive violent behavior among antisocial early alcoholics. *Molecular Psychiatry.*

Heston, L.L. (1966). Psychiatric disorders in foster-home reared children of schizophrenics. *British Journal of Psychiatry, 112,* 819–825.

Hibbeln, J.R., Linnoila, M., Umhau, J.C., Rawlings, R., George, D.T., & Salem, N. (1998). Essential fatty acids predict metabolites of serotonin and dopamine in cerebrospinal fluid among healthy control subjects, and early- and late-onset alcoholics. *Biological Psychiatry, 44,* 235–242.

Higley, J.D., Suomi, S.J., & Linnoila, M. (1992). A longitudinal assessment of CSF mono-amine metabolite and plasma cortisol concentrations in young Rhesus monkeys. *Biological Psychiatry, 32,* 127–145.

Higley, J.D., Thompson, W.W., Champoux, M., Goldman, D., Hasert, M.F., Kraemer, G.W., Scanlan, J.M., Suomi, S.J., & Linnoila, M. (1993). Paternal and maternal genetic and environmental contributions to cerebrospinal fluid monoamine metabolites in Rhesus monkeys. *Archives of General Psychiatry, 50,* 615–623.

Hodgins, S. (1992). Mental disorder, intellectual deficiency and crime: Evidence from a birth cohort. *Archives of General Psychiatry, 49,* 476–483.

Hodgins, S., Mednick, S.A., Brennan, P.A., Schulsinger, F., & Engberg, M. (1996). Mental disorder and crime: Evidence from a Danish birth cohort. *Archives of General Psychiatry, 53,* 489–496.

Kendell, R.E., & Kemp, I.W. (1989). Maternal influenza in the etiology of schizophrenia. *Archives of General Psychiatry, 46,* 878–882.

Kunugi, H., Takei, N., & Nanko, S. (1994). Head circumference at birth and schizophrenia. *British Journal of Psychiatry, 161,* 274–275.

Lappalainen, J., Long, J.C., Eggert, M., Ozaki, N., Robin, R.W., Brown, G.L., Naukkarinen, H., Virkkunen, M., Linnoila, M., & Goldman, M.D. (1998). Linkage of antisocial alcoholism to the serotonin 5-HT1B receptor gene in 2 populations. *Archives of General Psychiatry, 55,* 989–994.

Lindquist, P., & Allebeck, P. (1989). Schizophrenia and assaultive behavior: The role of alcohol and drug abuse. *Acta Psychiatrica Scandinavica, 82,* 191–195.

Linnoila, M., DeJong, J., & Virkkunen, M. (1989). Family history of alcoholism in violent offenders and impulsive fire setters. *Archives of General Psychiatry, 46,* 613–619.

Machon, R.A., & Mednick, S.A. (1994). Adult schizophrenia and early neurodevelopmental disturbances. In *Confrontations psychiatriques : Epidemiologie et psychiatrie, #35* (pp. 189–215). Paris: Specia Rhône-Poulenc Rorer.

Machon, R.A., Mednick, S.A., & Huttenen, M.O. (1997). Adult major affective disorder following prenatal exposure to an influenza epidemic. *Archives of General Psychiatry, 54,* 322–328.

Mednick S.A., Gabrielli W.F., & Hutchins, B. (1984). Genetic influences in criminal convictions: Evidence from an adoption cohort. *Science, 224,* 891–894.

Mednick, S.A., Machon, R.A., Huttunen, M.O., & Barr, C.E. (1990). Influenza and schizophrenia: Helsinki vs. Edinburgh. *Archives of General Psychiatry, 47,* 875–876.

Mednick, S.A., Machon, R.A., Huttunen, M.O., & Bonnet, D. (1988). Adult schizophrenia following prenatal exposure to an influenza epidemic. *Archives of General Psychiatry, 45,* 189–192.

Milberger, C., Biederman, J., Faraone, S.V., Chen, L., & Jones, J. (1996). Is maternal smoking during pregnancy a risk factor for attention deficit hyperactivity disorder in children? *American Journal of Psychiatry, 153,* 1138–1142.

Moffit, T.E. (1987). Parental mental disorder and offspring criminal behavior: An adoption study. *Psychiatry: Interpersonal and Biological Processes, 50,* 346–360.

Moffit, T.E. (1993). Adolescence-limited and life-course-persistent antisocial behavior: A developmental taxonomy. *Psychological Review, 100,* 674–701.

Monahan, J., & Steadman, H.J. (1983). Crime and mental disorder. In M. Tonry & N. Morris (Eds.), *Crime and justice: An annual review of the research (Vol. 4)*. Chicago: University of Chicago Press.

O'Callaghan, E., Sham, P., Takei, N., Glover G., & Murray, R.M. (1991). Schizophrenia after prenatal exposure to 1957 A2 influenza epidemic. *Lancet, 337*, 1248–1250.

Rantakallio, P., Laara, E., Isohanni, M., & Moilanen, I. (1992). Maternal smoking during pregnancy and delinquency of the offspring: An association without causation? *International Journal of Epidemiology, 21*, 1106–1113.

Schlesinger, M.J., Ashburner, M., & Tissieres, A. (1982). *Heat shock from bacteria to man*. Cold Spring Harbor, ME: Cold Spring Harbor Laboratory.

Selten, J.P., & Slaets, J.P. (1994). Evidence against maternal influenza as a risk factor for schizophrenia. *British Journal of Psychiatry, 164*, 674–676.

Susser, E., Lin, S.P., Brown, A.S., Lumey, L.H., & Erlenmeyer-Kimling, L. (1994). No relation between risk of schizophrenia and prenatal exposure to influenza in Holland. *American Journal of Psychiatry, 151*, 922–924.

Tehrani J.A., Brennan, P.A., Hodgins S., & Mednick, S.A. (1998). Mental illness and criminal violence. *Social Psychiatry and Psychiatric Epidemiology, 33*, 81–85.

Tehrani, J., & Mednick, S.A. (1999). *Violence and alcoholism: A possible genetic link*. Manuscript in preparation.

Teplin, L.A. (1984). Criminalizing mental disorder: The comparative arrest rate of the mentally ill. *American Psychologist, 39*, 794–803.

Virkkunen, M. (1974). Observations of violence in schizophrenia. *Acta Psychiatrica Scandinavica, 50*, 145–151.

Virkkunen, M., Eggert, M., Rawlings, R., & Linnoila, M. (1996). A prospective follow-up study of alcoholic violent offenders and fire setters. *Archives of General Psychiatry, 53*, 523–529.

Virkkunen, M., Nuutila, A., Goodwin, G., & Linnoila, M. (1987). Cerebrospinal fluid monoamine metabolite levels in male arsonists. *Archives of General Psychiatry, 44*, 241–247.

Virkkunen, M., Rawlings, R., Tokola, R., Poland, R., Guidotti, A., Nemeroff, C., Bissette, G., Kalgeras, K., Karonen, S., & Linnoila, M. (1994). CSF biochemistries, glucose metabolism, and diurnal activity rhythms in alcoholic, violent offenders, fire setters and healthy volunteers. *Archives of General Psychiatry, 51*, 20–27.

Waddington, J.L. (1992, June). *The declining incidence of schizophrenia controversy: A new approach in a rural Irish population*. Paper presented at the annual meeting of the Royal College of Psychiatrists, Dublin.

Welham, J.L., McGrath, J.J., & Pemberton, M.R. (1993). Schizophrenia: Birthrates and three Australian epidemics. *Schizophrenia Research, 9*, 142.

Wolfgang, M., Figlio, R.M., & Sellin, T. (1972). *Delinquency in a birth cohort*. Chicago: University of Chicago Press.

Wolfgang, M.E. (1977). Foreword. In S.A. Mednick & K.O. Christiansen (Eds.), *Biosocial bases of criminal behavior*. New York: Gardiner.

Jasmine A. Tehrani is a doctoral student in Clinical Psychology, University of Southern California, Los Angeles, California, USA, and Research Assistant, Social Science Research Institute, Los Angeles. Sarnoff A. Mednick is Professor of Psychology, Social Science Research Institute, Los Angeles, and Senior Research Associate, Institute of Preventive Medicine, Copenhagen, Denmark.

Authors' Note

This research was supported by a National Institute on Aging Forming Careers in Science Award (T32 AG00156) to Jasmine A. Tehrani, a National Institute of Mental Health Research Scientist Award (MH 00619) to Dr. Sarnoff A. Mednick, and a Guggenheim Foundation grant (W9600228) to Drs. Beatrice Golomb and Sarnoff A. Mednick.

Comments or queries may be directed to Jasmine A. Tehrani, Department of Psychology, University of Southern California, University Park, Los Angeles CA 90089 USA. Telephone: 213 740-4620. Fax: 213 740-7778. E-mail: <jtehrani@rcf.usc.edu>.

COMMENTARY

Tehrani and Mednick, "Etiological Factors Linked to Criminal Violence
and Adult Mental Illness"

MATTI VIRKKUNEN

I am glad to have the opportunity to comment on the review of Mednick's studies published during the 1980s and 1990s (Mednick, in press). I find this task rather daunting as the papers have been published in the best psychiatric journals. The reported studies related only in part to violence committed by mentally ill persons, and especially those with schizophrenia. They were more broadly concerned with violence among persons with personality disorder. The papers are based on studies with more than 14,000 Danish adoptees.

The first of the papers, published in *Science* in 1984 (Mednick, Gabrielli, & Hutchings, 1984), shows that genetic factors play a significant role in property offending but not in violent offending. When I read this I was astonished. These findings seemed to contradict much evidence showing the connection between violent alcoholic families—usually violent fathers—and aggressive conduct disorder in male offspring. Such cases, of course, meet Cloninger's criteria of type 2 alcoholism, which passes from fathers to sons and in which there is the tendency to behave violently under the influence of alcohol (Cloninger, Bohman, & Sigvardsson, 1981). Violence coupled with alcoholism has a genetic predisposition, but only among men. Even this early-onset alcoholism is thought to be secondary to early-onset conduct disorder, which precedes the development of antisocial personality disorder as it is defined in the DSM-IV (American Psychiatric Association, 1994).

It is possible that the reason for these astonishing early negative findings on violence is that alcoholism was not measured separately. Another reason may be the low frequency of violent crimes as compared to property crimes. In violent alcoholic families, much of the violence occurs when the father is intoxicated but it does not lead to prosecution, as the wife or sexual partner protects the aggressor and is not eager to report him to the police. However, it is relatively easy to obtain information on violence through structured psychiatric interviews.

Mednick has stated that the finding that a hereditary factor contributes to non-violent criminality may not be an anomaly, as it has been replicated in another adoption study (Bohman, Cloninger, Sigvardsson, & von Knorring, 1982). In this latter investigation, non-alcoholic petty criminals were found to have an excess of

77

S. Hodgins (ed.), Violence among the Mentally Ill, 77–87.
© 2000 *Kluwer Academic Publishers. Printed in the Netherlands.*

biological parents with a history of petty crime but not alcohol abuse. Further, type 2 alcoholism was found to be heritable and linked to violence. The latest paper from this research team suggests that a tendency to react abnormally under the influence of alcohol is inherited (Sigvardsson, Bohman, & Cloninger, 1996). Recent experimental evidence has shown that men diagnosed with ASPD behave violently under the influence of alcohol (Moeller, Dougherty, Lane, Steinberg, & Cherek, 1998).

Do Cloninger's and Mednick's Findings Converge?

The most recently published views of Mednick's group tend to converge with Cloninger's ideas when the former note a significant increase in the rate of violent offending among offspring whose biological parents were severely criminal (usually the father) or had been hospitalized one or more times for a psychiatric condition (typically the biological mother) (Figure 2) (Mednick, in press). These severely criminal fathers are, of course, often alcoholics with ASPD and typically impulsive, habitually violent tendencies. We must remember that these violent, antisocial individuals quite often marry psychotic women or have children with them. Mednick's latest findings are similar to Cloninger's: a significant relationship exists between alcohol-related problems and violent offending in the biological parents and violent offending and alcoholism in their adopted male offspring. Type 2 alcoholism, which is common among men with ASPD, could explain this result (Mednick). If I understand correctly, in this latter investigation "severe alcohol related problems" are defined as those associated with "court convictions for public intoxication" or "having been treated for alcoholism as a court-ordered condition of probation." Many people who behave impulsively and/or aggressively under the influence of alcohol would fulfil these criteria. It is a pity that Mednick's group was unable to examine the quantity and frequency of drinking among these individuals.

In some of their studies, Mednick's group seem to have excluded adoptees (and also their parents) who died or emigrated from Denmark before the age of 30. In the *Science* paper, Mednick et al. (1984) state that cases were excluded from the study if there was no record of place or date of birth or if the identity of the biological father could not be established. Antisocial alcoholics are usually very restless, and because of their criminal career they often travel from one country to another. Statistical power may have been diminished by the elimination of the "most severe" and most restless fathers and adoptees from the follow-up. It may also have been diminished by the fact that antisocial alcoholics die at an early age (due to suicide, murder, accidents, or other forms of violence, or as a result of alcoholism or drug dependence) (Martin, Cloninger, Guze, & Clayton, 1995; Rydelius, 1988). Mednick et al. (1984) state in the *Science* paper that the exclusion rates for the biological fathers were considerably higher than for the adoptive fathers. These were possibly recidivistic fathers. So it is possible that these fathers, in particular, had sons who became especially alcoholic and violent—thereby distorting the results.

Possible Genetic and Biochemical Aspects

Mednick believes that genetic factors may be associated with criminal violence, especially considering recent COMT (catechol-O-methyltransferase) polymorphism findings (Lachman, Nolan, Mohr, Saito, & Volavka, 1998; Strous, Bark, Parsia, Volavka, & Lachman, 1997). It is true that at present this is the only genetic polymorphism thought to be associated *with violence* (but not with violent crimes) *among persons with schizophrenia*. Two small studies have demonstrated an association between COMT gene polymorphism in chromosome 22 and violent behaviour among persons with schizophrenia. In question is the allele coding for the less active form of this enzyme (Lachman et al.; Strous et al.). However, these persons with schizophrenia had committed no violent crimes. We also do not know whether the low activity of COMT is linked to violent tendencies among persons who do not have schizophrenia. COMT renders catecholamines inactive. Preliminary findings with laboratory animals indicate that COMT may be linked to aggression (Gogos et al., 1998). At present the question is also whether this finding applies to individuals with schizophrenia. A recent study has shown that the low-activity allele thought to be associated with aggressivity is in fact associated with obsessive-compulsive traits. Furthermore, a very extensive mutation analysis of this gene in a large group of schizophrenic individuals revealed no mutations (Karayiorgou et al., 1998). We must also remember that DeLisi, in her critical review on genetics and schizophrenia, concludes that at present no gene can definitely be associated with schizophrenia (DeLisi, 1999).

The genetic factors that now seem to be linked to habitually violent and impulsive tendencies are the 5HT1B and TPH polymorphisms, both associated with abnormal serotonin metabolism (Lappalainen et al., 1998; Nielsen et al., 1998). The former is possibly associated with antisocial alcoholism and has already been replicated (New, Gelernter, Mitropoulou, Koenigsberg, & Siever, 1999). The latter is possibly associated with asocial tendencies as measured by the socialization subscale of the Karolinska Scales of Personality (KSP) (Nielsen et al.). A type of TPH polymorphism has also been found to be related to traits of aggressivity and anger (Manuck et al., 1999; New et al., 1998). However, these latter findings remain unclear. The KSP socialization subscale was originally constructed to assess psychopathic personality features (Gustavsson, 1997; Schalling, Asberg, Edman, & Oreland, 1987), but low scores characterize individuals with general pathology (Ekselius & von Knorring, 1999; Gustavsson). Preliminary findings indicate that the TPH polymorphism is not associated with violence among schizophrenic patients (Saito, Lachman, Mohr, Nolan, & Volavka, 1999). Serotonin receptors other than serotonin 1B do not appear to be involved, according to our studies conducted in collaboration with the US National Institute of Alcohol Abuse and Alcoholism (NIAAA). We need more information as to how these two polymorphisms relate to the findings of Mednick's group. The 5HT1B polymorphism may be central; 5HT1B knockout mice are characterized by excessive and impulsive aggression, inappropriate sexual activity, and increased alcohol and cocaine intake (Crabbe et al., 1996; Rocha et al., 1998; Saudou et al., 1994). These are, of course, very typical characteristics of individuals with ASPD. Knocking out only this 5HT1B gene profoundly changes behaviour, seemingly creating a disinhibitory syndrome, as described more than 20 years ago in relation to prefrontal cortical injury (Fuster, 1999).

There are genetic factors associated with attention-deficit and hyperactivity problems (Thaper, Holmes, Poulton, & Harrington, 1999), D4 and dopamine transporter polymorphisms. These seem to be linked to stimulus-seeking behaviour, and thus they may be the basis of attention deficit/conduct disorder problems and all kinds of recklessness behaviours. Current evidence indicates that many genetic factors other than COMT could explain the findings of Mednick's group.

There are also findings indicating that low serotonin and noradrenaline turnover is related to violent behaviour (Virkkunen, De Jong, Bartko, Goodwin, & Linnoila, 1989; Virkkunen, Eggert, Rawlings, & Linnoila, 1996). Although it is possible that serotonin turnover is inherited by sons from their fathers, Higley's studies with monkeys (Higley & Linnoila, 1997) show that the maternal contribution to serotonin turnover may also be important. We need research to determine whether low serotonin and noradrenaline turnover could explain Mednick's findings. For example, low noradrenaline turnover may lead to the low heart rate that Mednick's group have found to predict violent tendencies. This partly heritable trait is thought to reflect fearlessness and stimulus-seeking, which can be an early biological marker for aggressive behaviour (Raine, Venables, & Mednick, 1997).

Prenatal Factors (Other Than Smoking) and Criminality

I think Mednick's group is on the weakest ground when they attempt to link prenatal factors (other than smoking) to violence among males, and when they suggest that there is an etiological link between an influenza epidemic during the second trimester of pregnancy and violent tendencies in the offspring (Tehrani, Brennan, Hodgins, & Mednick, 1998). There is evidence from Mednick's group of an association between a second-trimester influenza epidemic and schizophrenia (Mednick, Machon, Huttunen, & Bonett, 1988), and even depression (Machon, Mednick, & Huttunen, 1997). It is important, however, to remember that we do not know if these mothers had the virus influenza during the epidemic. While many studies have replicated the finding of an association between second-trimester influenza epidemics and schizophrenia in the offspring, many have not. Those few studies that have had access to rare population samples of pregnant women for whom a history of actual influenza infection has been recorded at a prenatal clinic have failed to replicate the finding (Cannon et al., 1996; Crow & Done, 1992). Only Mednick's group has found some hint that these mothers had had influenza (Mednick, Huttunen, & Machon, 1994). As far as I know, no other group has replicated the association with depression—and no one has found an association with violent offending!

The authors state that when they interviewed the subjects who were in the second trimester of pregnancy during the influenza epidemic and who subsequently developed schizophrenia, these women differed from other persons with schizophrenia. The symptom picture of the former but not the latter group was dominated by suspiciousness and delusional ideation, which is possibly more often linked to violent behaviour (Tehrani et al., 1998). It is a little difficult for me to understand Figure 9 relating an influenza epidemic and violent tendencies. In this figure, even in the first and third trimesters of pregnancy the percentages of violent tendencies are as high as 20 to 25%. In their original paper (Tehrani et al.), the authors state that there was no relationship between property crime and period of gestation and exposure to the 1957 influenza epidemic. They do, however, note that the Finnish police register requires that records of less serious criminal convictions and arrests be discarded after 5 years. So it puzzles me as to how it is possible to reliably know anything about "old property crimes." To me, these findings are unclear.

Prenatal Smoking and Criminality

As to prenatal smoking, Mednick's group is on very solid ground (Brennan, Grekin, & Mednick, 1999). They provide figures showing that prenatal nicotine exposure could be a contributing factor in criminality and behavioural problems. Their findings are consistent with a number of studies that have demonstrated an association between maternal smoking and development of behaviour problems up to at least adolescence (Fergusson, Woodward, & Horwood, 1998; Millberger, Biederman, Faraone, Chen, & Joners, 1996; Orlebeke, Knol, & Verhulst, 1999; Rasanen et al., 1999; Wakslag et al., 1997). Mednick's group also found a linear dose-response relationship between the number of cigarettes the mother smoked per day and the percentage of the offspring who become violent offenders (Brennan et al., 1999). This relationship persisted despite controlling for various potential confounds such as socioeconomic status, parental psychiatric hospitalization, and paternal criminal history. It would be important for this group to examine the potential confounding factors such as attention deficit disorder, conduct disorder, and ASPD in the male offspring in all of their studies published in the years 1996–99.

It appears that the father's alcohol abuse, alcohol dependence, and violent tendencies under the influence of alcohol were not controlled for in many of these studies, confounding the variables in the logistic regression analyses (Brennan et al., 1999; Fergusson et al., 1998; Millberger et al., 1996; Rasanen et al., 1999). They were, however, somewhat controlled for concerning the mothers in the Wakslag et al. (1997) paper. This last study, however, found that smoking was an independent predictor of conduct disorder. Wakslag et al. found that maternal ASPD and maternal smoking were independent predictors of conduct disorder when other variables were controlled for. But even this research group says nothing about the fathers' problems.

One might ask how a father's alcoholism, violent tendencies, and ASPD could be connected with a mother's smoking during pregnancy. These ASPD males are very reckless, however, and they are likely to marry reckless women and have children with them. One aspect of a mother's recklessness is a tendency to smoke during pregnancy when it is commonly known that this can be harmful to the foetus.

Genetic Factors as Confounding Variables in Studies on Smoking

It is possible that the same genetic factors explain maternal prenatal smoking and conduct problems in male offspring. If Rasanen et al.'s (1999) finding that maternal prenatal smoking is associated with violent and persistent offending, but not with non-violent offending, is borne out, 5HT1B gene polymorphism is the most probable candidate (Lappalainen et al., 1998). These ideas parallel statements by Rantakallio, Laara, Isohanni, and Moilanen (1992), who also studied the association between maternal smoking and delinquency in the offspring. This group notes that even though the association between maternal smoking and delinquency in the offspring remained after adjustment for social and demographic factors, maternal smoking may be symptomatic of a certain lifestyle and abnormal behaviour likely to foster delinquency in children rather than being an agent with a direct causal role. This view is supported by the findings of Rantakallio et al. Their cohort, in contrast to the findings of Mednick's group (Brennan et al., 1999), showed no sign of the dose-response pattern. This finding was supported by the fact that cessation of smoking seemed to be of minor importance.

Mednick is interested in the timing of perinatal events, but it is possible that smoking, if a causal factor, affects the entire pregnancy, not only the second trimester. Fergusson et al. (1998) suggest that the effect of maternal smoking during pregnancy on externalizing behaviour is limited to male offspring. If the finding is gender-specific, why is this so?

Mednick's group points to "brain damage" as a possible explanation for the association between prenatal smoking and later criminality, but there may be others as well. Fergusson (1999), in commenting on the findings of Brennan et al. (1999), offers the following explanations: (a) foetal hypoxia, (b) changes in serotonin uptake, and (c) changes in dopaminergic systems. I believe insulin resistance linked to low birth weight could be a fourth possibility. There is clear evidence that maternal smoking during pregnancy is associated with low birth weight in the newborn (Mantzoros, Varvarigou, Kaklamani, Beratis, & Flier, 1997; van Baal & Boomsma, 1998), which is associated with later insulin resistance (Crowther, Cameron, Trusler, & Gray, 1998; McKeigue, Lithell, & Leon, 1998). There is some preliminary evidence suggesting that insulin resistance is common among men with ASPD who are habitual criminals. For instance, we have studied more than 100 ASPD violent offenders with insulin clamp/calorimetry, which measures insulin resistance (low glycogen formation) (Virkkunen et al., in preparation). This could be one mechanism linking maternal smoking to later criminality. However, it must be noted that there are also antisocial personalities who are very insulin-sensitive.

One other biological factor must be taken into account as a confounding variable in studies designed to clarify the importance of maternal smoking during pregnancy for behaviour problems in the offspring. Low cholesterol levels and lipid metabolism have been found to be associated with violent behaviour (Golomb, 1998; Hibbeln et al., 1998). During the 1970s and early 1980s, low cholesterol levels were found among habitually violent offenders with intermittent explosive disorder and violent ASPD (Virkkunen, 1979, 1983) and among males with aggressive conduct disorder (Virkkunen & Penttinen, 1984). These low cholesterol levels are, of course, usually associated with insulin-sensitive, not insulin-resistant, findings, and are suggestive of a low serotonin/cholesterol connection.

Summary and Importance of Mednick's Findings

Mednick's studies have many strengths. An important one is the adoption design, which makes it possible to separate, to a large extent, genetic from environmental factors. His project includes over 14,000 adoptions, which provides good statistical power to test hypotheses. The cohorts are from Denmark, whose homogeneous population makes it difficult to fully generalize the findings to more culturally diverse nations. They have used the stringent criterion of an alcohol-related criminal conviction or a psychiatric diagnosis of primary or secondary alcoholism, but no measurement of quantity or frequency of drinking to index alcohol-use disorders. Therefore, nothing is known about the severity of alcohol abuse. I think these studies by Mednick are critical because they point out the importance of interactions among several factors that contribute to violent and antisocial tendencies. Some risk factors may be significant only when coupled with another factor. It would be important to try and link Mednick's risk factors with other biological and even genetic factors about which there is some evidence, especially abnormal noradrenaline and serotonin turnover and genetic polymorphisms of dopamine 4 and dopamine transporter, serotonin 1B, and tryptophan hydroxylase. The COMT polymorphism requires more study.

CONNECTION BETWEEN THESE FINDINGS AND REPEATED VIOLENCE AND CRIMINALITY AMONG THE MENTALLY ILL

Because nearly all of the studies by Mednick's group involve all forms of violence, they cannot identify the factors that characterize habitually violent patients with schizophrenia. We do not know if specific biological factors are associated with repeated violence and criminal tendencies among individuals who develop schizophrenia. Only substance abuse and dependence have been shown to be associated with these behaviours in mentally ill persons (Citrome & Volavka, 1999; Rasanen et al., 1998; Steinert, Voellner, & Faust, 1998; Swartz et al., 1998).

It is important for us to understand why alcohol abuse and alcoholism play such a central role in violence among persons with schizophrenia. Is it only because alcohol makes them forget to take their antipsychotic medications, thus exacerbating their psychotic symptoms, hallucinations, and paranoia and leading to violent offending? Or do some individuals with schizophrenia have a tendency to behave violently under the influence of alcohol? Could such characteristics be identified among male relatives, as they have been among the relatives of ASPD violent offenders?

The findings of Hodgins's group describe two sets of offenders with major mental disorders: (a) those who commit their first offence before the onset of the disorder, and (b) those who commit their first offence after the onset of the disorder (Hodgins, Lapalme, & Toupin, 1999). The first group has, of course, early-onset conduct-disorder problems. These problems usually include early-onset alcohol problems—that is, type 2 alcoholism. Consequently, it will be important for future studies to clarify whether abnormal serotonin metabolism also plays a role.

There is little evidence to suggest that impulsivity and its biological basis, abnormal serotonin turnover, are central to the violence or repeated violence of individuals with schizophrenia. Few papers show that serotonin turnover may be somehow abnormal in schizophrenia. The problem has been that it is difficult to measure monoamine metabolites among violent schizophrenics because of the difficulty in arranging sufficiently long wash-out periods without medications. Psychiatric staff resist any decrease in or cessation of medication in such patients.

In order to present the complete picture, future studies of violent offenders with major mental disorders must include those variables that Mednick's group has found to be important, as well as the genetic and biological variables that I have described.

References

American Psychiatric Association. (1994). *Diagnostic and statistical manual of mental disorders, 4th Ed.* Washington: Author.

Bohman, M., Cloninger, C.R., Sigvardsson, S., & von Knorring, A.-L. (1982). Predisposition to petty criminality in Swedish adoptees. I: Genetic and environmental heterogeneity. *Archives of General Psychiatry, 39,* 1233–1241.

Brennan, P.A., Grekin, E.R., & Mednick, S.A. (1999). Maternal smoking during pregnancy and adult male criminal outcomes. *Archives of General Psychiatry, 56,* 215–219.

Cannon, M., Cotter, D., Coffey, V.P., Sham, P.C., Takei, N., Larkin, C., Murray, R.M., & O'Callaghan, E. (1996). Prenatal exposure to the 1957 influenza epidemic and adult schizophrenia: A follow-up study. *British Journal of Psychiatry, 168,* 368–371.

Citrome, L., & Volavka, J. (1999). Schizophrenia: Violence and comorbidity. *Current Opinion in Psychiatry, 12,* 47–51.

Cloninger, C.R., Bohman, M., & Sigvardsson, S. (1981). Inheritance of alcohol abuse: Cross-fostering analysis of adopted men. *Archives of General Psychiatry, 38,* 861–868.

Crabbe, J.C., Phillips, T.J., Feller, D.J., Hen, R., Wenger, C.D., Lessov, C.N., & Schafer, G.L. (1996). Elevated alcohol consumption in null mutant mice lacking 5-HT1B serotonin receptors. *Nature Genetics, 14,* 98–101.

Crow, T.J., & Done, D.J. (1992). Prenatal influenza does not cause schizophrenia. *British Journal of Psychiatry, 161,* 390–393.

Crowther, N.J., Cameron, N., Trusler, J., & Gray, J.P. (1998). Association between poor glucose tolerance and rapid post-natal weight gain in seven-year-old children. *Diabetologia, 41,* 1163–1167.

DeLisi, L.E. (1999). A critical overview of recent investigations into genetics of schizophrenia. *Current Opinion in Psychiatry, 12,* 29–39.

Ekselius, L., & von Knorring, L. (1999). Changes in personality traits during treatment with sertraline or citalopram. *British Journal of Psychiatry, 174,* 444–448.

Fergusson, D.M. (1999). Prenatal smoking and antisocial behavior. *Archives of General Psychiatry, 56,* 223–224.

Fergusson, D.M., Woodward, L.J., & Horwood, L.J. (1998). Maternal smoking during pregnancy and psychiatric adjustment in late adolescence. *Archives of General Psychiatry, 53,* 721–727.

Fuster, J.M. (1999). Synopsis of function and dysfunction of the frontal lobe. *Acta Psychiatrica Scandinavica* (Suppl 395), 51–57.

Gogos, J.A., Morgan, M., Luine, V., Santha, M., Ogawa, S., Pfaff, K., & Karayiorgou, M. (1998). Catechol-O-methyltransferase-deficient mice exhibit sexually dimorphic changes in catecholamine levels and behavior. *Proceedings of the National Academy of Sciences (USA), 95,* 9991–9996.

Golomb, B. (1998). Cholesterol and violence: Is there a connection? *Annals of Internal Medicine, 128,* 478–487.

Gustavsson, J.P. (1997). *Stability and validity of self-reported personality traits: Contributions to the evaluation of the Karolinska Scale of Personality.* Doctoral dissertation, Department of Clinical Neuroscience and Institute for Environmental Medicine, Karolinska Institute, Stockholm, Sweden.

Hibbeln, J.R., Umhau, J.C., Linnoila, M., George, D.T., Ragan, P.W., Shoaf, S.E., Vaughan, M.R., Rawlings, R., & Salem, N. Jr. (1998). A replication study of violent and nonviolent subjects: Cerebrospinal fluid metabolites of serotonin and dopamine as predicted by plasma essential fatty acids. *Biological Psychiatry, 44,* 243–249.

Higley, J.D., & Linnoila, M. (1997). A nonhuman primate model of excessive alcohol intake: Personality and neurobiological parallels of type I- and II-like alcoholism. In M. Galanter (Ed.), *Recent developments of alcoholism. Vol. 13: Alcohol and violence* (pp. 191–219). New York and London: Plenum.

Hodgins, S., Lapalme, M., & Toupin, J. (1999). Criminal activities and substance use of patients with major affective disorders and schizophrenia: A 2-year follow-up. *Journal of Affective Disorders, 55,* 187–202.

Karayiorgou, M., Gogos, J.A., Galke, B.L., Wolyniec, P.S., Nestadt, G., & Antonarakis, S.E. (1998). Identification of sequence variants and analysis of the role of the catechol-o-methyltransferase gene in schizophrenia susceptibility. *Biological Psychiatry, 43,* 425–431.

Lachman, H.M., Nolan, K.A., Mohr, P., Saito, T., & Volavka, J. (1998). Association between catechol-o-methyltransferase genotype and violence in schizophrenia and schizoaffective disorder. *American Journal of Psychiatry, 155,* 835–837.

Lappalainen, J., Long, J.C., Eggert, M., Ozaki, N., Robin, R.W., Brown, G.L., Naukkarinen, H., Virkkunen, M., Linnoila, M., & Goldman, D. (1998). Linkage of antisocial alcoholism to the serotonin 5HT1B receptor gene in 2 populations. *Archives of General Psychiatry, 55,* 989–994.

Machon, R.A., Mednick, S.A., & Huttunen, M.O. (1997). Adult major affective disorder after prenatal exposure to an influenza epidemic. *Archives of General Psychiatry, 54,* 322–328.

Mantzoros, C.S., Varvarigou, A., Kaklamani, V.G., Beratis, N.G., & Flier, J.S. (1997). Effect of birth weight and maternal smoking on cord blood leptin concentrations of full-term and preterm newborns. *Journal of Clinical Endocrinology and Metabolism, 82,* 2856–2861.

Manuck, S.B., Flory, J.D., Ferrell, R.E., Dent, K.M., Mann, J.J., & Muldoon, M.F. (1999). Aggression- and anger-related traits associated with a polymorphism of the tryptophan hydroxylase gene. *Biological Psychiatry, 45,* 603–614.

Martin, R.L., Cloninger, R., Guze, S.B., & Clayton, P.J. (1985). Mortality in a follow-up of 500 psychiatric outpatients. II: Cause-specific mortality. *Archives of General Psychiatry, 42,* 58–66.

McKeigue, P.M., Lithell, H.O., & Leon, D.A. (1998). Glucose tolerance and resistance to insulin-stimulated glucose uptake in men aged 70 years in relation to size at birth. *Diabetologia, 41,* 1133–1138.

Mednick, S.A. (in press). Early factors in violence. In S. Hodgins & R. Müller-Isberner (Eds.), *Violence, crime, and mentally disordered offenders: Concepts and methods for effective treatment and prevention.* London: Wiley.

Mednick, S.A., Gabrielli, W.F. Jr., & Hutchings, B. (1984). Genetic influences in criminal convictions: Evidence from an adoption cohort. *Science, 222,* 891–894.

Mednick, S.A., Huttunen, M.O., & Machon, R.A. (1994). Prenatal influenza infections and adult schizophrenia. *Schizophrenia Bulletin, 20,* 263–267.

Mednick, S.A., Machon, R.A., Huttunen, M.O., & Bonett, D. (1988). Adult schizophrenia following prenatal exposure to an influenza epidemic. *Archives of General Psychiatry, 45,* 189–192.

Millberger, B., Biederman, J., Faraone, S.V., Chen, L., & Joners, J. (1996). Is maternal smoking during pregnancy a risk factor for attention deficit hyperactivity disorder in children? *American Journal of Psychiatry, 153,* 1138–1142.

Moeller, F.G., Dougherty, D.M., Lane, S.D., Steinberg, J.L., & Cherek, D.R. (1998). Antisocial personality and alcohol-induced aggression. *Clinical and Experimental Research, 22,* 1898–1902.

New, A.S., Gelernter, J., Mitropoulou, V., Koenigsberg, H.W., & Siever, L. (1999). *Impulsive aggression associated with HTR1B genotype in personality disorders.* Abstracts of the meeting of the American Psychiatric Association, Washington, DC, May 15–20, p. 172.

New, A.S., Gelernter, J., Yovell, Y., Trestman, R.L., Nielsen, D.A., Siverman, J., Mitropoulou, V., & Siever, L.J. (1998). Tryptophan hydroxylase genotype is associated with impulsive-aggression measures: A preliminary study. *American Journal of Medical Genetics (Neuropsychiatric Genetics), 81,* 13–17.

Nielsen, D.A., Virkkunen, M., Lappalainen, J., Eggert, M., Brown, G.L., Long, J.C., Goldman, D., & Linnoila, M. (1998). A tryptophan hydroxylase gene marker for suicidality and alcoholism. *Archives of General Psychiatry, 55,* 593–602.

Orlebeke, J.F., Knol, D.L., & Verhulst, F.C. (1999). Child behavior problems increased by maternal smoking during pregnancy. *Archives of Environmental Health, 1,* 15–19.

Raine, A., Venables, P.H., & Mednick, S.A. (1997). Low resting heart rate at age 3 years predisposes to aggression at age 11 years: Evidence from the Mauritius Child Health Project. *Journal of the American Academy of Adolescent Psychiatry, 36,* 1457–1464.

Rantakallio, P., Laara, E., Isohanni, M., & Moilanen, I. (1992). Maternal smoking during pregnancy and delinquency of the offspring: An association without causation? *International Journal of Epidemiology, 21,* 1106–1113.

Rasanen, P., Hakko, H., Isohanni, M., Hodgins, S., Jarvelin, M.R., & Tiihonen, J. (1999). Maternal smoking during pregnancy and risk of criminal behavior among adult male offspring in the Northern Finland 1966 birth cohort. *American Journal of Psychiatry, 156,* 857–862.

Rasanen, P., Tiihonen, J., Isohanni, M., Rantakallio, P., Lehtonen, J., & Moring, J. (1998). Schizophrenia, alcohol abuse, and violent behavior: A 26-year followup study of unselected birth cohort. *Schizophrenia Bulletin, 24,* 437–441.

Rocha, B.A., Scearce-Levie, K., Lucas, J.J., Hiroi, N., Castanon, N., Crabbe, J.C., Nestler, E.J., & Hen, R. (1998). Increased vulnerability to cocaine in mice lacking the serotonin-1B receptor. *Nature, 14,* 175–178.

Rydelius, P.A. (1988). The development of antisocial behaviour and sudden violent death. *Acta Psychiatrica Scandinavica, 77,* 398–403.

Saito, T., Lachman, H., Mohr, P., Nolan, K., & Volavka, J. (1999). *Lack of association between violence in schizophrenia and polymorphisms in genes that regulate serotonin transmission.* Abstracts of the meeting of the American Psychiatric Association, Washington, DC, May 15–20, p. 92.

Saudou, F., Amara, D.A., Dierich, A., LeMeur, M., Ramboz, S., Segu, L., Buhot, M.C., & Hen, R. (1994). Enhanced aggressive behavior in mice lacking 5-HT1B receptor. *Science, 23,* 1875–1878.

Schalling, D., Asberg, M., Edman, G., & Oreland, L. (1987). Markers for vulnerability to psychopathology: Temperament traits associated with platelet MAO activity. *Acta Psychiatrica Scandinavica, 76,* 172–182.

Sigvardsson, S., Bohman, M., & Cloninger, C.R. (1996). Replication of the Stockholm Adoption Study of alcoholism: Confirmatory cross-fostering analysis. *Archives of General Psychiatry, 53,* 681–687.

Steinert, T., Voellner, A., & Faust, V. (1998). Violence and schizophrenia: Two types of criminal offenders. *European Journal of Psychiatry, 12,* 153–165.

Strous, R.D., Bark, N., Parsia, S.S., Volavka, J., & Lachman, H.M. (1997). Analysis of a functional catechol O-methyltransferase gene polymorphism in schizophrenia: Evidence for association with aggressive and antisocial behavior. *Psychiatry Research, 69,* 71–77.

Swartz, M.S., Swanson, J.W., Hiday, V.A., Borum, R., Wagner, H.R., & Burns, R.J. (1998). Violence and severe mental illness: The effects of substance abuse and nonadherence to medication. *American Journal of Psychiatry, 155,* 226–231.

Tehrani, J.A., Brennan, P.A., Hodgins, S., & Mednick, S.A. (1998). Mental illness and criminal violence. *Social Psychiatry and Psychiatric Epidemiology, 33*(Suppl 1), 81–88.

Thaper, A., Holmes, J., Poulton, K., & Harrington, R. (1999). Genetic basis of attention deficit and hyperactivity. *British Journal of Psychiatry, 174,* 105–111.

Van Baal, C.G., & Boomsma, D.I. (1998). Etiology of individual differences in birth weight of twins as a function of maternal smoking during pregnancy. *Twin Research, 1,* 123–130.

Virkkunen, M. (1979). Serum cholesterol in antisocial personality. *Neuropsychobiology, 5,* 27–30.

Virkkunen, M. (1983). Serum cholesterol levels in homicidal offenders: A low cholesterol level is connected with a habitually violent tendency under the influence of alcohol. *Neuropsychobiology, 10,* 65–69.

Virkkunen, M., De Jong, J., Bartko, J., Goodwin, F.K., & Linnoila, M. (1989). Relationship of psychobiological variables to recidivism in violent offenders and impulsive fire setters: A follow up study. *Archives of General Psychiatry, 46,* 600–603.

Virkkunen, M., Eggert, M., Rawlings, R., & Linnoila, M. (1996). A prospective follow-up study of alcoholic violent offenders and fire setters. *Archives of General Psychiatry, 53,* 523–529.

Virkkunen, M., & Penttinen, H. (1984). Serum cholesterol in aggressive conduct disorder: A preliminary study. *Biological Psychiatry, 19,* 435–439.

Wakslag, L.S., Lahey, B.B., Loeber, R., Green, S.M., Gordon, R.A., & Leventhal, B.L. (1997). Maternal smoking during pregnancy and the risk for conduct disorder in boys. *Archives of General Psychiatry, 54,* 670–676.

Matti Virkkunen, MD, PhD, is Professor of Forensic Psychiatry and is associated with the Psychiatric Clinic at Helsinki University Central Hospital, Helsinki, Finland.

Author's Note

Comments or queries may be directed to Matti Virkkunen, MD, PhD, Psychiatric Clinic, Helsinki University Central Hospital, Lapinlahdentie 00180, Helsinki 18, Finland. Telephone: 3589471811. Fax: 3589650326. E-mail: <mevirkku@cc.helsinki.fi>.

THE ETIOLOGY AND DEVELOPMENT OF OFFENDING AMONG PERSONS WITH MAJOR MENTAL DISORDERS

Conceptual and Methodological Issues and Some Preliminary Findings

SHEILAGH HODGINS

Introduction

Compelling evidence is presented in chapters 1, 2, and 3 of the criminality and violence of persons who suffer from major mental disorders. As noted, this phenomenon has been documented in recent years in many Western, industrialized countries, beginning at the time that mental health care was deinstitutionalized. Since then, little attention, and even less money, has been focused on the effective treatment and management of this population. Yet morality, professional ethics, and public accountability all require that care that prevents criminality and violence in this population be provided in a humane manner. Some lonely pioneers in the field have, as can be seen in the subsequent chapters of this book, even provided data showing that it can be successfully done!

This first chapter reviews research on the antecedents of illegal behaviours among persons who develop major mental disorders and discusses conceptual and methodological issues related to such investigations. The ultimate goal is to unravel the etiology so that primary prevention is possible. This is not a dream. As will be shown, persons who will develop a major mental disorder and offend in adulthood can be identified in childhood, as can some of the determinants of their illegal behaviours. In the meantime, the few programmes that have been shown to effectively prevent recidivism among mentally ill offenders await implementation, as well as further evaluation and refinement. This process can be facilitated by basing programme development on existing knowledge about the etiology and development of offending among persons with major mental disorders.

Current knowledge about mentally ill offenders suggests that effective treatment will have the following characteristics: (1) It will be long-term, often continuing from adolescence through old age. (2) It will address the multiple problems presented by mentally ill offenders. (3) It will involve short periods of hospitalization and long periods in the community. (4) It will have several components: clinical interventions (medications, behavioural and cognitive training, psychoeducational training) designed to reduce symptoms, eliminate illegal behaviours, and increase

89

S. Hodgins (ed.), Violence among the Mentally Ill, 89–116.
© 2000 *Kluwer Academic Publishers. Printed in the Netherlands.*

the skills necessary to live autonomously in the community; legal interventions, to be used restrictedly to ensure compliance with treatment; the social services necessary for independent community tenure; and various levels of supervision in the community. (5) It will be coordinated in a stable manner over the long term and will include outreach.

As with any treatment, it will be effective to the extent to which it matches the needs of the mentally ill offender. Mentally ill offenders do not constitute a homogeneous population with respect to treatment needs. In the past, two different strategies have been used to identify subgroups among the mentally ill that are homogeneous with respect to treatment needs. In two large security hospitals in Canada, Quinsey, Cyr, and Lavallé (1988) used cluster analyses of patient characteristics to identify subgroups. In a security hospital in Germany, Müller-Isberner (1993) identified subtypes based on Axis I and II diagnoses. Theoretically, subtypes identified on the basis of different etiologies and patterns of development should present advantages over these two methods. This strategy identifies historical factors more completely and accurately and should eventually describe the mechanisms involved in determining the disorder and the illegal behaviour. This strategy has another advantage: By identifying the etiology, and thereby the patients' deficits, it prevents the use of treatment strategies that require patients to do things they cannot do.[1] This should avoid causing patients additional difficulties and repeatedly putting them in situations in which they fail. Further, this strategy provides some indication of the degree to which specific characteristics may be modifiable. In addition, the subtypes that are homogeneous with respect to etiology and development are highly relevant for assessing the future risk of offending and/or violent behaviour, an ongoing, integral part of treatment.

Examining the Etiology of Illegal Behaviour Among Persons with Major Mental Disorders

It is presently unknown whether the illegal behaviours of persons with major mental disorders are a part of their disorder—symptoms or consequences of the neurobiological deficits—or are distinct problems. The concept of comorbid disorders currently used to describe the multiple problems presented by mentally ill offenders suggests that these behaviours are additional distinct problems. However, it is important to note that the concept of comorbid disorder is used only to facilitate communication among researchers and clinicians and to render the descriptions of the mentally ill offenders more objective. Identifying which aspects of the illegal behaviours are separate from the primary disorder and which are a part or a consequence of the disorder represents a major scientific challenge. It is unlikely that the relationship between the disorder and the offender is the same for all mentally ill offenders; for some the pattern of illegal behaviour may be a part of the disorder, while for others it may not be.

As noted above, mentally ill offenders are not all the same. As adults, they differ, among other things, as to: primary diagnoses; additional diagnoses; cognitive, emotional, and psychosocial functioning; personality traits; and onset, frequency, and type of offending. Consequently, it must be hypothesized that this population is constituted of subgroups, each with a distinct etiology. To test this hypothesis it is necessary to use the individual (and not the variable, as is usually the case) as the unit of measure, to presume until it is proven otherwise that all individuals are different, and to adopt a methodology and data-analysis strategy[2] that allows for identification of distinct subgroups. In addition, in order to understand the etiology and development of offending, one must adopt a developmental perspective in which biological, psychological, and social factors are measured to identify how and when during the course of development they interact to determine the disorder and/or the illegal behaviour (Hodgins, in press).

A Hypothesis

We have hypothesized that there are at least two subgroups among mentally ill offenders with distinct etiologies. The early-start offenders present a stable pattern of antisocial behaviour from a young age, while the late-start offenders present antisocial behaviour only after the onset of the major mental disorder (Hodgins, Côté, & Toupin, 1998). The results of our studies of three samples of male mentally ill offenders and one prospective, longitudinal investigation of a birth cohort including males and females have concurred, with one exception, in documenting similarities and differences between these two types. As among non-disordered offenders, among persons who develop a major mental disorder and offend there are more early-starters among the males and more late-starters among the females (Kratzer & Hodgins, 1999). The patterns of criminal offending distinguish the two groups. Early-starters, as the designation implies, begin offending in adolescence, and they are convicted of more violent and non-violent crimes than late-start offenders. The patterns of criminality of mentally ill early-start offenders have been found to be indistinguishable from those of non-mentally ill early-start offenders (Hodgins & Côté, 1993).

Our results concerning the principal diagnosis are inconsistent. In two studies we found no differences between the principal diagnoses of the early- and late-start offenders, but in one study it was found that half of the early-starters but only 20% of the late-starters suffered from delusional disorder (Côté, Lesage, Chawky, & Loyer, 1997). As discussed elsewhere, delusional disorder is very difficult to diagnose, and persons with this disorder as well as others with paranoid symptoms are unlikely to consent to participate in research projects. Further, they are not often seen in treatment and consequently little is known about them (Hodgins et al., 1998). Among offenders with schizophrenia and major affective disorders, early- and late-starters were not distinguished by patterns or severity of the symptoms of the primary disorder, but greater proportions of early-starters were found to have diagnoses of alcohol- and/or drug-use disorders.

In one study, the mentally ill early-start offenders were found to show fewer neurological soft signs than were mentally ill late-start offenders. Consistent with this surprising finding was the result that we and others obtained showing that early-start offenders with schizophrenia performed better than late-start offenders with the same disorder. There is some hint in our results and in those of two other investigations that early-starters with schizophrenia are also somewhat less impaired in psychosocial functioning than the late-starters (Hodgins et al., 1998). This despite the fact that they are much more likely to have comorbid diagnoses of alcohol and/or drug abuse/dependence.

Early-starters and late-starters, even with the same primary disorder, have been shown to differ as to the number and severity of personality traits of psychopathy. Finally, retrospective self-reports indicate that early-starters present behaviour problems at school and in the community from a young age. Retrospective self-reports have also shown that early-starters who develop a major mental disorder presented similar types and severity of antisocial behaviour in childhood and early adolescence as those who develop antisocial personality disorder and no mental illness (Hodgins et al., 1998).

My colleagues and I at the Karolinska Institute in Sweden have extended the characteristics of early- and late-start offenders with schizophrenia by examining a sample comprising 272 males referred for pre-trial psychiatric assessment. All have received a confirmed diagnosis of schizophrenia. The patterns of criminality of the early- and the late-start offenders with schizophrenia were similar to what we had previously observed. The early-starters had accumulated more total convictions, more convictions for non-violent offences, and more convictions for violent offences, and they were, on average, 10 years younger when first convicted for a serious violent crime ($M = 19.5$ ($SD = 4.8$), $M = 29.2$ ($SD = 8.2$), logt $= 7.18$, $p <.0001$). Also confirming previous results, we found that 76% of the early-starters and 42% of the late-starters had at least one diagnosis of substance abuse ($X^2 = (N = 267) = 23.71$, $p <.0001$) (alcohol abuse/dependence 61% early-starters, 32% late-starters; marijuana/hashish abuse/dependence 51% early-starters, 18% late-starters). Unlike previous researchers, we found that 72% of the early-starters as opposed to 36% of the late-starters had been intoxicated at the time of the index offence ($X^2(N = 222) = 28.12$, $p <.0001$) (Tengstrom, Hodgins, & Kullgren, 1999).

This hypothesis of the existence among persons who develop schizophrenia and major affective disorders[3] of subgroups who present a pattern of antisocial behaviour from a young age is consistent with etiological research on these disorders. This is important, because most of these data were collected before the relation between the major mental disorders and criminality was recognized, and because it was documented by scientists who for the most part were unaware of research on mental disorder and crime. Prospective longitudinal studies of children of parents with schizophrenia have identified a subgroup, larger among the males than the females, that show disruptive, aggressive behaviour from a young age (Asnarow, 1988). Further, a prospective longitudinal study of a Dutch general population sample found, like so many other studies, aggressive behaviour in childhood to be associated with aggressive behaviour in adulthood, but equally strongly predictive of thought disorder in adulthood (Ferdinand & Verhulst, 1995). A similar study in the United States found antisocial behaviour in childhood to be associated with the development of cluster A personality disorders (Bernstein, Cohen, Skodol, Bezirganian, & Brook, 1996).

Similarly, recent epidemiological investigations of community samples of children have documented relatively high rates of affective disorder comorbid with conduct disorder (see, for example, Angold & Costello, 1993). A prospective longitudinal study of children of parents with major affective disorders and investigations of children with affective disorders also documented significant comorbidity with conduct disorder, among both children with major depression and children with bipolar disorder (Carlson & Weintraub, 1993; Geller, Cooper, Watts, Cosby, & Fox, 1992; Harrington, Rutter, & Fombonne, 1996; Kovacs & Pollock, 1995). The prevalence of childhood conduct disorder is higher among adults with major depression than among the general population (Rowe, Sullivan, Mulder, & Joyce, 1996). In a longitudinal prospective study, we found that the sons and daughters of parents with bipolar disorder, as compared to children of parents with no mental disorder, were three and one half times more likely to present an externalizing disorder before age 12. Most also presented internalizing disorders (Hodgins & Lapalme, 1999). These findings are important, as previous work has shown that one in two children of parents with bipolar disorder are likely to develop a major affective disorder in adulthood (Hodgins, 1994). Children with depression and conduct disorder have been found to differ from those with only depression, by the absence of anxiety symptoms and the presence of impulsivity and delinquency, as well as having witnessed violence at home (Meller & Borchardt, 1996). Such boys have been described as disruptive and socially withdrawn (Kerr, Tremblay, Pagani, & Vitaro, 1997).

A recent investigation of a sample of patients concurs with our previous findings in demonstrating that conduct disorder in childhood is associated with violence among those who develop major mental disorders (Fulwiler & Ruthazer, 1999). Further, this study extends previous work in identifying a group of violent mentally ill subjects who presented substance-abuse problems before age 15, but not conduct disorder (Fulwiler, Grossman, Forbes, & Ruthazer, 1997). These results have two important implications. One, they concur with results of several previous investigations in showing that a subgroup of offenders with major mental disorders present conduct disorder in childhood or early adolescence and most subsequently develop substance-abuse problems. Two, substance abuse in childhood or early adolescence in the absence of conduct disorder may characterize a smaller, distinct subgroup of mentally ill offenders. This result is consistent with the conclusions drawn by Mueser, Drake, and Wallach (1998). These individuals, we hypothesize, inherit a vulnerability for abuse of specific substances due to a supersensitivity to the effects. Further, based on studies of adult samples, we hypothesize that early-start offenders with conduct disorder are more common among individuals with schizophrenia and that early-start substance abusers are more common among individuals with major affective disorders (Hodgins et al., 1998).

Etiology

Taking a developmental perspective, we are trying to identify the causal chains of factors that lead to the development of offending in persons who develop major mental disorders. We begin with the assumption that there are at least three subgroups: the early-starters with primary conduct disorder,[4] the early-starters with primary substance problems, and the late-starters.

HEREDITARY FACTORS

It is now well documented that the three major mental disorders are determined, in part, by hereditary factors. The combinations of genes that lead to each disorder do not, in and of themselves, determine the disorder. Rather, they contribute a vulnerability, which is strengthened and activated by other non-genetic factors, for the disorder.[5] In addition, hereditary factors may contribute a vulnerability for antisocial and/or violent behaviour per se, for abuse of different substances, and for other stable characteristics such as aggressive behaviour that are likely to lead to offending. This could function in two ways. The hereditary factors associated with each of the major mental disorders may increase central nervous system sensitivity to biological and/or psychosocial insult. The resulting insult or insults would form the neurobiological basis for behaviours associated with offending. Alternatively, some individuals who inherit vulnerabilities for a major mental disorder may also inherit vulnerabilities for other disorders or traits which increase the likelihood of criminal behaviour. Family studies, twin studies, and adoption studies have identified an inherited vulnerability for a stable pattern of antisocial behaviour across the life-span (Cadoret, Yates, Troughton, Woodworth, & Stewart, 1995; Lyons et al., 1995). Similarly, family studies, twin studies, and adoption studies, and in some cases molecular genetic studies, have identified heritable vulnerabilities for alcohol abuse/dependence (see, for example, Bierut et al., 1998; Lappalainen et al., 1998), drug abuse/dependence (Merikangas et al., 1998), major depression combined with alcohol dependence (Lin et al., 1996; Merikangas, Leckman, Prusoff, Pauls, & Weissman, 1985), aggressive behaviour (Coccaro, Silverman, Klar, Horvath, & Siever, 1994), novelty seeking (Ebstein et al., 1996), and impulsivity (Gottesman & Goldsmith, 1994). An allele associated with repetitive violent behaviour among men with schizophrenia has recently been identified (Lachman, Nolan, Mohr, Saito, & Volavka, 1998).

Early-starters with conduct disorder
We hypothesize that the early-starters with conduct disorder have inherited a vulnerability for antisocial behaviour as well as a vulnerability for a major mental disorder. There are few data available which test this hypothesis. In the sample of schizophrenic offenders described above (Tengstrom et al., 1999), we found that 56% of the early-start offenders and 26% of the late-start offenders had parents with substance-abuse problems.[6] In a sample of patients with major mental disorders, it was reported that among those with a stable pattern of antisocial behaviour from early adolescence, 82% had a father with an alcohol-use disorder and 27% a father with a drug-use disorder. The prevalence of these disorders among the other patients was significantly lower: no conduct disorder or antisocial disorder in adulthood, 52% and 6%; only childhood conduct disorder, 68% and 5%; only antisocial behaviour in adulthood, 46% and 18% (Mueser et al., 1999). In another sample of schizophrenic offenders, we found that one third of the early-starters, but only 4% of the late-starters, had a parent with a criminal record (Lapalme, Jöckel, Hodgins, & Müller-Isberner, 1999).

While there are few available findings which directly test our hypothesis, there are data which suggest criminality aggregates among the biological relatives of persons who develop schizophrenia, particularly among those with predominately positive symptoms (for a review, see Hodgins, Toupin, & Côté, 1996). For example, the Danish High Risk Study found that 35% of mothers with schizophrenia had a criminal record, as compared to 4.6% of mothers with no mental disorder. Equal proportions of the fathers had a criminal record. When the offspring were between 21 and 31 years old, 31% of those with mothers diagnosed with schizophrenia, as compared to 18% of those with mothers with no disorder, had a criminal record (Silverton, 1985). Providing stronger support for a hereditary contribution to criminality among the relatives of individuals with schizophrenia, two adoption studies (Heston, 1966; Silverton) found that the biological children of mothers with schizophrenia who had been adopted away at birth were at higher risk for criminality than the adopted-away offspring of mothers with no mental disorder. We hypothesize that it is the biological relatives of the early-start offenders and not those of the late-start offenders or the non-offenders who have criminal records.

Among the first-degree relatives of persons with major depression, the prevalence rate of antisocial personality disorder has been found to be elevated (Goldstein et al., 1994; Weissman et al., 1984). Two US studies have shown that the children of parents with major depression have a considerably increased risk of conduct disorder. In one study the risk was double that identified in the comparison group (Weissman, Fendrich, Warner, & Wickramaratne, 1992); in the other the risk was four times that of the comparison group (Hammen, Burge, Burney, & Adrian, 1990). Children with depression and conduct disorder have been found to be more likely than children with only depression to have a first-degree relative with a substance-abuse disorder (Meller & Borchardt, 1996; Weller et al., 1994). Among a small sample of depressed children, those with comorbid conduct disorder were found to be more likely than those without to have a father with alcohol problems. A recent study of siblings and twins showed that the association between the symptoms of depression and antisocial behaviour in adolescence is genetically mediated. Approximately half of the observed correlation was attributed to common genetic factors (O'Connor, McGuire, Reiss, Hetherington, & Plomin, 1998). The genetic factors common to both depression and antisocial behaviour have also been found to be responsible, in part, for the stability of the two disorders over time (O'Connor, Neiderhiser, Reiss, Hetherington, & Plomin, in press).

A comparison between children with bipolar disorder and children with both bipolar disorder and conduct disorder resulted in a not statistically significant elevation in the prevalence of antisocial personality disorder among the fathers of the latter group, and no differences among the mothers of the two groups (Kovacs & Pollock, 1995).

To conclude, based on results of epidemiological investigations of criminality of persons who develop major mental disorders, of studies of samples of mentally ill offenders, of prospective investigations of the precursors of each of the three major mental disorders, and of behavioural genetic studies, we hypothesize that there are two developmental pathways to conduct disorder. One involves a vulnerability for antisocial behaviour—that is, a failure to learn and follow rules—while the other involves craving for alcohol and/or certain drugs, which in turn leads to antisocial behaviour. The former type would be expected to present a stable pattern of antisocial behaviour from a young age and to then develop a substance-use disorder. Interestingly, a study of umbilical cord blood of newborns indicated that those with relatives with antisocial personality disorder had lower levels of 5-HIAA than those with non-disordered relatives (Constantino, Morris, & Murphy, 1997). The second type would be expected to develop a substance-use disorder in adolescence and subsequently to present a pattern of antisocial behaviour. We have been unable, as yet, to separate these two types of early-starters. However, in the 1953 Swedish birth cohort we observed that, among the men, 31% of the mentally ill offenders and only 7% of the non-offenders abused substances in childhood and/or early adolescence; among the females, this was true of 27% of the mentally ill offenders and 5% of the non-offenders.

Late-starters

Epidemiological findings indicate that some persons who develop major mental disorders, especially major affective disorders, commit violent crimes for the first time when in their thirties or forties (Brennan, Mednick, & Hodgins, in press; Hodgins et al., 1996). Similarly, those with alcohol-use disorders commit violent crimes only in mid-adulthood (Hodgins et al., 1996). Consequently, we hypothesize that some individuals may inherit vulnerabilities for both affective disorders and alcohol-use disorders. The persistent use of alcohol would lead to aggressive behaviour (Pihl & Peterson, 1993).

Currently there are few available findings which test this hypothesis. Further, the available findings are difficult to interpret, as antisocial behaviour and alcohol-use disorders co-occur at a high rate. Adoption studies suggest that the interaction between hereditary and environmental factors leading to major depression differ in males and females. Alcohol-use disorders in the biological parents are associated with major depression in females adopted away at birth (Cadoret et al., 1996). Other investigations (see, for example, Pickens, Svikis, McGue, & LaBuda, 1995) have identified hereditary factors common to major depression and alcohol-use disorders. A combination of antisocial behaviour and alcohol-use disorders in parents has been found to be associated with depression in their offspring as young adults (Chassin, Pitts, DeLucia, & Todd, 1999).

Conclusion

Studies of sibs and half-sibs and of twins are needed in order to identify hereditary factors that may contribute to the development of offending among persons who present major mental disorders. It is important to identify the cognitive and behavioural consequences of these vulnerabilities, because they could become the targets of treatment in early childhood. One notable problem is identifying and studying biological fathers with a history of antisocial behaviour.

PERINATAL FACTORS

Events occurring during pregnancy and birth have an impact on the developing brain of the foetus, some of which have lifelong consequences. These events may arise due to genetic factors or due to environmental factors acting on the foetus via the mother, such as nutrition, illness, hormonal functioning, maternal risk behaviours (substance use), and stress. Perinatal factors play a role in the etiology of schizophrenia (McNeil, 1988), major depression (Machón, Mednick, & Huttunen, 1997), and bipolar disorder (Kinney, Yurgelun-Todd, Tohen, & Tramer, 1998).

Complications occurring at birth and during the neonatal period have also been identified as precursors to violent offending among early-start non-disordered offenders and among the offspring of parents with mental disorders. The extant literature suggests that these specific associations, between obstetrical complications and violence and aggressive behaviour, are potentiated by poverty and adversity in the family of origin during early childhood, but that the association between obstetrical complications and impulsivity is not (for a review of this literature, see Hodgins, Kratzer, & McNeil, 1999). These conclusions are drawn from studies of obstetrical complications that have been observed and recorded by medical personnel caring for the pregnant woman and baby.

More recent investigations have focused on maternal risk behaviours unlikely to be reported in medical files. One in particular, smoking during pregnancy, has been repeatedly identified as a risk factor for a stable pattern of antisocial behaviour and violence in male offspring. A prospective investigation of a New Zealand birth cohort found maternal smoking during pregnancy to be specifically related to conduct disorder in late adolescence, even after the effects of socioeconomic disadvantage, poor parenting practices, and parental and family problems were controlled (Fergusson, Woodward, & Horwood, 1998). Similarly, in a Danish birth cohort and a Finnish cohort, maternal smoking during pregnancy has been found to significantly increase the risk of violent crime in adulthood among the male offspring (Brennan, Grekin, & Mednick, 1999; Räsänen, Helinä, Isohanni, Hodgins, & Tiihonen, 1999).

It is not easy to assess the role of perinatal factors in the development of either conduct disorder or offending. Longitudinal investigations in which information is collected prospectively are required. Both medical files and maternal reports are needed, as they provide different information. Further, the documentation of such an association requires detailed information on the timing of events that could be detrimental to the developing foetus.

It is important to note that damage to brain structures occurring during the perinatal period will become evident only when the structure in question becomes mature. This may be relatively late. For example, recent evidence indicates that the frontal lobes mature only at the end of adolescence and that inhibitory corrections to the amygdala are operative only after this occurs (Murray, 1998). Consequently, damage to this circuitry in the perinatal period may be apparent only in adulthood. Such a process could explain, at least in part, the development of late-start offenders.

Few data are available on the role of perinatal factors in the development of offending among persons who also present a major mental disorder in adulthood. We have examined information extracted from medical records entered during the pregnancies and births of the subjects included in the 1953 Swedish birth cohort. When we measured the number and severity of obstetrical complications, we found only a very weak association with offending among the mentally ill. However, when we measured complications taking account of the point in development at which they occurred (first, second, or third trimester of pregnancy; birth; neonatal period), we found a very significant association. Among the males who developed a major mental disorder in adulthood, 93% of the offenders and only 44% of the non-offenders had experienced complications during the neonatal period (Hodgins, Kratzer, & McNeil, 1999).

However, as with most etiological factors, it is unlikely that perinatal factors act alone. For example, an adoption study found that antisocial characteristics of the biological mother combined with alcohol abuse during the pregnancy were associated with the development of conduct disorder in the offspring (Cadoret et al., 1995). In interpreting this finding, it is important to remember that women with major mental disorders who become pregnant display more behaviours that endanger their foetus than do non-disordered women (Miller & Finnerty, 1996).

The hereditary factors associated with the major mental disorders may increase the likelihood, during the perinatal period, of maternal behaviours that lead to antisocial behaviour in the offspring. These same hereditary factors may also increase the foetus's sensitivity to the consequences of maternal behaviours. For example, in our prospective investigation comparing the development of children of parents with bipolar disorder to that of children of parents with no mental disorder we examined obstetrical complications rated from medical files and mothers' self-reports of risk behaviours. Of the offspring who were at super-high genetic risk for a major affective disorder (two parents diagnosed with a major affective disorder), 50% had a mother who smoked during the pregnancy. Of the offspring who were at high genetic risk (one parent diagnosed with bipolar disorder), 50% had a mother who smoked during the pregnancy. By contrast, among the offspring at low risk (both parents diagnosed as not having a mental disorder), only 13% had a mother who smoked during the pregnancy. Not only are the mothers of offspring at genetic risk for a major affective disorder more likely to smoke during the pregnancy, preliminary findings suggest that their foetuses may be more sensitive to the negative effects of smoking. Among the children at super-high genetic risk, 50% with mothers who smoked and 50% with mothers who did not smoke presented externalizing problems in childhood. Among the children at high genetic risk, 50% with mothers who smoked and 29% with mothers who did not smoke presented externalizing problems. By contrast, among the children at low genetic risk, 20% with mothers who smoked during the pregnancy and 6% with mothers who did not smoke presented externalizing problems (Hodgins, Tétreault, & McNeil, 1999). These are preliminary results based on only 94 families. While replication is required, they do suggest that mentally ill pregnant women are more likely than non-disordered pregnant women to engage in behaviours that may harm their foetus, and that the consequences of these behaviours may be more negative for foetuses at moderate genetic risk for a major mental disorder. If true, this would mean that other perinatal factors associated with the development of offending, such as exposure to low levels of lead (Needleman, Riess, Tobin, Biesecker, & Greenhouse, 1996), may have a more detrimental effect on foetuses at genetic risk for one of the major mental disorders.

Conclusion
Perinatal factors have been found to be particularly related to violent behaviour among the offspring in adulthood. Pregnant mentally ill women are more likely to

engage in behaviours which may damage their foetuses, and the effect of these be-haviours may be more negative for foetuses who are at genetic risk for a major mental disorder. While several studies have identified environmental pollutants such as lead (Needleman et al., 1996; Pihl & Ervin, 1990), cadium, and phthalate as pos-sible determinants of aggressive behaviour in non-disordered males, no investiga-tions have examined the effects of these substances on foetuses carrying the genes associated with a major mental disorder. The result of this sensitivity to environ-mental insult may be reflected by the finding that there are proportionately more early-start offenders among the mentally ill than among the non-disordered. For ex-ample, in the 1953 Swedish birth cohort, 30% of the mentally ill men and 12% of the non-disordered men became early-start offenders. By comparison, the propor-tions of late-start offenders were similar, 19% mentally ill and 12% non-disordered (Hodgins, 1992). In order to examine the role of perinatal factors in the offending of persons who develop major mental disorders, it is necessary to: (1) study foetuses at presumed genetic risk for a major mental disorder (as indexed by the presence of the disorder in the first-degree relatives), (2) measure perinatal factors prospectively using medical files and mothers' reports of risk behaviours, and (3) take account of the time during development when each factor is active.

EARLY CHILDHOOD FACTORS

Many investigations conducted in many different countries have identified approxi-mately 4–5% of males and less than 1% of females who present a stable pattern of antisocial behaviour across the lifespan (see, for example, Kratzer & Hodgins, 1999; Moffitt, 1993). Much more is known about the males than the females. In addition to conduct problems evident from the earliest age, the large majority of these boys are characterized by impaired verbal abilities, failure to learn age-appropriate social skills, impulsivity, and difficulty in delaying gratification (Moffitt, 1993, 1994). One study found that they showed low 5-HIAA measured in cerebral spinal fluid and that the low levels were stable over a 2-year period (Kruesi et al., 1992). By middle childhood, difficulties in school include both poor academic achievement and be-haviour problems. As Robins and McEvoy (1990) found, such children are exposed earlier than other children to alcohol and drugs. Abusive consumption becomes a pattern in adolescence. This population, we have hypothesized, is heterogeneous and includes several distinct subgroups. All present antisocial and criminal behaviour in adulthood, while specific subgroups develop schizophrenia, major depression, bipo-lar disorder, organic brain disorders, early-onset alcoholism, and drug dependence (Hodgins et al., 1998).

We have been able to observe the presence of antisocial behaviour among the early-start mentally ill offenders. In the Swedish cohort of offenders with schizo-phrenia, early-starters were found to differ significantly from late-starters as to be-haviour in childhood. While 50% of the early-starters presented behaviour problems at school, this was true of only 13% of the late-starters ($\chi^2(N = 170) = 24.68$, $p < 001$). Not only did proportionately more of the early-starters present behaviour problems, two thirds of them as compared to 27% of the late-starters earned marks below the average ($\chi^2(N = 199) = 28.12$, $p < .001$). Only 36% of the early-starters as compared to 82% of the late-starters presented no evidence of conduct disorder. Just over a third of the early-starters and 15% of the late-starters presented one or two symptoms, while 29% of the early-starters and 3% of the late-starters met full DSM-IV criteria for conduct disorder ($\chi^2(N = 176) = 43.45$, $p < .001$). The mean age at first substance abuse was lower for the early-starters ($M = 15.2$; $SD = 3.1$) as compared to the late-starters ($M = 18.6$; $SD = 5.3$) ($t = 4.12$, $p < .001$) (Tengstrom et al., 1999). These differences are striking given that all subjects were male, with a diagnosis of schizophrenia and a history of offending.

As noted previously, many of the parents of individuals who develop major mental disorders and offend may themselves present antisocial behaviour, evidence of substance abuse, and/or major mental disorders. Parents of antisocial children have been shown to engage in non-optimal parenting practices, failing to positively reinforce appropriate behaviours and failing to track and sanction inappropriate behaviour. If the child presents a specific behavioural problem, such as impulsivity or an academic deficiency, the parents do not intervene in a structured manner to resolve it, nor do they obtain professional help for the child. The quality of parenting practices may be diminished by the presence in the parents of antisocial traits, evidence of substance abuse, or impulsivity, and also the presence of a major mental disorder. While only one in 20 persons who develop schizophrenia have a parent with the disorder, 40% do have first-degree relatives with a schizophrenia spectrum disease characterized principally by social withdrawal and paranoia-like symptoms. Large proportions of persons who develop major affective disorders have a parent with a similar disorder and other first-degree relatives who are affected. Parenting skills are impaired not only during acute episodes but also during periods of remission (for a review, see Hodgins, 1994).

Again, it is important to remember that etiological factors interact with one another during development. For example, the Concordia Longitudinal Risk project found that of 2,000 females screened in elementary school the 5% who were the most aggressive had more offspring, and more offspring before age 20, than did the females who were not aggressive as children; further, they were far more likely than the other females who became pregnant to smoke during the pregnancy (Serbin, personal communication, 1999). In this case, the offspring will have experienced a perinatal factor—maternal smoking during the pregnancy—associated with conduct disorder in childhood and violent offending in adulthood and be exposed to a mother who models aggressive behaviour. Thus, individuals who offend and develop a major mental disorder are likely born with specific behavioural tendencies and with vulnerabilities resulting from inherited factors and events which occurred during the perinatal period. They may have a central nervous system which is overly sensitive to environmental insults, either biological or psychological. Already compromised, they often are raised in families that provide less than optimal parenting.

An Attempt to Study the Development of Offending Among Men Who Present Major Mental Disorders in Adulthood

In an effort to begin identifying the developmental trajectories of persons who develop major mental disorders and offend, we used a person approach and analysed data from the 1953 Swedish birth cohort.[7]

SUBJECTS

The Metropolitan birth cohort is composed of all persons (N = 15,117) born in Stockholm in 1953 (Jansen, 1984). Ninety-four percent of these individuals were still alive and residing in Sweden at the end of the 30-year follow-up period. All of the male subjects were included in the present study. Of the 7,362 men who were still living in Sweden in 1983, those with mental retardation and those admitted on a psychiatric ward for reasons other than having a major mental disorder were further excluded from the analyses (n = 348).

The 7,014 remaining men were divided into three groups according to their criminal record at the age of 30, which was extracted from the Swedish National Police Register. Non-offenders included all those with no record of criminal convictions, early-start offenders included those who had been first convicted before the age of 18, and late-start offenders included those first convicted after the age of 18. The subjects were further classified on the basis of their mental status; those who had been admitted to a psychiatric ward and discharged with a diagnosis of schizophrenia, major affective disorder, paranoid state, or other non-organic psychoses were classified in the Major Mental Disorder (MMD) group and all the others in the Non-disordered (NO md) group.

MEASURES OF CHILDHOOD AND ADOLESCENT CHARACTERISTICS

Obstetrical complications
Obstetrical complications were documented from medical files that were transcribed and coded in the early 1970s. For the present study, obstetrical complications were considered as present if two or more of the following had been reported in the medical file: premature pelvic contractions, maternal illness, mother's hospitalization or surgery, presence of rhesus factor, length of pregnancy one standard deviation below or above the mean for the cohort, abnormal mode of presentation, neonatal asphyxia, rupture of membranes prior to onset of labour, duration of labour one standard deviation longer than the mean for the cohort, and birth weight one standard deviation below the mean for the cohort.

Family problems
Family problems were rated for three time periods based on the subject's age: from birth to age 6, from age 7 to 12, and from age 13 to 18. Family problems were rated as present if the parents had received social welfare for 1 year or more during the period or if the Child Welfare Committee had intervened (therapy, supervision, placement of the child) because of inadequate parental care.

Intellectual performance
Global intelligence test scores were obtained using the Härnqvist Swedish Intelligence Test when the subjects were 12 years old. Intellectual performance was rated as poor if the standardized global test score was more than one standard deviation below the cohort mean.

School performance
The subject's academic performance was recorded from their school files when they were 12 (Grade 6) and 15 years of age (Grade 9). School performance was rated as poor if the average overall mark fell more than one standard deviation below the mean for the males in the cohort.

Behaviour problems
Behaviour problems were documented for two time periods: ages 7 to 12 and 13 to 18. Behaviour problems were rated based on information extracted from the record of the Child Welfare Committee. For the time period when the subjects were 7 to 12 years old, behaviour problems were rated as present if one or more of the following behaviours were noted in the Child Welfare Committee records: disorderly conduct in the community, vandalism, and theft. During the later time period, when subjects were 13 to 18, behaviour problems were rated as present if one or more of the following behaviours were noted in the Child Welfare Committee records: disorderly conduct in the community, vandalism, assault, theft, substance abuse, traffic accidents due to alcohol or drug use, and other traffic offences.

STATISTICAL ANALYSIS

The SLEIPNER statistical package for person-oriented analyses was used (Bergman & El-Khouri, 1998). The first step in the analyses focused on the identification of cross-sectional patterns of risk factors. Four such analyses were conducted covering the time periods of infancy (birth to 6 years), childhood (7 to 12 years), adolescence (13 to 18 years), and adulthood (19 to 30 years). For this purpose, configural frequency analyses (CFA) were conducted (Krauth & Lienert, 1982; von Eye, 1990). Initially, all the different possible patterns of risk, or configurations, were listed. Then, the observed and expected frequencies of each pattern were compared assuming a model of independence of the factors that constituted the pattern. The importance of the difference between the expected and observed frequencies was tested based on the binomial distribution, as explained by Krauth and Lienert.

The next step in the person-oriented analyses focused on the relations between the patterns of risk factors identified at each developmental period and at age 30. Cross-tabulations were calculated using the patterns of risk identified at one time period as one of the two categorical variables, and the patterns of risk identified at a subsequent time period as the other categorical variable. Then, each cell in the contingency table was tested in order to establish whether the observed frequency significantly differed from what could be expected if the variables were independent (for a detailed description of this rationale, see Bergman, 1998; Lienert & Bergman, 1985). The significance test was based on the hypergeometric distribution, following the Fisher rationale as implemented in the EXACON computer programme (see Bergman & El-Khouri, 1987)

Levels of significance

In the present context, as in most others, the large number of (dependent) significance tests that were performed created a validity problem by increasing the chance of spurious significant findings, the so-called mass significance problem. To safeguard against this threat to the validity of our results, the Bonferroni correction was used. However, the application of this stringent correction would lead to very low power in the analyses involving the MMD group, which includes only 81 subjects. Therefore, the nominal level of significance was used in cases where clear expectations of types or antitypes were present beforehand, and the Bonferroni correction was applied to all other tests. This was done for each analysis separately and for each group separately.

Treatment of missing data

Like other multivariate analyses, pattern analysis requires complete data-sets. Twenty percent of the subjects had one missing value and 5% two missing values. For these subjects, an imputation procedure was used. For each subject with one or two missing values, a twin subject with the same values on all other variables was identified. Then, the value of the twin was imputed to the subject with a missing value (for a discussion of this procedure, see Bergman & El-Khouri, 1992). Subjects with three or more missing values were excluded. Thus, the analyses were carried out with the 6,193 subjects for whom complete data were available after application of the imputation procedure. (For further details, see Lapalme, Hodgins, & Bergman, 1999.)

In contrast to results obtained when looking at relations between single-risk factors and outcomes at age 30, use of a CFA allowed us to identify patterns of risk factors from infancy through adolescence that are related to mental illness and criminal offending in adulthood. In effect, these analyses identified subgroups of subjects who were homogeneous with respect to patterns of risk factors. The developmental trajectories from infancy to adulthood were then calculated for each subgroup.

RESULTS

In the interests of clarity, the developmental trajectories are presented in two separate figures. Figure 1 presents the trajectories for subjects who had no risk factors in infancy and those who had experienced obstetrical complications. Figure 2 presents the trajectories for subjects whose families had problems during their first 6 years of life and the trajectories for subjects who both experienced obstetrical complications and were raised in problem families. Only the trajectories that are statistically significant at the .01 level are illustrated in Figures 1 and 2.

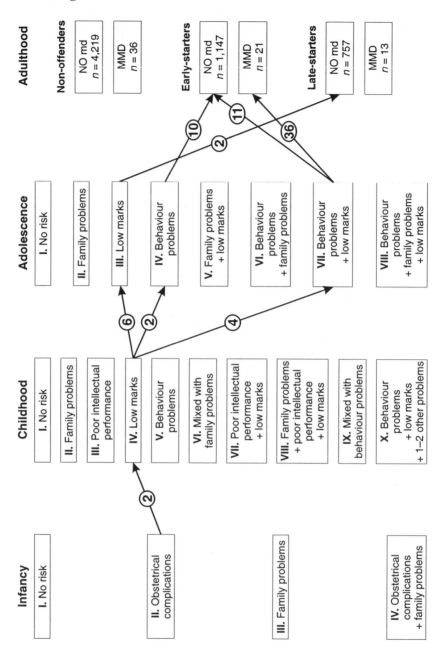

Figure 1. Typical developmental trajectories for Groups I and II from infancy to childhood. (*Note:* The numbers on the arrows indicate the number of times these subjects, as compared to those from the no-risk group, are likely to follow this pathway. Only significant types are shown [*p* < .01 after Bonferroni correction]. Levels of significance are based on exact cell-wise hypergeometric probability tests.)

Figure 1 presents the developmental trajectories for boys who presented no risk factors during their first 6 years of life and those who experienced obstetrical complications. As can be observed, children with no risk factors in their first 6 years of life typically continued to be free of problems during childhood and adolescence and are typically members of the non-offender and non-mentally disordered group in adulthood. The trajectory characterized by behaviour problems paired with low school marks in adolescence (Group VII) is the only pathway related to early-start offending among males with a major mental disorder. The association between having both behaviour problems and low marks in adolescence and early-start offending and mental illness is strong, with an odds ratio of 36. It is interesting to note that this association is much stronger for the mentally ill subjects than for the non-mentally ill early-start offenders. Further, the trajectory characterized by obstetrical complications, then poor intellectual performance in childhood, and behaviour problems alone or in combination with behaviour problems during adolescence was observed among non-disordered but not mentally ill early-start offenders.

Figure 2 presents the developmental trajectories that characterized the boys who were raised in problematic families during their first 6 years of life. Family problems during the first 6 years of life increased by 15 to 20 times the risk of continuing to be raised in such families in childhood, and increased by 6 to 12 times the risk of presenting behaviour problems in addition to other problems. These five groups of boys were then very likely to present multiple problems during adolescence, most often including behaviour problems. These adolescents are 11 to 12 times more likely than those from the no-risk group to be convicted of a criminal offence before the age of 18, and 34 to 58 times more likely to develop, in addition, a major mental disorder by the age of 30.

Two developmental trajectories are noteworthy. They both start with family problems during the first 12 years of life. During adolescence, some of these subjects present both family problems and low marks at school, and some persistent family problems, poor academic performance, and behaviour problems. The outcomes at age 30 associated with one or the other pattern of risk in adolescence are quite different. Family problems paired with low school marks are more likely to lead to late-start offending among non-disordered men, whereas family problems paired with behaviour problems are more likely to lead to early-start offending among men both with and without major mental disorders.

Finally, the results illustrated in Figure 2 indicate that obstetrical complications do not notably add to the risk already conveyed by family problems that are present during early childhood. In fact, boys who had experienced both obstetrical complications and problem families did not develop behaviour problems in middle childhood. Further, none of the early-start offenders with a major mental disorder had been part of this subgroup during infancy.

The results obtained underline the necessity of examining combinations of risk factors and how they change during development. Indeed, the same patterns of risk in childhood may have different outcomes in adulthood depending on the antecedents in infancy and/or transitions in adolescence. Moreover, many patterns of risk that were not statistically significant when related bivariately to early-start offending

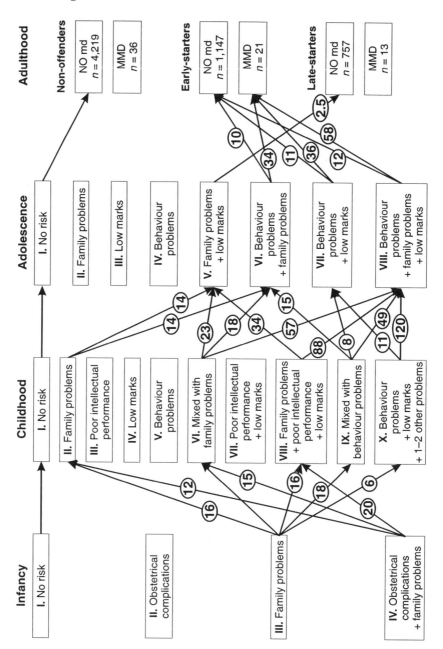

Figure 2. Typical developmental trajectories for Groups III and IV from infancy to childhood. (*Note:* The numbers on the arrows indicate the number of times these subjects, as compared to those from the no-risk group, are likely to follow this pathway. Only significant types are shown [*p* < .01 after Bonferroni correction]. Levels of significance are based on exact cell-wise hypergeometric probability tests.)

among men with major mental disorders were found to be a part of developmental trajectories that were highly statistically significant. Indeed, in most cases early-start offenders with and without major mental disorders followed similar developmental trajectories.

METHODOLOGICAL ISSUES

While the investigation described above has made an attempt to identify the developmental trajectories of etiologically homogeneous subgroups of offenders with major mental disorders, it has many weaknesses which need to be corrected in future investigations. In order to identify how and why offending develops among persons who present major mental disorders in adulthood, investigations will need to have the following characteristics: (1) Large samples of both males and females. As noted above, although we had a birth cohort of more than 15,000 persons, we did not have sufficient mentally ill female offenders by age 30 to allow us to conduct analyses. (2) Follow-up of subjects at least into their forties. Current epidemiological information indicates that large proportions of mentally ill offenders—especially among females—commit their first crime after age 30. (3) Data collected prospectively. (4) Data collected to take account of the point in development at which each factor or event occurred. This is essential. Using the Swedish 1953 birth cohort and obstetrical data extracted from medical files, we obtained two very different results, depending on whether or not we took account of the timing of perinatal events. (5) Many different factors and their interactions need to be measured simultaneously. As noted above, bivariate analyses provided misleading results concerning developmental trajectories. Further, studies must be designed to take account of possible inherited vulnerabilities. Presently, this means using family history information to index possible genetic risk. (6) Probably most important is the notion that for any outcome there will be more than one developmental pathway. Consequently, data analyses must be undertaken so as to allow the homogeneous subgroups among the subjects to be identified and tracked separately.

A Cohort Effect

As can be noted in chapters 1, 2, and 3, all of the epidemiological data which are available on the increased prevalence of offending among persons with major mental disorders, as compared to persons with no disorders, are for subjects born between 1944 and 1966. The possibility of a cohort effect cannot presently be excluded. If such an effect exists, it is important for unravelling the etiology of offending among the mentally ill, as it suggests that the search for the determinants should focus on factors that distinguish this cohort from previous and subsequent ones. The cohort born between 1944 and 1966 includes the first generation of persons with major mental disorders to be treated in the era of deinstitutionalization. The type and quality of mental health care affect both the early- and late-start mentally ill offenders. This can be seen in the rapid increases in the proportions of mentally ill persons who committed offences in the years following deinstitutionalization (for a discussion, see Hodgins & Lalonde, 1999). However, the type and quality of mental health care would have no effect on the initial offending of the early-starters. This cohort also includes the first generation of mentally ill persons treated with neuroleptics. Again, this would not influence the initial offending of the early-starters. Another impact of the deinstitutionalization era is that persons with major mental disorders live longer. While precise data are unavailable, some facts are known. In the asylums of the mid-20th century as many as 10% of patients died annually from infections. Consider, for example, persons with bipolar disorder. In addition to death by infection, one in five suicided and a sizeable number died from exhaustion during manic episodes (Hodgins & Lalonde). While rates of premature death among the mentally ill still far exceed those among non-disordered persons (Hodgins, 1998), especially in countries with low HIV infection rates, persons with mental illness may live longer than was the case in previous generations. One of the consequences of this longevity may be antisocial behaviour. The proportional increase in the numbers of mentally ill persons results not only from the decrease in premature death rates, but also from the increase in the prevalence of the major affective disorders (cf. Kessler et al., 1994).

However, the cohort (born 1944–1966), which includes a significant proportion of offenders among the mentally ill, may include a disproportionate number of persons who exhibited a stable pattern of antisocial behaviour since early childhood. The Epidemiological Catchment Area study in the US suggests that the proportion of such persons has been increasing since the beginning of the 20th century (Robins, Tipp, & Przybeck, 1990). This increase could result from exposure to specific perinatal and early childhood events which did not affect previous, and maybe subsequent, generations. Such factors could include maternal smoking and alcohol consumption during pregnancy, exposure to low levels of lead, and specific obstetrical practices that have been associated with negative adult outcomes.

Conclusion

Investigations on the etiology and development of offending in the mentally ill are conducted with a view to developing primary prevention programmes and to improving treatment efficacy by identifying subgroups of mentally ill offenders who are homogeneous with respect to etiology and development. The results of such investigations will also be useful in increasing the accuracy of predictions of offending and/or violent behaviour among the mentally ill. In the investigations of the 1953 Swedish birth cohort, 21 of the 26 early-start mentally ill offenders were identified before age 13. Surprisingly, 47% of the mentally ill late-start offenders were identified before the age of 13 and 60% by age 18. Not only can these mentally ill offenders be identified long before they have committed a crime or developed a major mental disorder, but they can be identified by non-invasive means. In fact, what distinguishes them is that they are having difficulty coping with life. Thus, early-childhood intervention is justified because it would directly address the difficulties that these children present, and would also, we hypothesize, act to prevent the development of offending in later life.

Etiological investigations provide information which can be used to improve the effectiveness of treatment and management. Information about the developmental patterns associated with each subtype of mentally ill offender contributes to more precise identification of treatment needs, individual strengths and weaknesses, and deficits. Not only is this information necessary for accurately matching patient needs and treatment; it is also useful for making decisions concerning management and security and for identifying conditions under which the individual can live in the community without committing an offence.

Notes

1. The history of the treatment of schizophrenia, for example, is replete with instances of treatments which required persons with the disorder to do what today we know they cannot do. The brain abnormalities which characterize schizophrenia explain why individuals with the disorder have difficulty with the abstract thinking that is necessary in, for example, psychotherapy, have difficulty coping with emotionally charged interpersonal situations and thereby often need to live apart from their families, and have limited concentration and the planning abilities often necessary for employment. Asking these patients to participate in psychotherapy, to live with their families, and to work in regular jobs leads to failures and immeasurable suffering, because they simply do not have the necessary capacities.
2. This is a major problem. The most commonly used statistical procedures presume that groups of subjects are homogeneous, and, if they are not—if they are in fact constituted by distinct subgroups—these procedures will hide them and not allow them to emerge. For example, consider a series of comparisons between a group of men with schizophrenia who have committed homicide and a group of non-disordered homicide offenders, in which the strength of the observed differences is measured using t-tests or analyses of variance. The presumption is made that the distributions of the characteristics being compared are similar in the two groups. If this presumption is not true, the results of the comparisons are erroneous and misleading. If, in addition, the populations of schizophrenic and non-disordered homicide offenders are not homogeneous but rather each includes several different subgroups, then different samples of schizophrenic and non-disordered homicide offenders would likely include different proportions of each subgroup. This would lead not only to erroneous results, but also to results that vary from one study to another. (For further discussion, see Bergman & Magnusson, 1997.)
3. The need for further descriptive, epidemiological studies of mentally ill offenders is illustrated by the present confusion concerning criminality and violent behaviour among persons with major affective disorders. Consider the following. (1) The diagnostic criteria for major depression identify a heterogeneous group of persons. (2) The diagnosis is not understood and used in the same way in Europe and North America. (3) It has been estimated that less that one third of persons with either major depression or bipolar disorder consult a mental health professional (Weissman, Bruce, Leaf, Florio, & Holzer, 1991). Males are less likely to consult than females (Rutz, 1996). (4) Because such a small proportion of persons with major affective disorders are diagnosed, it is very difficult to estimate the rate of suicide. However, a number of studies suggest that these disorders are the principal cause of suicide and that more than 80% of suicide victims meet diagnostic criteria for a major affective disorder. Among persons with major affective disorders, those most likely to suicide show stable patterns of impulsive and aggressive behaviour (Brådvik & Ber-

glund, 1993; Bronisch, 1996). Similarly, among depressed children and adolescents the risk of suicide is highest among those with a comorbid diagnosis of conduct disorder (Myers et al., 1991). (5) Adolescents with conduct problems have an increased risk of premature death (Hodgins, 1994). These findings suggest two conclusions. First, among persons with major affective disorders the risk factors for suicide and for criminality and/or violence are the same. Second, because the risk of premature death by suicide or accident is elevated among those with major affective disorders and suicide, those most at the risk to offend are likely to die young. Third, because few of these persons come to the attention of mental health professionals, the association between these disorders and offending is difficult to document.

4. While we view antisocial behaviour or conduct disorder in childhood as a category, we accept that these behaviours may in fact represent only the extreme of a continuum of what is observed in the general population. "...CD may not necessarily be a discrete entity but rather an extreme of the normal variation in conduct-disordered behaviour found in the general population...the risk factors for and correlations and consequences of normal-range or subclinical forms of childhood antisocial behaviours are the same as though for CD. This is consistent with reports from the Epidemiological Catchment Area Study (Robins & Regier, 1991), in which the number of childhood CD symptoms functioned as a continuum in predicting adult antisocial behaviours (Robins & Price, 1991; Robins, Tipp, & Przybeck, 1991), drug use (Robins & McEvoy, 1990), age of onset of alcohol and drug use (Robins & McEvoy, 1990), substance abuse (Robins & McEvoy, 1990), alcohol and drug use and dependence (Robins & Price, 1991), somatization disorder (Robins & Price, 1991), depression (Robins & Price, 1991), and schizophrenia (Robins & Price, 1991)." (Slutske et al., 1997, p. 273)

5. These findings do not preclude the possibility of the existence of non-genetic forms of the major mental disorders.

6. Family aggregation of a characteristic does not necessarily mean that the characteristic is genetically determined. Clearly, more research designed specifically to identify hereditary factors is required to test this hypothesis.

7. This work was done by M. Lapalme, S. Hodgins, and L. Bergman.

References

Angold, A., & Costello, E.J. (1993). Depressive comorbidity in children and adolescents: Empirical, theoretical, and methodological issues. *American Journal of Psychiatry, 150*(12), 1779–1791.

Asnarow, J R. (1988). Children at risk for schizophrenia: Converging lines of evidence. *Schizophrenia Bulletin, 14,* 613–631.

Bergman, L.R. (1998). A pattern oriented approach to studying individual development: Snapshots and processes. In R.B. Cairns, L.R. Bergman, & J. Kagan (Eds.), *Methods and models for studying the individual.* New York and Thousand Oaks, CA: Sage.

Bergman, L.R., & El-Khouri, B.M. (1987). EXACON: A Fortran 77 program for the exact analysis of single cells in a contingency table. *Educational and Psychological Measurement, 476,* 155–161.

Bergman, L.R., & El-Khouri, B.M. (1992). *M-PREP: A Fortran 77 computer program for the preparatory analysis of multivariate data* (Report #1). Stockholm: Stockholm University, Department of Psychology.

Bergman L.R., & El-Khouri, B.M. (1998). *Spleiner: A computer package for person oriented analyses of developmental data* (Version II). Stockholm: Stockholm University, Department of Psychology.

Bergman, L.R., & Magnusson, D. (1997). A person-oriented approach in research on developmental psychopathology. *Development and Psychopathology, 9,* 291–319.

Bernstein, D.P., Cohen, P., Skodol, A., Bezirganian, S., & Brook, J.S. (1996). Childhood antecedents of adolescent personality disorders. *American Journal of Psychiatry, 153,* 907–913.

Bierut, L.J., Dinwiddie, S.H., Begleiter, H., Crowe, R.R., Hesselbrock, V., Nurnbreger, J.I., Porjesz, B., Schuckit, M.A., & Reich, T. (1998). Familial transmission of substance dependence: Alcohol, marijuana, cocaine, and habitual smoking. A report from the Collaborative Study on the Genetics of Alcoholism. *Archives of General Psychiatry, 55,* 982–988.

Brådvik, L., & Berglund, M. (1993). Risk factors for suicide in melancholia: A case-record evaluation of 89 suicides and their controls. *Acta Psychiatrica Scandinavica, 87,* 306–311.

Brennan, P.A., Grekin, E.R., & Mednick, S.A. (1999). Maternal smoking during pregnancy and adult male criminal outcomes. *Archives of General Psychiatry, 56,* 215–224.

Brennan, P.A., Mednick, S.A., & Hodgins, S. (1999). Psychotic disorders and criminal violence in a total birth cohort. *Archives of General Psychiatry.*

Bronisch, T. (1996). The relationship between suicidality and depression. *Archives of Suicide Research, 2,* 235–254.

Cadoret, R.J., Winokur, G., Langbehn, D., Troughton, E., Yates, W.R., & Stewart, M.A. (1996). Depression spectrum disease. I: The role of gene-environment interaction. *American Journal of Psychiatry, 153*(7), 892–899.

Cadoret, R.J., Yates, W.R., Troughton, E., Woodworth, G., & Stewart, M.A. (1995). Genetic-environmental interaction in the genesis of aggressivity and conduct disorders. *Archives of General Psychiatry, 52,* 916–924.

Carlson, G.A., & Weintraub, S. (1993). Childhood behavior problems and bipolar disorder—relationship or coincidence? *Journal of Affective Disorders, 28,* 143–153.

Chassin, L., Pitts, S.C., DeLucia, C., & Todd, M. (1999). A longitudinal study of children of alcoholics: Predicting young adult substance use disorders, anxiety, and depression. *Journal of Abnormal Psychology, 108*(1), 106–119.

Coccaro, E.F., Silverman, J.M., Klar, H.M., Horvath, T.B., & Siever, L.J. (1994). Familial correlates of reduced central serotonergic system function in patients with personality disorders. *Archives of General Psychiatry, 51,* 318–324.

Constantino, J.N., Morris, J.A., & Murphy, D.L. (1997). CSF 5-HIAA and family history of antisocial personality disorder in newborns. *American Journal of Psychiatry, 154*(12), 1771–1773.

Côté, G., Lesage, A., Chawky, N., & Loyer, M. (1997). Clinical specificity of prison inmates with severe mental disorders: A case-control study. *British Journal of Psychiatry, 170,* 571–577.

Ebstein, R.P., Novick, O., Umansky, R., Priel, B., Osher, Y., Blaine, D., Bennett, E.R., Nemanov, L., Katz, M., & Belmaker, R.H. (1996). Dopamine D_4 receptor (D_4DR) exon lll polymorphism associated with the human personality trait of novelty seeking. *Nature Genetics, 12,* 78–82.

Ferdinand, R.F., & Verhulst, F.C. (1995). Psychopathology from adolescence into young adulthood: An 8-year follow-up study. *American Journal of Psychiatry, 152,* 1586–1594.

Fergusson, D.M., Woodward, L.J., & Horwood, L.J. (1998). Maternal smoking during pregnancy and psychiatric adjustment in late adolescence. *Archives of General Psychiatry, 55,* 721–727.

Fulwiler, C., Grossman, H., Forbes, C., & Ruthazer, R. (1997). Early-onset substance abuse and community violence by outpatients with chronic mental illness. *Psychiatric Services, 48,* 1181–1185.

Fulwiler, C., & Ruthazer, R. (1999). Premorbid risk factors for violence in adult mental illness. *Comprehensive Psychiatry, 40*(2), 96–100.

Geller, B., Cooper, T.B., Watts, H.E., Cosby, C.M., & Fox, L.W. (1992). Early findings from a pharmacokinetically designed double-blind and placebo-controlled study of lithium for adolescents comorbid with bipolar and substance dependency disorders. *Progress in Neuropsychopharmacology and Biological Psychiatry, 16,* 281–299.

Goldstein, R.B., Weissman, M.M., Adams, P.B., Horvath, E., Lish, J.D., Charney, D., Woods, S.W., Sobin, C., & Wickramatne, P.J. (1994). Psychiatric disorders in relatives of probands with panic disorder and/or major depression. *Archives of General Psychiatry, 51,* 383–394.

Gottesman, I.I., & Goldsmith, H.H. (1994). Developmental psychopathology of antisocial behavior: Inserting genes into its ontogenesis and epigenesis. In C.A. Nelson (Ed.), *Threats to optimal development* (pp. 69–104). Hillsdale, NY: Erlbaum.

Hammen, C., Burge, D., Burney, E., & Adrian, C. (1990). Longitudinal study of diagnoses in children of women with unipolar and bipolar affective disorder. *Archives of General Psychiatry, 47,* 1112–1117.

Harrington, R., Rutter, M., & Fombonne, E. (1996). Developmental pathways in depression: Multiple meanings, antecedents, and endpoints. *Development and Psychopathology, 8,* 601–616.

Heston, L.L. (1966). Psychiatric disorders in foster home reared children of schizophrenic mothers. *British Journal of Psychiatry, 112,* 819–825.

Hodgins, S. (1992). Mental disorder, intellectual deficiency and crime: Evidence from a birth cohort. *Archives of General Psychiatry, 49,* 476–483.

Hodgins, S. (1994). *A critical review of the literature on children at risk for major affective disorders.* Report commissioned by the Minister of Health of Canada.

Hodgins, S. (1998). Epidemiological investigations of the associations between major mental disorders and crime: Methodological limitations and validity of the conclusions. *Social Psychiatry and Epidemiology, 33*(1), 29–37.

Hodgins, S. (in press). Studying the etiology of crime and violence among persons with major mental disorders: Challenges in the definition and measurement of interactions. In L. Bergman & B. Cairns (Eds.), *Developmental science and the holistic approach.* Mahwah, NJ: Erlbaum.

Hodgins, S., & Côté, G. (1993). The criminality of mentally disordered offenders. *Criminal Justice and Behavior, 28,* 115–129.

Hodgins, S., Côté, G., & Toupin, J. (1998). Major mental disorders and crime: An etiological hypothesis. In D. Cooke, A. Forth, & R.D. Hare (Eds.), *Psychopathy: Theory, research and implications for society* (pp. 231–256). Dordrecht: Kluwer.

Hodgins, S., Kratzer, L., & McNeil, T.F. (1999). *Is there a relationship between obstetrical complications and crime? A longitudinal investigation of an unselected birth cohort.* Manuscript submitted for publication.

Hodgins, S., & Lalonde, N. (1999). Major mental disorders and crime: Changes over time? In P. Cohen, C. Slomkowski, & L.N. Robins (Eds.), *Historical and geographical influences on psychopathology* (pp. 57–83). Mahwah, NJ: Erlbaum.

Hodgins, S., & Lapalme, M. (1999). *The offspring of parents with bipolar disorder.* Manuscript submitted for publication.

Hodgins, S., Tétreault, I., & McNeil, T.F. (1999). *An etiological factor for violence among the mentally ill?* Manuscript submitted for publication.

Hodgins, S., Toupin, J., & Côté, G. (1996). Schizophrenia and antisocial personality disorder: A criminal combination. In L.B. Schlesinger (Ed.), *Explorations in criminal psychopathology: Clinical syndromes with forensic implications* (pp. 217–237). Springfield, IL: Charles C. Thomas.

Janson, C.-G. (1984). *A longitudinal study of a Stockholm cohort* (Research Report #21). Stockholm: University of Stockholm, Department of Sociology.

Kerr, M., Tremblay, R.E., Pagani, L, & Vitaro, F. (1997). Boys' behavioral inhibition and the risk of later delinquency. *Archives of General Psychiatry, 54,* 809–816.

Kessler, R.C., McGonagle, K.A., Zhao, S., Nelson, C.B., Hughes, M., Eshleman, S., Wittchen, H.-U., & Kendler, K.S. (1994). Lifetime and 12-month prevalence of DSM-III-R psychiatric disorders in the United States. *Archives of General Psychiatry, 51,* 8–19.

Kinney, D.K., Yurgelun-Todd, D.A., Tohen, M., & Tramer, S. (1998). Pre- and perinatal complications and risk for bipolar disorder: A retrospective study. *Journal of Affective Disorders, 50,* 117–124.

Kovacs, M., & Pollock, M. (1995). Bipolar disorder and comorbid conduct disorder in childhood and adolescence. *Journal of the American Academy of Child and Adolescent Psychiatry, 34*(6), 715–723.

Kratzer, L., & Hodgins, S. (1999). A typology of offenders: A test of Moffitt's theory among males and females from childhood to age 30. *Criminal Behaviour and Mental Health, 9,* 57–73.

Krauth, J., & Lienert, G.A. (1982). Fundamentals and modifications of configural frequency analysis (CFA). *Interdisciplinaria, 3.*

Kruesi, M.J.P., Hibbs, E.D., Zahn, T.P., Keysor, C.S., Hamburger, S.D., Bartko J.J., & Rapoport, J.L. (1992). A 2-year prospective follow-up study of children and adolescents with disruptive behavior disorders. *Archives of General Psychiatry, 49,* 429–435.

Lachman, H.M., Nolan, K.A., Mohr, P., Saito, T., & Volavka, J. (1998). Association between catechol O-Methyltransferase genotype and violence in schizophrenia and schizoaffective disorder. *American Journal of Psychiatry, 155*(6), 835–837.

Lapalme, M., Hodgins, S., & Bergman, L. (1999). *Developmental patterns of risk associated with criminal offending and major mental disorders: A prospective, longitudinal investigation of an unselected birth cohort.* Manuscript submitted for publication.

Lapalme, M., Jöckel, D., Hodgins, S., & Müller-Isberner, R. (1999). *Treatment and management of mentally disordered offenders: Relevance of co-morbid antisocial personality disorder.* Manuscript submitted for publication.

Lappalainen, J., Long, J.C., Eggert, M., Ozake, N., Tobin, R.W., Brown, G.L., Naukkarinen, H., Virkkunen, M., Linnoila, M., & Goldman, D. (1998). Linkage of antisocial alcoholism to the serotonin 5-HT1B receptor gene in two populations. *Archives of General Psychiatry, 55,* 989–995.

Lienert, G.A., & Bergman, L.R. (1985). Longisectional interaction structure analysis (LISA) in psychopharmacology and developmental psychopathology. *Neuropsychobiology, 14,* 27–34.

Lin, N., Eisen, S.A., Scherrer, J.F., Goldberg, J., True, W.R., Lyons, M.J., & Tsuang, M.T. (1996). The influence of familial and non-familial factors on the association between major depression and substance abuse/dependence in 1874 monozygotic male twin pairs. *Drug and Alcohol Dependence, 43,* 49–55.

Lyons, M.J., True, W.R., Eisen, S.A., Goldberg, J., Meyer, J.M., Faraone, S.V., Eaves, L.J., & Tsuang, M.T. (1995). Differential heritability of adult and juvenile antisocial traits. *Archives of General Psychiatry, 52,* 906–915.

Machón, R.A., Mednick, S.A., & Huttunen, M.O. (1997). Adult major affective disorder after prenatal exposure to an influenza epidemic. *Archives of General Psychiatry, 54,* 322–328.

McNeil, T.F. (1988). Obstetric factors and perinatal injuries. In M.T. Tsuang & J.C. Simpson (Eds.), *Handbook of schizophrenia. Vol. 3: Nosology, epidemiology and genetics.* New York: Elsevier.

Meller, W.H., & Borchardt, C.M. (1996). Comorbidity of major depression and conduct disorder (research report). *Journal of Affective Disorders, 39,* 123–126.

Merikangas, K.R., Leckman, J.F., Prusoff, B.A., Pauls, D.L., & Weissman, M.M. (1985). Familial transmission of depression and alcoholism. *Archives of General Psychiatry, 42,* 367–372.

Merikangas, K.R., Stolar, M., Stevens, D.E., Goulet, J., Preisig, M.A., Fenton, B., Zhang, H., O'Malley, S.S., & Rounsaville, B.J. (1998). Familial transmission of substance disorders. *Archives of General Psychiatry, 55,* 973–979.

Miller, L.J., & Finnerty, M. (1996). Sexuality, pregnancy, and childrearing among women with schizophrenia-spectrum disorders. *Psychiatric Services, 47,* 502–506.

Moffitt, T.E. (1993). Adolescence-limited and life-course-persistent antisocial behavior: A developmental taxonomy. *Psychological Review, 100,* 674–701.

Moffitt, T.E. (1994). Natural histories of delinquency. In E.G.M. Weitekamp & H.-J. Kerner (Eds.), *Cross-national longitudinal research on human development and criminal behavior* (pp. 3–61). Dordrecht: Kluwer.

Mueser, K.T., Drake, R.E., & Wallach, M.A. (1998). Dual diagnosis: A review of etiological theories. *Addictive Behaviors, 23*(6), 717–734.

Mueser, K.T., Rosenberg, S.D., Drake, R.E., Miles, K.M., Wolford, G., Vidager, R., & Carrieri, K. (1999). Conduct disorder, antisocial personality disorder, and substance use disorders. *Journal of Studies on Alcohol , 60,* 278–284.

Müller-Isberner, R. (1993). Managing insane offenders: The practice of hospital order treatment in the forensic psychiatric hospital. *International Bulletin of Law and Mental Health, 4,* 28–30.

Murray, B. (1998, August). Research reveals potential cause of youthful impulsiveness. *Monitor, American Psychological Association,* p. 9.

Myers, K., McCauley, E., Calderon, R., Mitchell, J., Burke, P., & Schloredt, K. (1991). Risks for suicidality in major depressive disorder. *Journal of the American Academy of Childhood and Adolescence, 30,* 86–94.

Needleman, H.L., Riess, J.A., Tobin, M.J., Biesecker, G.E., & Greenhouse, J.B. (1996). Bone lead levels and delinquent behavior. *Journal of the American Medical Association, 275*(5), 363–369.

O'Connor, T.G., McGuire, S., Reiss, D., Hetherington, E.M., & Plomin, R. (1998). Co-occurrence of depressive symptoms and antisocial behavior in adolescence: A common genetic liability. *Journal of Abnormal Psychology, 107*(1), 27–37.

O'Connor, T.G., Neiderhiser, J.M., Reiss, D., Hetherington, E.M., & Plomin, R. (in press). Genetic contributions to continuity, change, and co-occurrence of antisocial and depressive symptoms in adolescence. *Journal of Child Psychology and Psychiatry and Allied Disciplines.*

Pickens, R.W., Svikis, D.S., McGue, M., & LaBuda, M.C. (1995). Common genetic mechanisms in alcohol, drug, and mental disorder comorbidity. *Drug and Alcohol Dependence, 39,* 129–138.

Pihl, R.O., & Ervin, F. (1990). Lead and cadmium levels in violent criminals. *Psychological Reports, 66,* 839–844.

Pihl, R.O., & Peterson, J.B. (1993). Alcohol/drug use and aggressive behavior. In S. Hodgins (Ed.), *Mental disorder and crime.* Newbury Park, CA: Sage.

Quinsey, V.L., Cyr, M., & Lavallé, Y.J. (1988). Treatment opportunities in a maximum security psychiatric hospital: A problem survey. *International Journal of Law and Psychiatry, 11,* 179-194.

Räsänen, P., Helinä, H., Isohanni, M., Hodgins, S., & Tiihonen, J. (1999). Maternal smoking during pregnancy and risk of criminal behavior in the Northern Finland 1966 birth cohort. *American Journal of Psychiatry, 156,* 857–862.

Robins, L.N., & McEvoy, L. (1990). Conduct problems as predictors of substance abuse. In L.N. Robins & M. Rutter (Eds.), *Straight & deviant pathways from childhood to adulthood* (pp. 182–204). Cambridge: Cambridge University Press.

Robins, L.N., & Price, R.K. (1991). Adult disorders predicted by childhood conduct problems: Results from the NIMH Epidemiologic Catchment Area project. *Psychiatry, 54,* 116–132.

Robins, L.N., & Regier, D.A. (1991). *Psychiatric disorders in America: The Epidemiologic Catchment Area study.* New York: Macmillan/Free Press.

Robins, L.N., Tipp, J., & Przybeck, T. (1991). Antisocial personality. In L.N. Robins & D. Regier (Eds.), *Psychiatric disorders in America: The Epidemiologic Catchment Area study* (pp. 258–290). New York: Macmillan/Free Press.

Rowe, J.B., Sullivan, P.F., Mulder, R.T., & Joyce, P.R. (1996). The effect of a history of conduct disorder in adult major depression. *Journal of Affective Disorders, 37,* 51–63.

Rutz, W. (1996). Prevention of suicide and depression. *Nordic Journal of Psychiatry, 50*(suppl. 37), 61–67.

Silverton, L. (1985). *Crime and the schizophrenia spectrum: A study of two Danish cohorts.* Doctoral dissertation, University of Southern California.

Slutske, W.S., Heath, A.C., Dinwiddie, S.H., Madden, P.A.E., Bucholz, K.K., Dunne, M.P., Statham, D.J., & Martin, N.G. (1997). Modeling genetic and environmental influences in the etiology of conduct disorder: A study of 2,682 adult twin pairs. *Journal of Abnormal Psychology, 107*(2), 266–279.

Tengstrom, A., Hodgins, S., & Kullgren, G. (1999). *Early- and late-start offenders with schizophrenia.* Manuscript submitted for publication.

Von Eye, A. (1990). *Introduction to configural frequency analysis: The search for types and antitypes in cross classification.* New York: Cambridge University Press.

Weissman, M.M., Bruce, M.L., Leaf, P.J., Florio, L.P., & Holzer, C. III. (1991). Affective disorders. In L.N. Robins & D. Regier (Eds.), *Psychiatric disorders in America: The Epidemiologic Catchment Area study* (pp. 53–80). New York: Macmillan/Free Press.

Weissman, M.M., Fendrich, M., Warner, V., & Wickramaratne, P. (1992). Incidence of psychiatric disorder in offspring at high and low risk for depression. *Journal of the American Academy of Child and Adolescent Psychiatry, 31*(4), 640–648.

Weissman, M.M., Gershon, E.S., Kidd, K.K., Prusoff, B.A., Leckman, J.F., Dibble, E., Hamovit, J., Thompson, D., Pauls, D.L., & Guroff, J.J. (1984). Psychiatric disorders in relatives of probands with affective disorders: The Yale University-National Institute of Mental Health Collaborative Study. *Archives of General Psychiatry, 41,* 13–21.

Weller, R.A., Kapadia, P., Weller, E.B., Fristad, M., Lazaroff, L.B., & Preskorn, S.H. (1994). Psychopathology in families of children with major depressive disorders. *Journal of Affective Disorders, 31,* 247–252.

Sheilagh Hodgins is a professor at the Université de Montréal, Montreal, Quebec, Canada, and a foreign adjunct professor at the Karolinska Institute, Stockholm, Sweden.

Author's Note

Comments or queries may be directed to Sheilagh Hodgins, Departément de psychologie, Faculté des arts et des sciences, CP 6128, Succursale Centre-ville, Montreal QC H3C 3J7 Canada. Telephone: 514 343-7875. Fax: 514 343-2285. E-mail: <sheilagh.hodgins@umontreal.ca>.

Section II

ASSESSMENT, EFFECTIVE TREATMENT, AND MANAGEMENT

CAPTURING CHANGE

An Approach to Managing Violence and Improving Mental Health

CHRISTOPHER D. WEBSTER
KEVIN S. DOUGLAS
HENRIK BELFRAGE
BRUCE G. LINK

Recently colleagues of ours discoursed on the topic of treatment effectiveness as it relates to persons with serious mental and personality disorder (Harris & Rice, 1997). They introduced their piece by pointing out that, although they had never encountered a fully effective intervention programme, they would in all likelihood recognize one such if they were to see it. Our present outlook is similar to that of Harris and Rice but goes a step further. We suggest that even if a programme is actually effective, chances are that behavioural and attitudinal changes will be indexed so haphazardly, if at all, that they will not be captured and so will not enter the record. And if positive changes are not pinned down during treatment or intervention the result can be to the great detriment of the individual patient, prisoner, or parolee. By the same token, if absence of changes or negative changes are not taken into account, innocent members of society can be placed at risk for violence. It will be argued here that, despite the almost mesmerizing abundance of validated, semi-validated, and unvalidated tests and scales for risk assessment on the market, there exist in fact few clinically relevant, procedurally fair devices for measuring changes in risk-relevant "dynamic" factors on an interdisciplinary basis. This would apply to measurements both in institutions and in the community. We would also like to posit that serious attempts to document dynamic changes could very possibly have salutary effects, meaning that the mere focus on indexing changes may play an important if minor role in inducing them.

The notion of "dynamic" change requires some comment. Later in the chapter, especially as we discuss the Historical, Clinical Risk (HCR-20) Scheme (Webster, Douglas, Eaves, & Hart, 1997), we draw a distinction between static, more-or-less demographic, largely unchangeable, file-based factors and dynamic, alterable, mainly clinical variables. In this chapter emphasis is placed much more on the latter than on the former. We are interested in exploration of variables known to have the potential to elevate or reduce risk of violence in institutions and in the community. If these variables can be agreed upon, defined, and measured, there is at least some

S. Hodgins (ed.), Violence among the Mentally Ill, 119–144.

chance that persons suffering from mental and personality disorders (including drug and alcohol abuse) can be shown to have reduced likelihood of future aggression and violence (and can be demonstrated to have achieved improvements in mental health functioning). Quinsey, Coleman, Jones, and Altrow (1997) make our point for us very aptly when they state: "There is thus a pressing need to develop a predictive scheme involving temporally varying (dynamic) predictors. Continuously varying predictors (e.g., an offender's mood state) are useful in determining when an offender may be more or less likely to reoffend in the immediate future, but because of their very nature, they are not relevant to long-term predictions" (p. 797).

It needs to be understood at the outset that the present approach to the topic of measuring attitudinal and behavioural change is by way of the now older literature on "dangerousness" (e.g., Shah, 1978). We suggest that of late the conceptual disaggregation of dangerousness into risk prediction, risk assessment, and risk management allows for important conceptual, methodological, and day-to-day practical clinical advances. On this basis, our plea is for renewed interest in measuring the kinds of change that may be useful for both research and clinical practice.

It is likely true that researchers and clinicians approach the topic of measurement quite differently. By and large, researchers want, as their "standard of truth," to be able to demonstrate alteration in one or more measures over time as a result of defined interventions. Generally, they expect to be able to demonstrate "statistical significance." With important exceptions (e.g., Patterson, 1979), they approach their task nomothetically. At best they see the overall picture; at worst they overlook the importance of "outliers" or fail to consider the rare ground-breaking example or case. Clinicians are more ideographically inclined. They focus, as they must, on the patients and prisoners who show up for assessment and treatment. At best they see the effects of their labour in the individual case; at worst they have neither the time nor the means to extract the important general principles which might be synthesized from their daily rounds. The time-honoured theoretical debate as to whether two such distinct viewpoints are actually needed to provide a truly comprehensive and satisfactory model of humankind is of course relevant to this matter (e.g., Medawar, 1967).

Whatever the eventual result of this philosophical debate, there can be no doubt that from an everyday, practical angle researchers and clinicians have, at least until recently, engaged insufficiently in conversations of mutual benefit and that the enormous volume of published research has affected daily practice rather little (Borum, 1996; Webster & Cox, 1997). Similarly, clinical experience all too rarely has inspired sustained and committed research. There is also the fact that administrators have often failed to encourage, and indeed to insist on, effective and balanced working relationships between clinicians and researchers. Too frequently, they are driven to encourage and to accept superficial assessments which, though possibly "looking good," come nowhere close to meeting sound standards of professional practice. Dietz (1985) makes the point that, given the high stakes around risk assessments, it is a pity they do not receive the kinds of financial investment that are made routinely in most areas of medical practice.

The discussion so far allows us to state our general theme: The time is ripe for clinicians, researchers, and administrators collectively to devise the kinds of means of measuring dynamic change that will help promote mental health in prisoners and patients. Indeed it may well be that those who receive services should also be vitally included in these attempts at collaboration (see, generally, Spaniol, Gagne, & Koehler, 1997).

The chapter opens with a few comments on what might be considered "administrative issues." These are included to frame the subsequent discussion. Next comes a section dealing with the "attribution" of "dangerousness" or violence potential. It serves to remind the reader that, unless care is taken, decisions about patients and prisoners might be made on the basis of the kinds of "static" characteristics that can actually be discriminatory. Although these complex difficulties have recently been explored in the literature (Mathiesen, 1998; Webster, 1998), the issue is so important that it warrants treatment early in the chapter. Then follows a very brief review on the prediction, assessment, and management of violence in mentally and personality disordered individuals. This review is short, partly because it is only incidental to the main points of interest and partly because it is well dealt with by other contributors to this volume. Then comes a brief outline of the HCR-20 (Webster et al., 1997) and associated instruments. This allows us to concentrate on explicating a general approach to clinical research on measuring change. The subsequent section gives some concrete examples of how behavioural change was measured in three separate projects. These findings are encouraging, since they apparently document what good clinical sense would expect. The final section points to what we think needs to be done to promote effective collaboration among clinicians, researchers, and administrators.

Administrative Issues

Throughout the Western world we are witnessing a seemingly new phenomenon: Large psychiatric hospitals, mostly built in Victorian times, lie empty and abandoned, while new forensic psychiatric units have very often risen on the same grounds. The general psychiatric population continues to decline, but health ministries find themselves trying to accommodate seemingly endless numbers of new forensic patients. This remarkable shift over recent years in the way resources have been redistributed from general psychiatric to "mentally disordered and addicted offenders" seems attributable to many influences.

Since space precludes a discussion of the present state of affairs in any detail, it may suffice to observe in the most general way possible that this "labelling" trend rests on an assumption by legislators that mental patients, including those suffering from various kinds of addictions, require an appreciable degree of supervision and support in the community if the risks of antisocial conduct they present are to be kept within containable bounds. Since new law in so many jurisdictions is bound to be informed to some degree by the opinions and experiences of mental health clinicians and researchers, it seems probable that the new outlook referred to above has gone some way towards establishing systems of supervision and control. As the mental health professions have asserted their competence, mostly on demonstrably solid grounds (Stoff, Breiling, & Maser, 1997), so have they become even more centrally involved in risk prediction, assessment, and management.

Canada provides a useful example of the rapid rate at which the forensic system is expanding (often at the expense of civil psychiatric beds). In 1992, the law surrounding persons found Not Guilty by Reason of Insanity (NGRI) (now Not Criminally Responsible by Reason of Mental Disorder, NCRMD) and Not Fit to Stand Trial (NFST) was altered. The details of the changes are too complex to be dealt with here. Suffice to say that the revised law allows the use of NCRMD in relatively minor, summary conviction, cases. Because of this and other factors, the number of such patients in Canada has at least doubled since 1992. Many of these persons were previously treated as ordinary civil psychiatric patients. Now, having been processed through the courts, they tend to be placed under the more-or-less final authority of a specially constituted review board. They are held on a fully indeterminate basis subject to annual review. Mental health evidence at their hearings is critical and plays a major role in determining whether privileges are increased, a conditional discharge allowed, or an absolute discharge granted. Whereas entry to this "Disposition Order" system under the Criminal Code is the result of a mental disorder that rendered individuals "incapable of appreciating the nature and quality of the act [committed] or omission or of knowing that it was wrong" or that renders them incapable of defending themselves at present, exit from the system depends on quite other grounds. To progress towards the goal of absolute discharge, individuals must be able to demonstrate that they are "not a significant threat to the safety of the public." At least some of the new Disposition Order patients in Canada would have previously been "ordinary" civil psychiatric patients. The 1992 changes to the law allow application of long-term detention provisions to persons accused of committing appreciably less serious criminal offences. Under civil commitment, it is the physician who has the power to decertify; under the Disposition Order system, it is the review board which determines if and when a patient is to be released absolutely or under conditions. The Disposition Order procedure is much more complicated, formal, and subject to check than the civil route. Risk of violence, never an easy issue for the individual clinician to deal with, becomes much more difficult to determine when various parties like prosecutors, hospital administrators, and defence lawyers enter the arena. Some of these parties have a vested interest in the patient's continued detention (usually, of course, with the patient's best interest in mind). This means that, to an extent at any rate, "dangerousness" or "risk" must be demonstrated to exist or be "constructed" (cf. Menzies, 1989; Pfohl, 1978). In Canada, it was planned at the time of introduction of the new 1992 legislation that persons who had been accused of minor crimes would not be held beyond certain stipulated limits. But the "capping" safeguard has yet to be proclaimed, with the result that all patients, in order to obtain release, must be able to show that they no longer constitute a "significant threat" to the public. This can be a tall order. Certainly, the present state of affairs calls for the application of impartial, disinterested assessments of risk for violence potential. It also requires attention to how risk can best be contained or managed.

It is instructive to observe review boards at work. With so many vested interests, it sometimes seems miraculous that any decision comes to be made. Certainly, the decision-making process itself needs to be taken more seriously than it is as an object of scientific study (cf. Esses & Webster, 1988; Quinsey & Ambtman, 1979;

Whittemore, 1999). Some clinicians, as they sit on the board, favour an impression-istic approach with main reliance on professional judgement and experience; others have been greatly influenced by the accumulated scientific evidence on risk predic-tion. At these hearings, points of view can vary dramatically, discussion can come to centre on one or a few issues, and comprehensiveness can be forsaken in favour of a drive to implicate the apparent key factor or factors. Not uncommonly, decisions seem to be made on the basis of what information is available rather than on what information could be made available (cf. Dietz, 1985). This can be problematic for some Disposition Order patients such as recent immigrants (who may be dispropor-tionately represented in the current Canadian Disposition Order population). Cer-tainly—and this ties to the central theme of this chapter—the heterogeneity of these forensic patients, in terms of presenting clinical status, is not helped by the near ab-sence of a working vocabulary, one which could be used and agreed on by members of different mental health disciplines as a basis for measuring change.

The Attribution Problem

A standard dictionary definition of the word attribute is: "ascribe to or regard as the effect of (a stated cause)" (Concise Oxford Dictionary). With respect to the pre-diction and assessment of violence potential, a central concern is that some current predictive schemes may have unanticipated adverse consequences for patients and prisoners. Although such consequences will likely be unintended by those who de-sign devices and scales, the plain fact is that such a state of affairs would hardly be without precedent. The history of mental health service delivery is, in fact, replete with examples. The well-meaning actions of the Jeffersonian-era reformers who created "asylums," away from the strife of modern urban life, yielded results which would have dismayed them. "Asylums" became "snakepits." Similarly, the policy of "deinstitutionalization" of mental patients seems not fully to have anticipated "homelessness." There should of course be no particular surprise about the way unimpeachably sensible actions too often give way to perverse consequences. Robert Merton made it evident that no action occurs in a "social vacuum" and that actions have unanticipated consequences, because their effects "ramify into other spheres of value and interest" (Merton, 1934, p. 902).

With these remarks as general background, it would be prudent for us to con-sider what might be the unanticipated consequences of developing risk assessment tools like the HCR-20 (Webster et al., 1997). To what extent is evaluation under these schemes "risky assessment"? To what extent ought researchers, clinicians, and administrators to be attempting to consider and anticipate counter-productive effects, especially during the current phase in which such instruments are being devised and proliferated? It is argued here, of course, not that such efforts should cease, only that as researchers and citizens we should be alert to potentially pernicious effects.

When instruments like the HCR-20 are used, even if used thoroughly and com-petently, they still usually find their applications within a context of coercion and control. And it has to be recognized that judicial, correctional mental health, social welfare, and other systems do not treat all people equally. Generally speaking, it is better to be a member of the dominant group. Few willingly eschew wealth, power, and prestige. The risk assessment, like the courts and other such processes, is almost bound to have unequal applications to individuals of different races, classes, and genders. Recently, in a well-publicized case, a Canadian woman shot her husband six times in an apparent attempt to kill him. Placed on a Disposition Order as NCRMD, she achieved an absolute discharge after 3 and a half years mostly spent in the community. Although the facts of the decision-making process are not available, it would seem likely that her secure economic position and social connections did her no harm. It could be, too, that 3 and a half years of supervision amply sufficed to ensure that she would no longer be a "significant threat." Of interest is the observation that this time served was brief relative to that served by many persons who have committed far less serious offences. Most people of course are not nearly as fortunate. They face problems of unemployability, lack of education, poverty, membership in minority groups, and so on. It is important that, to the extent possible, such characteristics not further stigmatize people whose lives have already been unduly circumscribed and disadvantaged.

One of the ascriptions most difficult to conceptualize is mental disorder. Monahan (1981) deemed it a "non-correlate" of violence in his influential 1981 book. As readers will know, this position was revised by him (Monahan, 1992) and later in his work with Steadman (Monahan & Steadman, 1994). The consensus now seems to be that there likely is some, albeit modest, correlation between mental disorders of different kinds and violence variously defined. Some would even have it that, relative to contrast populations, persons with previous diagnoses of major mental disorder are at reduced risk for violence (Quinsey, Harris, Rice, & Cormier, 1998). The published scientific literature seems to be changing quite rapidly in this area (though whether the views of experienced mental health clinicians working on a day-to-day basis have cause to change may be another matter—meaning that just because normative, statistically inclined researchers have not detected for certain the mental disorder/violence association in the aggregate does not mean that the connection does not exist, at least in particular, important individual cases). What this indicates, and it is a point emphasized in the concluding section of the chapter, is that clinical assessment guides may need frequent revision on this point. The current HCR-20 (Webster et al., 1997) seems to summarize matters quite well: "There is little evidence that most DSM-IV (or DSM-III, or DSM-III-R, etc.) conditions are strongly and almost invariably associated with violent conduct. Even sophisticated mental health workers may commonly over-emphasize the connection between violence and mental disorder..." (p. 9).

As structured clinical guides like the HCR-20 are developed, they will need to incorporate not only "clinical realities" but also "community realities." There is a place for epidemiological study. Clinical samples themselves do not suffice. There is every reason to want to know whether and to what extent people with certain disorders are at elevated risk for violence. It is necessary to find out whether such persons are more likely than their counterparts to be violent in the community when matched for age, gender, socioeconomic status, and other such variables, because eventual discharge will be to the community. There can be no question that the eventual validity of risk assessment guides must be founded in part on community comparison groups and that the present rather overweighted emphasis on clinical and institutional samples requires correction. This, then, is a matter of relative risk. The individual can be assessed relative to his or her cohort of patients and prisoners (i.e., as being at high or low risk relative to similarly situated persons), or the individual's level of risk can be projected relative to a community cohort (i.e., as being in line with or not in line with typical members of that community). Both aspects are clearly important and get back to the basic issue of establishing baseline levels of violence (e.g., Monahan, 1981).

Mental disorder is not the only potentially problematic "attributional variable." Race and class affect diagnosis, treatment, and the sifting and sorting of people to different destinations within mental health, correctional, and related spheres (Rosenfield, 1984). Several studies have indicated that African Americans are often inappropriately diagnosed with schizophrenia (Pavkov, Lewis, & Lyons, 1989). Also, people of relatively low social status are apt to receive coercive and less desirable forms of treatment (Hollingshead & Redlick, 1958). African-American youths are likely to be shunted to juvenile justice settings, whereas their white counterparts are likely to be treated in mental health settings. A difficulty with this is that these events and characteristics are prone to be entered in administrative records. Once in the file, they tend to be indelibly fixed there and indeed are often carried forward, sometimes erroneously (Konechni, Mulcahy, & Ebbensen, 1980). It needs to be conceded that, if this "objective" information is thoughtlessly used, risk assessors can be unduly influenced by it. All of this is to say that a person who has been the victim of such previous discrimination is inclined to be treated as more of a violence risk than he or she should be.

Certain groups are at markedly enhanced risk of being arrested. Members of these groups can achieve long records. Yet close examination of the file may reveal that few, if any, such arrests mean much. In one study, race was unrelated to violence once incidents involving the police were excluded (Link, Andrews, & Cullen, 1992). Differential police processing may be a reason for elevated arrest rate. If arrest rate stands as a proxy for "violence," persons with long arrest records are likely to be confined and receive coercive treatment. The point to be taken from this is that risk assessment should, to the extent humanly possible, exclude variables that are the result of social processing. That is why the emphasis should be on obtaining valid measures of actual dangerous and violent behaviour. At the very least, a risk assessment guide should stipulate clearly what is meant by violent behaviour. (The HCR-20 defines violence as "actual, attempted, or threatened harm to a person or persons. Threats of harm must be clear and unambiguous...rather than vague statements of hostility" [Webster et al., 1997, p. 24].)

The problem of "attribution"—the idea that bias can enter risk assessment through convenient proxies like age, gender, class, and, perhaps to a lesser degree, diagnosis, clinical states, or even "likeability" (Day, 1998)—is a topic which deserves renewed scientific attention in its own right. That pieces of information, none of which would come close to meeting ordinary evidentiary standards, can be unwittingly "laundered" into fact is an idea that has been with us for some time (Monahan, 1981). If airline pilots can be taught to screen out the irrelevancies and to concentrate on the essentials, it is to be hoped that a new generation of mental health professionals can educate themselves to avoid making what can be little more than moral condemnations (e.g., Eisenman, 1987). A first step in this direction may be to distinguish among the functions of risk prediction, risk assessment, and risk management.

The Prediction, Assessment, and Management of Violence

We have already alluded to the idea that the notion of "dangerousness," which was still prevalent in the 1970s and early 1980s, has given way to an emphasis on risk prediction, risk assessment, and risk management. The notion of the "dangerous individual" has been around a long time (Petrunic, 1982). It is in fact firmly embedded in such statutes as the Canadian Dangerous Offender and Long Term Offender legislation, which is paralleled in many US states (cf. Moore, Estrich, McGillis, & Spelman, 1984). Clinical thinking has to mirror these statutes in the sense that practitioners consider it their duty to aid the courts in their quest to understand such abstruse concepts as "brutality" and "evil" (as found, for example, in the Canadian Criminal Code provisions related to Dangerous Offenders). Little current research is centred on the idea of "dangerousness." What has substituted is an emphasis on sheer actuarial prediction, the process of risk assessment, and the challenge of risk management (see Heilbrun, 1997).

Added to this—and, though important, not dealt with in much detail here—is the notion of immediate crisis intervention. By this we mean the way in which professionals like police officers, psychiatric nurses, and prison officers deal with potentially calamitous incidents in the community, on the wards, and the like. This would include such serious and threatening incidents as hostage-takings and riots. Even though such dramas often take place over seconds, and even though they too have precipitators that can be isolated and analyzed, they are best left for consideration elsewhere (e.g., Rice, Harris, Varney, & Quinsey, 1989).

PREDICTION

The kinds of variables which are important in the prediction of violence likely depend critically on the interval over which the predictions are made. If predictions are to be made over the short term, in a matter of hours or days, it may be well to consider the kinds of variables included in the little known and used Interview Assessment Scale (IAS, Menzies & Webster, 1995, p. 768), or even the Dangerous Behavior Rating Scheme (DBRS, Menzies, Webster, & Sepejak, 1985a; see also Megargee, 1976). Such variables centre on items like eye contact, affect, posturing, agreeability, pace, tension, and rapport (IAS), and passive aggression, hostility, anger, rage, guilt, capacity for empathy, tolerance, and manipulativeness (DBRS). If, at the other extreme, the prediction is to be tailored to the long term (i.e., years), there seems little doubt that basic, "static," more-or-less unchanging variables can yield surprisingly accurate predictions of violence. This has been shown most convincingly, perhaps, via the so-called Violence Risk Appraisal Guide (VRAG, Quinsey et al., 1998) and also in studies by Menzies and Webster (1995) and Steadman et al. (in press). The important point about prediction is that, at its simplest, it concerns only two time points: when the prediction was made and when eventual follow-up information on aggression or violence was obtained. All else, all that occurs between Time 1 (T1) and Time 2 (T2), is excluded. The results of modern studies on prediction, perhaps especially those by Quinsey et al., have been clear in showing that variables like psychopathy (whether measured by the Psychopathy Checklist-Revised [PCL-R, Hare, 1991] or the Child and Adolescent Taxon Scale [CATS—see Quinsey et al., 1998, p. 167]), early school maladjustment, marital status, and the like have appreciably more long-range predictive power than had been thought earlier (see Menzies, Webster, & Sepejak, 1985b). There can be no doubt that having a conscientiously coded VRAG score, or perhaps a total H score from the HCR-20, can be an invaluable aid in decision-making once it has been deemed appropriate for use in a given sample. This is perhaps particularly so in cases where scores are relatively high or relatively low.

ASSESSMENT

Clinicians will sometimes have the benefit of a VRAG or other type of actuarially based score. Yet, helpful though this will usually be, ordinarily it will not in and of itself suffice for assessment. Someone, most often a mental health professional, must face the task of matching the individual's possible future actions with the situation in which that person could or will exist. While T2, in prediction, may remain an important focal point for the purposes of planning, evaluation, and research, the assessor must take into account the many factors that might arise at any number of unspecifiable intermediate times between T1 and T2. The assessor must also take a stab at how these largely uncontrollable factors will likely interact with one another. Such assessment entails a process of identifying risks and specifying the likelihood of violence over defined periods. It encourages a step towards the goal of preventing violence (a process which, if successful, will disprove the prediction and hence reduce the predictive accuracy). The "linear" approach described under PREDICTION above may or may not work and may apply to some individuals better than others (Bem & Allen, 1974; Mischel, 1968). The overall level of risk of violence in some people will likely decrease for a specified kind of violence, maintain a steady level for others, and show increased propensity for yet others (see Krause, Howard, & Lutz, 1998). The clinical challenge, one that often necessitates a considerable amount of theorizing and speculation at the case level, is to figure out which persons in which situations will likely fare most prosocially or most antisocially. The problem is that a fair amount of variability can be expected in terms of the exigencies presented by different physical, social, and cultural circumstances. We do not think that clinicians can step over this complexity through a sole or even main reliance on static prediction. Would that it were otherwise.

MANAGEMENT

According to the present formulation, risk management is the task of constructing social and physical environments that, in combination with knowledge of the individual's assets and liabilities, will likely lead to substantial reduction in violence potential. With creative engineering, overall level of violence should drop for a particular individual or a group of persons characterized and treated in a similar way. This of course is the essence of intensive community supervision programmes, which, though conceivably effective, tend to be insufficiently researched or administratively monitored on a day-to-day basis. The success of such programmes doubtless depends in part on the ability of case managers, parole officers, "boundary spanners," and the like not just to isolate "risk factors" but to address the actual needs of clients (Rice, Harris, Quinsey, & Cyr, 1990; Webster, Hucker, & Grossman, 1993).

The HCR-20

The HCR-20 first appeared in 1995 (Webster, Eaves, Douglas, & Wintrup, 1995). It was intended as a broad-spectrum instrument which might constructively be applied to psychiatric patients, forensic patients, and, on the correctional side, inmates and parolees in cases where mental or personality disorder is a consideration. The device was based on extensive consultation with clinicians in a variety of mental health disciplines, and it aimed to incorporate up-to-date information gleaned from the formal scientific literature. Two years later it was revised (Webster et al., 1997) in an attempt to tighten and clarify the various definitions. A certain amount is now known about the characteristics of the guide (Douglas, Cox, & Webster, 1999; Douglas & Webster, 1999a, 1999b), how best to implement it (Belfrage, 1998), and how aspects of it stack up against other prediction devices (Polvi, 1999).

The predictive aspects of the HCR-20 are largely covered by 10 items labelled as "historical." Following Hare (1991), these items are scored as 0 (not present), 1 (possibly applicable), and 2 (definitely applicable). The items are identified as follows: H1 – previous violence; H2 – young age at first violent incident; H3 – relationship instability; H4 – employment problems; H5 – substance-abuse problems; H6 – major mental illness; H7 – psychopathy; H8 – early maladjustment; H9 – personality disorder; and H10 – prior supervision failure. It should be evident that these items derive loosely from Monahan (1981), that they are similar to items in the VRAG of Quinsey et al. (1998), and that they overlap partially with the kind of items now being studied by Steadman et al. (in press). Since prediction on the basis of prior historical variables is not the main focus of this chapter, these 10 variables will not be dealt with further. More detail is available in Douglas, Cox, and Webster (1999). It is acknowledged that, unless care is taken in the coding of these items, attributional bias can enter in the scoring of some of the H variables (see section on attribution above).

The five dynamic clinical items, C1 – lack of insight; C2 – negative attitudes; C3 – active symptoms of mental illness; C4 – impulsivity; and C5 – unresponsive to treatment, are intended to cover, mainly but not exclusively, aggressive conduct in the fairly immediate future (e.g., as in an intensive-care psychiatric unit). The five dynamic risk variables are expected to cover the indefinite future. These variables are: R1 – plans lack feasibility; R2 – exposure to destabilizers; R3 – lack of personal support; R4 – noncompliance with remediation attempts; and R5 – stress. Although they are generally cast towards life in the community, the manual is so constructed that clinicians can opt to rate the individual on the basis of possible continued confinement in an institution or on the presumption that the person will be released to the community under some form of supervision. Actual experience with the guide shows that some colleagues choose to rate the individual in both contexts. To date, in conformity with expectations, C variables perform better than H and R variables when tested on patients held on an intensive-care unit of a psychiatric hospital (Ross, Hart, & Webster, 1998). Also as anticipated, the R variables yielded their highest correlations with post-discharge assaultive behaviour in the community (Ross et al.). Generally, there is some support for the predictive power of C and R variables (see Strand, Belfrage, Fransson, & Levander, 1999).

Although the HCR-20—being patterned, at least in terms of structure, on the 20-item Hare (1991) PCL-R—can function as a scale, there are, at this early stage, no formally published norms. Some clinicians simply use the 20 headings of the HCR-20 as they prepare reports for courts, boards, committees, and tribunals. Recently it has come to our attention that some practising colleagues use the C and R variables of the HCR-20 to monitor the individual's progress in treatment or rehabilitation. When high scores are allotted, the clinician is immediately challenged with the task of finding ways to reduce the level of risk. Moreover, he or she has, with previous C and R scores in hand, a baseline against which to evaluate progress in treatment. This point is elucidated in the next section.

Evaluating Change over Time Using the HCR-20

This section has as its main goal the demonstration of change in the Clinical and Risk Management Scales of the HCR-20. Of course, the basic treatment-related logic underlying these and other ostensibly dynamic violence risk factors is that, because they are prone to change, they ought to be targeted for violence-reducing treatment strategies. We describe existing research evaluating whether scores on the C and R scales do in fact change over time. The studies that have addressed this question, or at least that have collected data that permit the analysis of this question, have been situated within institutional (e.g., civil psychiatric, forensic psychiatric) contexts. We will briefly describe these research efforts, and focus on portraying data on the change within the C and R scales and the items within them.

In carrying out violence risk assessments, it is important that dynamic, or changeable, risk factors be identified and evaluated. A dynamic violence risk factor, for the present purposes, can be identified as a variable that relates to violence, that may fluctuate with time, and that can be changed as a function of deliberate intervention. Both in risk assessments of institutional violence and in assessments of risk for violent criminality after discharge from institutional care, some recent studies have suggested that these dynamic factors have a strong predictive validity (Douglas, Ogloff, Nicholls, & Grant, 1999; Strand et al., 1999). This further stresses the importance of having these factors targeted for violence-reducing strategies.

RESEARCH STUDY 1: CIVIL PSYCHIATRIC PATIENTS

In the first sample, data were coded from the files of 193 civilly psychiatric patients who were involuntarily committed to a large psychiatric hospital in western Canada. The HCR-20 was coded from extensive hospital files. The sample and study are more fully described in Douglas, Ogloff, et al. (1999). In summary, most participants were male (117 of 193; 60.6%) and the mean age at admission was 38.1 years (*SD* = 14.9). The majority of the sample were Caucasian (*n* = 152; 79%) and were unemployed at the time of admission (*n* = 180; 93%). More than half of the sample had not completed high school (*n* = 107; 55%).

Many patients (*n* = 123; 64%) had previous convictions or arrests for any type of criminal offence, and 78 (40%) had been arrested or convicted for violence offences; 120 patients (62%) had documented histories of physical violence against others. Most patients (*n* = 184; 95%) had prior hospitalizations. The mean duration of the index hospitalization was 272 days (*SD* = 558.3). Many patients (*n* = 145; 75%) had a history of substance abuse. Diagnostically, the most common Axis I diagnosis was schizophrenia (*n* = 85; 44%), followed by affective disorders (*n* = 31; 16%). Twenty-seven patients (14%) were diagnosed with antisocial personality disorder or traits, 43 (22%) with some other personality disorder or traits. It was possible to code the C scale of the HCR-20 both at admission and at discharge. The following analyses pertain to this issue. Correlations between scores at admission and at discharge were in the moderate to large range, as shown in Table 1. Intraclass correlation coefficients (ICC) were calculated along with Pearson *r*, because ICC takes into account differences in "anchor points" between ratings, whereas Pearson *r* does not. However, in the present case, the magnitude of correlation is similar. These correlations demonstrate that, while C-scale item scores are related to one another at different times, this relationship is, as might be expected, far from perfect.

Table 1. Change in mean C-scale and item scores between admission and discharge

Clinical-scale items	ICC_1	R	Admission score	Discharge score	Change score	t	p
C1. Lack of insight	.39***	.40***	1.75 (0.51)	1.18 (0.62)	0.57 (0.63)	12.42	.000
C2. Negative attitudes	.57***	.57***	1.31 (0.68)	0.75 (0.59)	0.56 (0.59)	12.97	.000
C3. Active symptoms	.44***	.45***	1.65 (0.63)	0.69 (0.72)	0.96 (0.71)	18.67	.000
C4. Impulsivity	.50***	.51***	0.92 (0.63)	0.41 (0.52)	0.51 (0.58)	12.32	.000
C5. Unresponsive to treatment	.47***	.47***	1.58 (0.56)	1.01 (0.60)	0.57 (0.60)	13.31	.000
C-scale total	.44***	.44***	7.21 (1.59)	4.05 (1.91)	3.06 (1.87)	23.51	.000

Notes: Partial correlation holds time constant. *** = $p \leq .001$

Table 1 also shows mean scores. These dropped significantly for the Total Score as well as for every item. For the Total Score, this drop was in the magnitude of 3 points out of 10 (i.e., from approximately 7 to 4). The distribution of C-scale scores was negatively skewed at admission and closer to normal, though positively skewed, at discharge. This pattern is to be expected. Patients who arrive at the psychiatric hospital tend to be quite disorganized, psychotic, and hard to manage. At discharge, they are more stable.

To illustrate more specifically the nature of change in the specific items, the reader is referred to Table 2, which displays the number and proportion of patients who scored 2/2 on each C-scale item. As can be seen, at admission many patients scored high on the items. Three of the items were rated 2/2 for more than half of the sample. At discharge, in contrast, four of five items were rated 2/2 in fewer than 20% of cases and for two of the items in fewer than 10% of cases. At admission close to half of the patients ($n = 93$) scored in the 8 to 10 range on the C scale. At discharge only seven patients scored in this upper range.

Table 2. Proportion of patients scoring high (2/2) on clinical-scale items at admission and discharge

Clinical-scale items	Admission	Discharge
	n (%)	*n* (%)
C1. Lack of insight	152 (78.8)	58 (30.2)
C2. Negative attitudes	83 (43.0)	15 (7.8)
C3. Active symptoms	142 (73.6)	29 (15.0)
C4. Impulsivity	31 (16.1)	3 (1.6)
C5. Unresponsive to treatment	119 (61.7)	35 (18.1)
C-scale total (8, 9, or 10)	93 (48.2)	7 (3.4)

This pattern is evident in percentile ranks for total scores. Generally, the same score at discharge results in a much higher percentile rank than at admission. For instance, at admission a score of 5/10 was at the 10th percentile. At discharge the same score of 5/10 was at the 70th percentile. At admission a score of 7 would place the patient no higher than the 50th percentile. At discharge the same score of 7 would place the patient in the 95th percentile.

The above data reflect a seeming change in the clinical make-up of the sample at two different times. At admission the majority of patients displayed a marked lack of insight into their mental illness, violence proneness, and lack of understanding of the effects of medication and other treatments on their disorders (C1). Most patients displayed active symptoms of major mental illness such as hallucinations, delusions, or cognitive disorganization (C3). Again, the bulk of patients were rated as unresponsive to treatment at the time of admission (C5). Just under half of the patients displayed some sort of manifest negativity in attitude (C2). A small minority were considered highly impulsive (C4). At discharge, while up to 30% of patients were still with little if any insight (C1), the other clinical states had been reduced to at least moderate levels. Although data of this sort do not show convincingly how particular interventions affected particular patients, there is no reason to assume that the documented changes were not at least partly attributable to treatments patients received while hospitalized. At a practical, clinical level, it would be most helpful to be able to pinpoint, by way of data graphed for individual patients over multiple, successive periods, how change was related to various interventions. Essentially, this means a renewed call for a baseline-treatment-baseline, individual participant study. The HCR-20's contribution to this would be the mere supplying of outcome definitions (i.e., C1, C2, etc.). There is also the point that the C variables function as a clinical risk assessment device designed for use over the relatively short run. They centre, more than H variables do, on conditional probabilities (Mulvey & Lidz, 1995). In principle, this change can likely be attributed to treatment received in hospital.

RESEARCH STUDY 2: FORENSIC PSYCHIATRIC PATIENTS (CANADA)

In a sample of 175 forensic psychiatric patients who had been found NCRMD, Douglas, Hart, Webster, and Eaves (1998) analyzed the psychometric properties of the HCR-20, including change on C- and R-scale scores. The sample represents approximately 1 year of data from a maximum security forensic inpatient facility in western Canada. Psychiatrists completed the C and R scales of the HCR-20 for patients who appeared before a criminal review board seeking conditional or absolute discharge. Although some patients appeared only once, others appeared multiple times. Thus it was possible to analyze C- and R-scale scores across time.

The sample was primarily male (*n* = 154; 88%), with a mean age at admission of 33.0 (*SD* = 9.4). Most participants were unemployed (*n* = 163; 93%) and unmarried (*n* = 126; 72%) at admission. Schizophrenia was the predominant Axis I diagnosis at time of review board appearance (*n* = 97; 55%), followed by mood disorders (*n* = 21; 12%), other psychotic disorders (*n* = 20; 11.%), substance-use disorders (*n* = 14; 8%), schizoaffective disorders (*n* = 12; 7%), and other disorders (*n* = 12; 7%). Twenty-eight patients (16%) were diagnosed with personality disorder. These diagnoses were made by attending psychiatrists according to criteria of the *Diagnostic and Statistical Manual of Mental Disorders, 4th Edition* (DSM-IV; American Psychiatric Association, 1994). Most patients (*n* = 151; 86%) had been hospitalized in the past, and the majority (*n* = 95; 54%) had previous charges for violent offences. Finally, most patients (*n* = 148; 86%) had a violent index offence.

The results of these analyses are displayed in Table 3. The pattern of results is comparable to that found among the civil psychiatric patients. All C- and R-scale scores were significantly lower at the last assessment than at the first. The magnitude of drop on the total scores is not as great as for the previous sample. Again, Pearson *r* correlations for the C scale ranged from moderate (.33) to large (.63) in magnitude, with the C-scale total scores correlating at .56. Use of ICC reduced the correlations only very slightly. For the R scale, the correlations were smaller, averaging in the moderate (.30) range. One exception is for R2, which was not correlated across assessments. The smaller and less consistent nature of these correlations suggests that release plans are changed across assessment times. In fact, poor release plans may play a role in the review board's decision to refuse discharges at the first hearing. By the last assessment, social workers and patient advocates may have worked to improve these plans, resulting in low correlations across assessments.

Perhaps it is worth noting that R scores are, in a sense, reflective not only of the patients' or prisoners' state of preparedness for release but also of the clinicians' and administrators' imaginativeness in creating opportunities for safe re-integration into the community.

Table 3. Correlation between and change in C- and R-scale and item scores across first and last assessment times (Canadian forensic psychiatric sample)

HCR-20 scale and item	ICC_1	r	Time 1 M score (SD)	Time 2 M score (SD)	Difference score (SD)	t (p)
C Scale						
C1	.39***	.43***	1.51 (.60)	1.29 (.64)	0.22 (.66)	3.88 (.000)
C2	.29***	.33***	1.17 (.59)	0.96 (.60)	0.22 (.69)	3.69 (.000)
C3	.59***	.63***	1.09 (.81)	0.85 (.80)	0.24 (.70)	4.01 (.000)
C4	.50***	.53***	0.93 (.69)	0.75 (.78)	0.18 (.72)	2.97 (.004)
C5	.29***	.34***	1.21 (.61)	0.96 (.67)	0.25 (.74)	4.05 (.000)
Total	.48***	.56***	5.90 (2.31)	4.80 (2.56)	1.10 (2.30)	5.62 (.000)
R Scale						
R1	.09	.24**	1.53 (.62)	0.99 (.82)	0.54 (.90)	6.72 (.000)
R2	.04	.08	1.41 (.69)	1.15 (.73)	0.26 (.97)	2.99 (.003)
R3	.25**	.30***	1.34 (.64)	1.04 (.71)	0.30 (.79)	4.31 (.000)
R4	.29***	.33***	1.32 (.56)	1.11 (.67)	0.20 (.72)	3.27 (.001)
R5	.21**	.23**	1.36 (.54)	1.22 (.60)	0.14 (.71)	2.22 (.028)
Total	.25**	.30**	6.18 (2.17)	5.19 (2.62)	0.99 (2.86)	3.12 (.002)

Notes: Partial correlation holds time constant. ** $= p \le .01$ *** $= p \le .001$.
Adapted from Douglas et al. (2000).

RESEARCH STUDY 3: FORENSIC PSYCHIATRIC PATIENTS (SWEDEN)

This sample contains 42 forensic psychiatric patients who were sentenced to forensic psychiatric care according to the Swedish penal code (i.e., found guilty but sentenced to psychiatric treatment). The sample represents approximately 1 year of data from a special maximum security forensic psychiatric hospital in Northern Sweden (Sundsvall). Patients at special, secure units are considered the most dangerous of Sweden's forensic psychiatric patients. Such units house about 30% of all forensic psychiatric patients in Sweden; the balance are contained in medium secure or civil psychiatric hospitals. Every 6 months the patients at Sundsvall appear before a criminal review board seeking conditional or absolute discharge. In addition to these reviews, the patients are assessed by a team consisting of psychiatrists, psychologists, social workers, and other members of the staff using the Swedish-authorized version of the HCR-20 and the PCL:SV. The HCR-20 has, since 1997, been fully implemented into clinical practice at Sundsvall, a process which is described in detail in Belfrage (1998).

The sample was all male, with a mean age at the time of the first assessment of 37.1 (*SD* = 10.90). Seventeen patients (40%) were diagnosed with psychotic disorders, 20 (48%) with personality disorder, and five (12%) with other disorders. The diagnoses were made by psychiatrists according to the DSM-IV (APA, 1994). All patients had committed violent crimes; 13 (31%) were sentenced for homicide, five (12%) for violent sexual criminality, and seven (17%) for arson. At the time of the first assessment, the patients had been hospitalized for an average of 3 years (*MDN*

= 3 years), with a range of 1 to 19 years (a fraction of a year was counted as a full year—e.g., 1 year, 3 months, was scored as 2 years).

Table 4. Correlation between and change in C- and R-scale and item scores across first and last assessment times (Swedish forensic psychiatric sample)

HCR-20 scale and item	ICC_1	r	Time 1 M score (SD)	Time 2 M score (SD)	Difference score (SD)	t (p)
C scale						
C1	.71	.71***	1.43 (0.59)	1.36 (0.62)	0.07 (0.46)	1.00 (.323)
C2	.87	.89***	1.19 (0.74)	1.05 (0.76)	0.14 (0.35)	2.61 (.012)
C3	.76	.77***	0.45 (0.63)	0.48 (0.71)	0.03 (0.47)	−0.33 (0.74)
C4	.67	.66***	0.67 (0.61)	0.69 (0.64)	0.02 (0.52)	−0.30 (0.77)
C5	.60	.60***	1.10 (0.76)	0.98 (0.81)	0.12 (0.71)	1.10 (0.28)
Total	.83	.83***	4.83 (2.29)	4.55 (2.55)	0.29 (1.47)	1.26 (.215)
R scale (in)						
R1	.73	.79***	1.00 (0.71)	0.71 (0.72)	0.29 (0.46)	2.83 (0.01)
R2	.61	.61***	0.67 (0.48)	0.57 (0.51)	0.10 (.044)	1.00 (0.33)
R3	.80	.79***	1.38 (.074)	1.33 (0.80)	0.05 (0.50)	0.44 (0.67)
R4	.37	.49***	1.38 (0.67)	0.95 (0.67)	0.43 (0.68)	2.91 (0.01)
R5	.02	.00	1.00 (0.45)	0.95 (0.50)	0.05 (0.67)	0.33 (0.75)
Total	.63	.69***	5.43 (1.99)	4.52 (2.18)	0.90 (1.64)	2.53 (.020)
R scale (out)						
R1	.72	.71***	0.96 (0.77)	1.00 (0.80)	0.04 (0.60)	−0.33 (0.75)
R2	.78	.79***	1.35 (0.49)	1.31 (0.55)	0.04 (0.34)	0.57 (0.75)
R3	.53	.52***	1.00 (0.80)	0.96 (0.77)	0.04 (0.77)	0.57 (0.55)
R4	.78	.77***	0.77 (0.76)	0.80 (0.80)	0.03 (0.53)	0.25 (0.80)
R5	.70	.70***	1.19 (0.75)	1.19 (0.69)	0.00 (0.57)	−0.37 (0.71)
Total	.77	.76***	5.27 (3.01)	5.27 (3.11)	0.00 (2.14)	0.00 (1.00)

Notes: Partial correlation holds time constant. *** $= p \leq .001$

The data are portrayed in Table 4 in a format similar to that used for the other samples. As can be seen, there is less change in scores than found with the other samples. Analysis of the Pearson correlations and ICCs shows that, overall, the relationship between total scale scores at the different assessment times was very strong (*range* = 0.63 to 0.83). It is apparent that in this sample there was no significant reduction over time in size of total C-scale score. Only one item, C2 (negative attitudes), yielded an effect. Such knowledge could be useful to clinicians at the site. The programme appears successful in reducing negative attitudes but shows less effectiveness in other spheres. Although it could well be that the C variables are too broadly conceived to detect precise changes in attitudes and behaviour, it could also be that the negative result should be taken seriously and that some aspects of the programme deserve review or carefully contrived alteration. The point is that even simple data of the kind shown in Table 4 can help clinicians, researchers, and administrators in thinking as a group about programme planning and intervention. Even a relatively crude score, such as is obtainable from the C scale of the HCR-20, can help invigorate planning.

The R-scale data presented in Table 4 require some additional description. The R variables in the HCR-20 can be scored as if the individual is expected to be retained in the institution for the foreseeable future (In) or as if he or she is about to be released to the community (Out). Assessors sometimes provide both types of rating. It can be seen that the Swedish assessors discerned some positive change when they reacted on the basis of continued detention but not when they assumed fairly imminent release. Since all of the individuals in the sample had committed serious violent offences, and since for many of them release was an unlikely option, it is perhaps not surprising that change in R scores could not be detected when some form of conditional release was offered as the criterion.

Two further comments about the lack of change in the C scale, in Research Study 3, are warranted. One is that, as noted, the Sundsvall sample was a selective high-risk group. The other stems from the characteristics of the sample. In Canada patients are often very acutely psychotic upon admission to forensic and civil psychiatric institutions. However, due to differences in legal structure between Sweden and Canada, comparable persons admitted to forensic institutions in Sweden would likely have been routed through the criminal justice system in Canada. Although some 40% of patients in this sample were psychotic, close to half were personality disordered. It may be expected, then, that the Swedish forensic psychiatric sample is less acutely mentally ill than the Canadian samples. As such, the R-scale items may be prone to change more in this sample than the C-scale items. Yet it may simply be that the C scale in this sample is not picking up clinical factors that are targeted for intervention among this group of patients. What is clear from this and other samples in Sweden, however, is that the C and R scales do distinguish between patients and prisoners who are and are not violent (Belfrage, Fransson, & Strand, 1999; Douglas, Ogloff, et al., 1999, for R scale; Strand et al., 1999). This implies that treatment strategies may benefit from targeting C-and-R-scale sorts of constructs.

At a more general level, the present data are useful in illustrating a point which, though obvious, is often overlooked. Whereas researchers can usually define time frames as they design and conduct studies (or can impose them on data already collected), clinicians have to make projections over widely different periods. The factors that influence the prediction of violence on the psychiatric ward over minutes or seconds is a topic that is little examined (though see Rice et al., 1989) and in urgent need of exploration, because C-scale type variables may have little or no pertinence to this issue. The C-scale variables do seem to have some power for predicting over days or weeks under such reasonably controlled circumstances as those of an inpatient ward. Similarly, R-scale type variables would appear helpful in forecasting community violence (and in planning successful integration).

Part of the process of violence risk assessment involves planning treatment strategies. Effective treatment takes advantage of dynamic violence risk factors, because they give some hope of change. The logic, and a premise of the HCR-20, is that if there are variables which relate to violence, and these can be changed, perhaps there will be an ameliorative effect on risk. For the three samples described above, there generally was a drop in scores across assessment or rating times. This was particularly so for two of the samples, with the third sample showing a significant drop for the R scale only. It would seem that attitudes and behaviours covered

by the 10 dynamic violence risk factors contained in the HCR-20 are indeed changeable, and hence logical targets for intervention. Although it was not possible to analyze specified causes of the changes in scores, a reasonable inference is that the
treatment and management in psychiatric and correctional institutions are responsible for change. At the very least, persons are recruited into regular medication regimes, hence many of their C-scale symptoms are stabilized; and social workers
devise release plans, hence the risk associated with R-scale variables is reduced. Our
hope is that greater reduction of these HCR-20 scores can be obtained through focused targeting of the scale's 10 dynamic factors.

The Next Steps

If the HCR-20 is to have any eventual, deservedly wide, influence in the practicali-
ties of everyday clinical, forensic, and correctional life, its limits will have to be
determined. The same could be said for a device called the Spousal Assault Risk
Assessment guide (SARA; Kropp, Hart, Webster, & Eaves, 1995, 1999), the Sexual
Violence Risk-20 guide (SVR-20; Boer, Hart, Kropp, & Webster, 1998), and the
Early Assessment Risk List for Under 12 Boys (EARL-20B; Augermeri, Webster,
Koegle, & Levene, 1998). They need rigorous evaluation in several settings—mental
health, corrections, forensic, addictions, and so on. To an extent, this is well under-
way (see Douglas & Webster, 1999a; Douglas, Ogloff, et al., 1999). Presumably the
HCR-20 will be found to be more helpful in some decision-making settings than
others. It has also become apparent that validation of instruments takes time and
that, to be convincing, they need to be authenticated by different researchers in different contexts. Related to this point is the one made above concerning attributional
bias: Since the eventual goal of most treatment and intervention programmes is the
release of patients and prisoners to the usual world, it is imperative that norms be
established in the pertinent communities.

Much more needs to be learned about how best to incorporate guides like the
HCR-20 into practice (see Belfrage, 1998). In our experience, it takes much determination, care, and patience to draw a basic guide such as the HCR-20 into routine
clinical practice and, importantly, routine research practice. This is a topic of serious
scientific interest and one that deserves close attention over the next few years. The
matter of routine research practice is important for several simple reasons: (1) clinicians are often much better placed than researchers to collect standard follow-up
data; (2) clinicians are often well situated to appreciate the clinical significance of
follow-up data once they are obtained; and (3) properly organized research-inspired
data can help clinicians see the "trajectories" of their individual patients, make the
necessary adjustments, and plan the required interventions (Greenland, 1985).

Standards for training must be established and maintained. Although the path is
not yet clear in this direction, it may pay to note that the predictive success of the
Hare PCL-R very likely depends on whether those who use it are trained in its application. Hare (1998) has wisely been insistent on this matter. At some point relatively
soon this must be addressed. It is hard to see how the present HCR-20 could, or

should, survive without assurance that its application across jurisdictions is supported scientifically.

If the HCR-20 has caught the attention of an appreciable number of clinicians and researchers in different jurisdictions in various parts of the world (Canada, Sweden, the US, Germany, Britain), as it appears to have done, the development of some kind of intervention-oriented guide seems urgently necessary. Such a guide might help alert the attention of clinicians and correctional professionals to concrete possibilities with respect to violence reduction. It is perhaps not sufficient to publish a guide outlining risk factors. What is needed is some kind of "approachable" text which users would find helpful as they struggle to reduce risk of violence (and which would, more broadly, help people to cope with mental and personality disorders). Such a guide is in fact in draft form (see Douglas, Webster, Eaves, Hart, & Ogloff, 2000). The idea is to expound material relevant to each of the five C items and five R items. In constructing this document, variously conceived as an aide-mémoire, companion guide, and supplement, the editors are being careful to include ideas from the fields of corrections, addictions, and developmental criminology.

The fact that the R items have definite connections to situational variables, and oblige the assessor to think contextually, should not take away from the idea that there will now likely be an advantage in developing an HCR-20 type of instrument that is based on situations rather than individuals (see, e.g., Shumow, Vandell, & Posner, 1998, who stress the importance of neighbourhood characteristics). That is, there ought to be some way of encouraging thinking about how different settings, such as schools, religious orders, the military, airports, prisons, and so on, have the capacity to elicit violence. Obviously, in the light of enormous variability across contexts, this will not be easy to do. Yet such a task merits consideration. It is surely necessary to isolate and attend to "toxic" settings—custodial, educational, and others (e.g., Garbarino, 1999).

Even if the HCR-20, or a future version of it, does achieve a fairly standard place in the clinical and research armamentarium, it may well be that some kind of auxiliary version will be needed to deal with front-line decision-making and recording. The findings and views of practitioners who are in daily contact with patients, prisoners, parolees, and others enter the record in great volume. There is very likely considerable over-recording of incidents, and yet, when examined closely, those entries often offer information that is vague and even unduly attributional. The sheer amount of recorded material often stands in the way of obtaining data which would assist in decision-making at the level of the interdisciplinary team. The HCR-20 vocabulary would seem to be in need of some extension or reworking at this level. It will, of course, be important to ensure that the concepts connect well and that there is minimal slippage from one form of use to the other.

More effort needs to be made to include the views of persons who have experienced mental and personality disorder. To date, the attempt to establish risk assessment devices appears to have focused on forming alliances between clinicians and researchers. It now seems important to refine these guides in light of the opinions formed by persons who have at some time been subject to these kinds of assessment. One advantage of stipulating factors and defining them in manuals like the HCR-20 is that individuals under assessment can, if they wish, gain a clear appreciation of what conduct is required of them if they are to obtain privileges, releases, discharges, and the like. This "transparency" (Baker, 1993) should help set the stage for educational and training programmes (see Bellack, Mueser, Gingerick, & Agresta, 1997).

If attitudinal and behavioural changes are indeed to be captured in the course of day-to-day life in institutions and community agencies, much more attention will have to be devoted to the measurement of those changes. This may be accomplished in part through the use of the conventional T1 to T2 approach noted above. But new data-gathering systems will have to be developed as well. Conceivably, these might entail approaches as yet only partially envisioned (e.g., Marks-Tarlow, 1993), but it could be that researchers and clinicians concerned principally with risk management will benefit from a reconsideration of long-available and well-understood single-subject designs (e.g., Webster et al., 1978). An excellent recent extension of such an approach is offered by Nishith, Hearst, Mueser, and Foa (1995). These authors used a technique based on classical test theory as explained by Yarnold (1988). The advantage of such an approach is evident: It permits focus on the individual case at hand while allowing statistical confirmation of effects which may or may not be evident "by eye." This kind of measurement precision can show how treatment programmes or other interventions might benefit some patients but not others (Mueser, Yarnold, & Foy, 1991). This type of individual-statistical design can, of course, be applied to pharmacological, cognitive-behavioural, or other approaches. The question "What works?" (Martinson, 1974) is now, perhaps, altogether too general. Of interest for the future is the question "What works for which individual patients and how can change be demonstrated unambiguously?" Gaining facility with Yarnold-type or similar approaches would seem an important next step. Unless care is taken, too much attention will be focused on "front end" assessment considerations (as with VRAGs, HCR-20s, and the like) without a parallel focus on "back end' intervention applications and analysis. It is now vital that we find ways not only of attenuating violence in individual patients and mentally and personality-disordered prisoners but also of devising and applying the means of measurement. Review boards, courts, and tribunals rely heavily on mental health professional opinion as they make their decisions. One way of assisting them is to use research-based clinical trials conducted at the level of the individual. Without such an effort, it can only be assumed that the size of the forensic population will continue to grow in a more-or-less uncontrolled fashion.

The foregoing discussion raises another point. In the core of this chapter we pointed to the seeming power of the C and R variables of the HCR-20 to demonstrate change from T1 to T2. Yet it must be noted that although care has been taken in defining these 10 variables, the content of the items is in fact quite broad. Each of the items could undoubtedly be made more precise through the inclusion of any number of readily available, well-researched, properly standardized instruments.

Throughout this chapter the emphasis has been on adults suffering from mental and personality disorder and drug and alcohol dependence. We have tried to make the point that over the past 2 decades much has been learned on the assessment front (e.g., Litwack & Schlesinger, in press) and on the treatment front (e.g., Stoff et al., 1997). As for application to forensic psychiatric patients, and probably psychiatric patients in general, the advances have perhaps been greater in assessment than in intervention. Yet despite the obvious importance of the topic, and despite the recent publication of abundant high-quality longitudinal studies (see Day, 1998; also, generally, Loeber & Farrington, 1998a), the literature on assessment and intervention with children and adolescents appears to lag (though the present state of affairs is admirably summarized by Kazdin, 1997; Loeber & Farrington, 1998b; and Rutter, Giller, & Hagell, 1998). This is an area which invites much effort and innovation.

Summary

The importance of relatively static, more-or-less demographic predictors of violence in mentally and personality disordered adults has become increasingly apparent over the past 2 decades. This has come about mainly because of studies which have followed large cohorts over appreciable periods of time. We view such prediction as an important topic but emphasize the processes entailed in risk management, arguing that insufficient attention has been paid to the problem of how biases and even moral judgements are transmitted during routine assessments. The point is that "dangerousness" and "risk" are, at least under some circumstances, more-or-less ascribed or attributed on the basis of characteristics with no known relevance to aggression and violence. One partial solution is "guided clinical decision-making." The HCR-20 system, involving 10 defined static and 10 defined dynamic variables, is offered by way of example. Recent information bearing on conventional reliability and validity support this approach. The current clinical (C) and future risk (R) variables not only have some predictive power beyond that supplied by the historical (H) variables, but can be used to index change over time.

The measurement of attitudinal and behavioural change, during treatment or as a result of planned intervention, is a major challenge for mental health professionals. Unless positive changes are detected, individuals are obliged to live under conditions of undue restrictions (and, by the same token, unless negative changes are discernible, members of society are placed at unnecessary risk). There is a need for intervention programmes that are based on individual cases (with statistical verification where necessary and appropriate). In the most general terms, we need assessment and treatment that place roughly equal weight on the normative, group-statistical approach and the ideographic, conventionally clinical point of view. The time-honoured actuarial versus clinical distinction can be distracting in the sense that future work in this area will surely demand tight integration of both approaches.

References

American Psychiatric Association. (1994). *Diagnostic and statistical manual of mental disorders, 4th Ed. (DSM-IV)*. Washington: Author.

Augermeri, L., Webster, C.D., Koegle, C., & Levene, K. (1998). *The early assessment of risk list for boys' (EARL-20B), Version 1, Consultation Edition*. Toronto: Earlscourt Child and Family Centre.

Baker, E. (1993). Dangerousness, rights, and criminal justice. *Modern Law Review, 56,* 528–547.

Belfrage, H. (1998). Implementing the HCR-20 scheme for risk assessment in a forensic psychiatric hospital: Integrating research and clinical practice. *Journal of Forensic Psychiatry, 9,* 328–338.

Belfrage, H., Fransson, G., & Strand, S. (1999). *Prediction of violence within the correctional system using the HCR-20 risk assessment scheme.* Manuscript under review.

Bellack, A.S., Mueser, K.T., Gingerick, S., & Agresta, J. (1997). *Social skills training for schizophrenia: A step-by-step guide.* New York: Guilford.

Bem, D., & Allen, A. (1974). On predicting some of the people some of the time: The search for cross-situational consistencies in behaviors. *Psychological Review, 81,* 506–520.

Boer, D.P., Hart, S.D., Kropp, P.R., & Webster, C.D. (1998). *The SVR-20 manual.* Vancouver: Family Violence Institute.

Borum, R. (1996). Improving the clinical practice of violence risk assessment: Technology, guidelines, and training. *American Psychologist, 51,* 945–956.

Day, D.M. (1998). Risk for court contact and predictors of an early age for a first court contact among a sample of high risk youths: A survival analysis approach. *Canadian Journal of Criminology, 40,* 421–443.

Dietz, P.E. (1985). Hypothetical criteria for the prediction of individual criminality. In C.D. Webster, M.H. Ben-Aron, & S.J. Hucker (Eds.), *Dangerousness: Probability and prediction, psychiatry and public policy* (pp. 87–102). New York: Cambridge University Press.

Douglas, K.S., Cox, N.D., & Webster, C.D. (1999). Empirically validated violence risk assessment. *Legal and Criminological Psychology, 4,* 149–184.

Douglas, K.S., Hart, S.D., Webster, C.D., & Eaves, D. (1998). *HCR-20 violence risk assessment scheme: Psychometric properties in a sample of forensic patients.* Manuscript under review.

Douglas, K.S., Ogloff, J.R.P., Nicholls, T.L., & Grant, I. (1999). Assessing risk for violence among psychiatric patients: The HCR-20 violence risk assessment scheme and the psychopathy checklist: Screening version. *Journal of Consulting and Clinical Psychology, 17,* 917–930.

Douglas, K.S., & Webster, C.D. (1999a). The HCR-20 violence risk assessment scheme: Concurrent validity in a sample of incarcerated offenders. *Criminal Justice and Behavior, 26,* 3–19.

Douglas, K.S., & Webster, C.D. (1999b). Predicting violence in mentally and personality disordered individuals. In R. Roesch, S.D. Hart, & J.R.P. Ogloff (Eds.), *Psychology and law: The state of the discipline* (pp. 175–239). New York: Kluwer/Plenum.

Douglas, K.S., Webster, C.D., Eaves, D., Hart, S.D., & Ogloff, J.R.P. (2000). *Risk management: A companion guide to the HCR-20.* Manuscript in preparation.

Eisenman, R. (1987). Sexual acting out: Diagnostic category or moral judgment? *Bulletin of the Psychonomic Society, 25,* 387–388.

Esses, V.M., & Webster, C.D. (1988). Physical attractiveness, dangerousness, and the Canadian Criminal Code. *Journal of Applied Social Psychology, 18,* 1017–1031.

Garbarino, J. (1999). *Lost boys: Why our sons turn violent and how we can save them.* New York: Free Press.

Greenland, C. (1985). Dangerousness, mental disorder, and politics. In C.D. Webster, M.H. Ben-Aron, & S.J. Hucker (Eds.), *Dangerousness: Probability and prediction, psychiatry and public policy* (pp. 25–40). New York: Cambridge University Press.

Hare, R.D. (1991). *Manual for the Hare Psychopathy Checklist—Revised.* Toronto: Multi-Health Systems.

Hare, R.D. (1998). The Hare PCL-R: Some issues concerning its use and misuse. *Legal and Criminological Psychology, 3,* 99–119.

Harris, G.T., & Rice, M.E. (1997). Mentally disordered offenders: What research says about effective service. In C.D. Webster & M.A. Jackson (Eds.), *Impulsivity: Theory, assessment and treatment* (pp. 361–393). New York: Guilford.

Heilbrun, K. (1997). Prediction versus management models relevant to risk assessment: The importance of legal decision-making context. *Law and Human Behavior, 21,* 347–359.

Hollingshead, A.B., & Redlich, F.C. (1958). *Social class and mental illness.* New York: Wiley.

Kazdin, A.E. (1997). A model for developing effective treatments: Progression and interplay of theory, research and practice. *Journal of Clinical Child Psychology, 26,* 114–129.

Konechni, V., Mulcahy, E., & Ebbensen, E. (1980). Prison or mental hospital: Factors affecting the processing of persons suspected of being "mentally disordered offenders." In P. Lipsitt & B. Sales (Eds.), *New directions in psychological research* (pp. 87–124). New York: Van Nostrand Reinhold.

Krause, M.S., Howard, K.I., & Lutz, W. (1998). Exploring individual change. *Journal of Consulting and Clinical Psychology, 66,* 838–845.

Kropp, P.R., Hart, S.D., Webster, C.D., & Eaves, D. (1995). *Manual for the Spousal Assault Risk Assessment Guide, 2nd Ed.* Vancouver: British Columbia Institute on Family Violence.

Kropp, P.R., Hart, S.D., Webster, C.D., & Eaves, D. (1999). *Manual for the Spousal Assault Risk Assessment Guide, 3rd Ed.* Toronto: Multi-Health Systems.

Link, B.G., Andrews, H., & Cullen, F.T. (1992). The violent and illegal behavior of mental patients reconsidered. *American Sociological Review, 57,* 275–292.

Litwack, T.R., & Schlesinger, L.B. (in press). Dangerousness risk assessments: Research findings, legal considerations, and clinical guidelines. In I. Weiner & A. Hess (Eds.), *Handbook of forensic psychology, 2nd Ed.* New York: Wiley.

Loeber, R., & Farrington, D.P. (Eds.). (1998a). *Serious and violent juvenile offenders: Risk factors and successful interventions.* Thousand Oaks, CA: Sage.

Loeber, R., & Farrington, D.P. (1998b). Never too early, never too late: Risk factors and successful interventions for serious and juvenile offenders. *Studies on Crime and Crime Prevention, 7,* 7–30 (National Council for Crime Prevention).

Marks-Tarlow, T. (1993). A new look at impulsivity: Hidden order beneath apparent chaos? In W.G. McCown, J.L. Johnson, & M.B. Shure (Eds.), *The impulsive client: Theory, research and treatment* (pp. 119–138). Washington: American Psychological Association.

Martinson, R. (1974). What works? Questions and answers about prison reform. *Public Interest, 35,* 22–54.

Mathiesen, T. (1998). Selective incapacitation revisited. *Law and Human Behavior, 22,* 453–467.

Medawar, P.B. (1967). *The art of the soluble.* London: Methuen.

Megargee, E.I. (1976). The prediction of dangerous behavior. *Criminal Justice and Behavior, 3,* 3–22.

Menzies, R.J. (1989). *Survival of the sanest: Order and disorder in a pretrial psychiatric clinic.* Toronto: University of Toronto Press.

Menzies, R.J., & Webster, C.D. (1995). Construction and validation of risk assessments in a six-year follow-up of forensic patients: A tridimensional analysis. *Journal of Consulting and Clinical Psychology, 63,* 766–778.

Menzies, R.J., Webster, C.D., & Sepejak, D.S. (1985a). The dimensions of dangerousness: Evaluating the accuracy of psychometric predictions of violence among forensic patients. *Law and Human Behavior, 9,* 35–36.

Menzies, R.J., Webster, C.D., & Sepejak, D.S. (1985b). Hitting the forensic sound barrier: Predictions of dangerousness in a pre-trial psychiatric clinic. In C.D. Webster, M.H. Ben-Aron, & S.J. Hucker (Eds.), *Dangerousness: Probability and prediction, psychiatry and public policy* (pp. 115–143). New York: Cambridge University Press.

Merton, R.K. (1934). The unanticipated consequences of purposive social action. *American Sociological Review, 1,* 894–904.

Mischel, W. (1968). *Personality and assessment.* New York: Wiley.

Monahan, J. (1981). *Predicting violent behavior: An assessment of clinical techniques.* Beverly Hills, CA: Sage.

Monahan, J. (1992). Mental disorder and violent behavior. *American Psychologist, 47,* 511–521.

Monahan, J., & Steadman, H.J. (Eds.). (1994). *Violence and mental disorder: Developments in risk assessment.* Chicago: University of Chicago Press.

Moore, M.H., Estrich, S.R., McGillis, D., & Spelman, W. (1984). *Dangerous offenders: The elusive target of justice.* Cambridge, MA: Harvard University Press.

Mueser, K.T., Yarnold, P.R., & Foy, D.W. (1991). Statistical analysis for single-case designs: Evaluating outcome of chronic PTSD. *Behavior Modification, 15,* 134–155.

Mulvey, E.P., & Lidz, C.W. (1995). Conditional prediction: A model for research on dangerousness to others in a new era. *International Journal of Law and Psychiatry, 18,* 129–143.

Nishith, P., Hearst, D.E., Mueser, K.T., & Foa, E.B. (1995). PTSD and major depression: Methodological and treatment considerations in a single case design. *Behavior Therapy, 26,* 319–335.

Patterson, G.R. (1979). *Living with children.* Champaign, IL: Research Press.

Pavkov, T.W., Lewis, D.A., & Lyons, J.S. (1989). Psychiatric diagnoses and racial bias: An empirical investigation. *Professional Psychology: Research and Practice, 20,* 364–368.

Petrunic, M. (1982). The politics of dangerousness. *International Journal of Law and Psychiatry, 5,* 225–253.

Pfohl, S.J. (1978). *Predicting dangerousness: The social construction of psychiatric reality.* Lexington, MA: Lexington Books.

Polvi, N. (1999). *Predicting violence: Actuarial and clinical considerations.* Unpublished doctoral dissertation, Simon Fraser University, Vancouver, British Columbia.

Quinsey, V.L., & Ambtman, R. (1979). Variables affecting psychiatrists' and teachers' assessments of mentally ill offenders. *Journal of Consulting and Clinical Psychology, 47,* 353–362.

Quinsey, V.L., Coleman, G., Jones, B., & Altrow, I. (1997). Proximal antecedents of eloping and reoffending among mentally disordered offenders. *Journal of Interpersonal Violence, 12,* 794–813.

Quinsey, V.L., Harris, G.T., Rice, M.E., & Cormier, C.A. (1998). *Violent offenders: Appraising and managing risk.* Washington: American Psychological Association.

Rice, M.E., Harris, G.T., Quinsey, V.L., & Cyr, M. (1990). Planning treatment programs in secure psychiatric facilities. In D. Weisstub (Ed.), *Law and mental health: International perspectives* (pp. 162–230). New York: Pergamon.

Rice, M.E., Harris, G.T., Varney, G.W., & Quinsey, V.L. (1989). *Violence in institutions: Understanding, prevention and control.* Toronto: Hans Huber.

Rosenfield, S. (1984). Race differences in involuntary hospitalization: Psychiatric versus labeling perspectives. *Journal of Health and Social Behavior, 25,* 14–23.

Ross, D.J., Hart, S.D., & Webster, C.D. (1998). *Aggression in psychiatric patients: Using the HCR-20 to assess risk for violence in hospital and in the community.* Unpublished manuscript.

Rutter, M., Giller, H., & Hagell, A. (1998). *Antisocial behavior by young people.* New York: Cambridge University Press.

Shah, S.A. (1978). Dangerousness: A paradigm for exploring some issues in law and psychology. *American Psychologist, 33,* 224–238.

Shumow, L., Vandell, D.L., & Posner, J. (1998). Perceptions of danger: A psychological mediator of neighborhood demographic characters. *American Journal of Orthopsychiatry, 68,* 468–478.

Spaniol, L., Gagne, C., & Koehler, M. (Eds.). (1997). *Psychological and social aspects of psychiatric disability.* Boston: Center for Psychiatric Rehabilitation, Boston University.

Steadman, H.J., Silver, E., Monahan, J., Applebaum, P.S., Robbins, P.C., Mulvey, E.P., Grisso, T., Roth, L., & Banks, S. (in press). A classification tree approach to the development of actuarial violence risk assessment tools. *Law and Human Behavior.*

Stoff, D.M., Breiling, J., & Maser, J.D. (Eds.). (1997). *Handbook of antisocial behavior.* New York: Wiley.

Strand, S., Belfrage, H., Fransson, G., & Levander, S. (1999). Clinical and risk management factors in risk prediction of mentally disordered offenders—more important than historical data? A retrospective study of 40 mentally disordered offenders assessed with the HCR-20 violence risk assessment scheme. *Legal and Criminological Psychology, 4,* 67–76.

Webster, C.D. (1998). Comment on Mathiesen. *Law and Human Behavior, 22,* 471–476.

Webster, C.D., & Cox, D.N. (1997). Integration of nomothetic and ideographic positions in risk assessment: Implications for practice and the education of psychologists and other mental health professionals. *American Psychologist, 52,* 1245–1246.

Webster, C.D., Douglas, K.S., Eaves, D., & Hart, S.D. (1997). *The HCR-20: Assessing risk for violence, Version 2.* Vancouver: Mental Health, Law and Policy Institute, Simon Fraser University.

Webster, C.D., Eaves, D., Douglas, K.S., & Wintrup, A. (1995). *The HCR-20 scheme: The assessment of dangerousness and risk.* Vancouver: Simon Fraser University and Forensic Psychiatric Services Commission of British Columbia.

Webster, C.D., Hucker, S.J., & Grossman, M.G. (1993). Clinical programmes for mentally ill offenders. In K. Howells & C.R. Hollier (Eds.), *Clinical approaches to the mentally disordered offender* (pp. 87–109). Chichester: Wiley.

Webster, C.D., Somjen, L., Sloman, L., Bradley, S., Mooney, S., & Mack, J. (1978). The child care worker in the family: Some case examples and implications for the design of family-centered programs. *Child Care Quarterly, 8,* 5–18.

Whittemore, K.E. (1999). *Releasing the mentally disordered offender: Disposition decisions for individuals found unfit to stand trial and not criminally responsible.* Unpublished manuscript.

Yarnold, P.R. (1988). Classical test theory methods for repeated measures $N = 1$ research designs. *Educational and Psychological Measurement, 48,* 913–919.

Christopher D. Webster is Professor of Criminology and Psychiatry, University of Toronto, Ontario, Canada, Professor Emeritus of Psychology, Simon Fraser University, Vancouver, British Columbia, Canada, and Senior Research Consultant, Earlscourt Child and Family Centre, Toronto. Kevin S. Douglas is associated with the Department of Psychology, Simon Fraser University, Vancouver, British Colum-

bia, Canada. Henrik Belfrage is associated with the Forensic Psychiatric Centre, Research Unit, Växjö, Sweden, and the Karolinska Institute, Stockholm, Sweden. Bruce G. Link is associated with the Columbia School of Public Health, New York, New York, USA.

Authors' Note

Comments or queries may be directed to Christopher D. Webster, Centre of Criminology, University of Toronto, 8th Floor, Robarts Library, 130 St. George Street, Toronto ON M6J 1H4 Canada. Telephone: 416 532-8817. Fax: 416 532-5041. E-mail: <pdmac@ibm.net>.

TREATMENT IMPLICATIONS OF THE ANTECEDENTS OF CRIMINALITY AND VIOLENCE IN SCHIZOPHRENIA AND MAJOR AFFECTIVE DISORDERS

JOSEPH D. BLOOM
KIM T. MUESER
RÜDIGER MÜLLER-ISBERNER

Introduction

MEDICATING THE MENTALLY ILL

Since last January, when Kendra Webdale was pushed in front of a Manhattan subway train by a man with a history of mental problems, politicians in Albany have been debating whether to make it easier to force people with mental illness to take their medication. Andrew Goldstein, the man accused of shoving Ms. Webdale to her death, had been repeatedly hospitalized for schizophrenia, but seemed to have a pattern of dropping out of his treatment programs and neglecting to take his medicine.

Now, Attorney General Eliot Spitzer has proposed legislation that would make it possible for courts to order some of the mentally ill to follow their outpatient treatment programs or face institutionalization. Proposing a new law in the wake of a widely publicized tragedy is such a knee-jerk reaction for politicians that Mr. Spitzer's bill deserves special scrutiny. But the idea has real merit.

The bill would apply only to people who have been hospitalized due to a failure to follow a treatment program. When such patients are released, hospitals or care givers could apply to the court for a special order requiring that they take their medication and follow their outpatient program. Petitioners would have to demonstrate that the patients' history showed a particular danger that they would fail to take care of themselves, and that their conditions were serious enough to justify court supervision. If patients ignored an order and failed to take medication, care givers could ask that they be recommitted to the hospital for re-evaluation.

Civil libertarians worry that such a law could be used to force medication or commitment on someone with borderline mental problems. Mr. Spitzer and the Legislature must be sensitive to those concerns. But they must also

S. Hodgins (ed.), Violence among the Mentally Ill, 145–169.
© 2000 *Kluwer Academic Publishers. Printed in the Netherlands.*

listen to families of the mentally ill who too often see their loved ones' refusal to take medication lead to recurrent psychotic symptoms. The result of that sort of tailspin is seldom the kind of violence that led to the Webdale tragedy. But it almost always takes a terrible toll on the patient, the family and the community. That was just the pattern described last week by the parents of a man shot while brandishing a sword on a commuter train. He had been repeatedly treated for mental problems but failed to follow through on his outpatient care. If the Legislature can make it easier to avoid these crises, it should act promptly. ("Medicating," 1999)

This editorial appeared in one of the most prestigious newspapers in the United States following a shocking incident of unprovoked violence committed by an individual reported to be suffering from chronic schizophrenia. This is just one in a series of reports and editorials that have appeared in US newspapers over the last decade chronicling such events. The editorial links an often repeated situation: A chronic schizophrenic person with frequent hospitalizations and poor compliance with community treatment, particularly in the area of medication, commits an irrational act of violence. As stated in the editorial, a potential legal solution to this problem is legislation in the form of an outpatient commitment statute requiring medication compliance.

The editorial sets the stage for this paper to examine what we believe are the proximal and distal factors of criminality and violence among persons suffering from severe mental illness, schizophrenia, and bipolar disorder. Once the factors are defined, the paper will examine their treatment implications and suggest treatment approaches.

The Proximal and Distal Antecedents of Criminality and Violence

PROXIMAL ANTECEDENTS

In this section we will focus on mental illness modified by comorbid conditions and mental status factors that appear to form a pattern of factors associated with criminality and violence. A symptomatic schizophrenic person with a history of substance abuse and/or antisocial personality disorder, complicated by an under-appreciation of the fact that he or she may be ill, is the person most likely to engage in a violent act or to become a candidate for entry into the criminal justice system.

SCHIZOPHRENIA OR MAJOR AFFECTIVE DISORDER—UNTREATED OR UNDER-TREATED

A middle-aged, single, homeless male lived among abandoned vehicles in the industrial area of a large western US city. He came to a homeless shelter for the first time in years following acute medical care and the surgeon's recommendations that he be monitored for several days while he took antibiotics. During lunch on the second day, he stood up, picked up a meat cleaver, walked across the room, and attacked and killed another resident. He said he did this because the man was smacking his lips—a signal from the "aliens" that they wanted to turn him into a homosexual. He said he did this deliberately. He was found to be profoundly mentally ill, suffering from chronic paranoid schizophrenia. He had received no treatment in years.

We focus on acute or chronic illness, untreated or under-treated, as the critical factor linking the patient population suffering from these conditions to many negative social outcomes, including violence, various types of criminality (Lindqvist & Allebeck, 1990b) and other forms of morbidity and increased mortality.

Unfortunately the case presented is somewhat typical of a subgroup of homeless schizophrenic individuals. A person who has not had psychiatric treatment for years becomes involved in an extremely irrational and violent criminal act. Researchers have now examined the relationship of acute and chronic illness to criminality and violence (Hodgins, Mednick, Brennan, Schulsinger, & Engberg, 1996). Taylor (1993) examined a cohort of violent and non-violent prisoners, some suffering from schizophrenia, and found an association in the schizophrenic group between psychotic symptomatology and violence.

Another way of looking at the effects of acute illness on violence relates to hospital admission. Studies in this area have made a link between severe mental illness and violence that occurs immediately preceding or shortly following admission (Beck, White, & Gage, 1991; McNiel, Binder, & Greenfield, 1988). In contrast, violence that occurs after discharge, when, presumably, the acute illness has been treated, has been linked more to personality disorder (Tardiff, Marzuk, Leon, & Portera, 1997).

Investigators are now looking at possible links between specific symptoms or symptom clusters in relation to delusions (Tardiff, 1989; Taylor et al., 1994), hallucinations in general (McNiel, 1994), and command hallucinations in particular. Link and Stueve (1994) define the "principle of rationality-within-irrationality" as a subgroup of psychotic symptomatology derived from Dohrenwend, Shrout, Egri, and Mendelsohn (1980).

Comorbid conditions

This is a critical component in understanding the relationship among mental illness, criminality, and violence. Two conditions, substance abuse and antisocial personality, have been linked to criminality and violence in individuals suffering from schizophrenia and bipolar disorder.

Substance abuse. Substance abuse is common in schizophrenia, with 10 to 70% comorbidity, depending upon criteria and the group studied (Mueser et al., 1990). The Epidemiologic Catchment Area study found that 47% of all individuals with a lifetime diagnosis of schizophrenia met criteria for some form of substance abuse or dependence (Regier et al., 1990). Studies now also clearly link schizophrenia and violence to alcoholism and/or substance abuse (Abram & Teplin, 1991; Cuffel, Shumway, Chouljian, & MacDonald, 1994; Drake, Bartels, Teague, Noordsy, & Clark, 1993; Drake, Mueser, Clark, & Wallach, 1996; Lindqvist & Allebeck, 1990a). Borum, Swanson, Swartz, and Hiday (1997) examined the relationship between medication compliance and arrest in a sample of severely ill individuals. They found that substance abuse alone or medication non-compliance alone did not predict violent behaviour but that the two together significantly predicted criminality and/or violent behaviour. Steadman et al. (1998) recently reported on the association among substance abuse, mental illness, and violence.

Antisocial personality disorder. Schizophrenic individuals who are comorbid with antisocial personality disorder or childhood conduct disorder have been found to have, as expected, increased rates of substance abuse, aggression, and legal problems (Mueser et al., 1997). Hodgins (1993) found that criminal activity in individuals with major mental disorders followed two distinct patterns: that committed by those whose criminal history predated the onset of illness; and that committed by those whose criminal history post-dated the onset of symptoms. From a clinical point of view we might speculate that these divergent patterns will segregate according to the presence or absence of comorbid conditions.

Mental status factors

The role of insight.

A civil case was brought by the personal representative of an individual who had been killed in an automobile accident. At the time of the accident the defendant was on conditional release, granted by the Oregon Psychiatric Security Review Board, from the state forensic psychiatric hospital where he had been incarcerated for a criminal offence involving reckless driving. A week prior to the accident concerns had developed about his mental state and he was hospitalized briefly in a community hospital. When the accident took place he was following an ambulance through a traffic signal in order to get to the scene of a previous accident in order to help. (*Cain v. Rijken,* 1985, 1986)

At the time of the accident this man's insight and judgement were severely affected by his schizoaffective disorder. The violence occurred partially as a result of his lack of insight into the fact that he was becoming increasing more ill and his lack of judgement surrounding the use of a motor vehicle, a potentially dangerous instrument.

Mental status factors are a cornerstone of psychiatric assessment, and insight is being increasingly recognized as an important component of the evaluation. Hales and Yudofsky (1999) define insight as the capacity to be aware of and understand that one has a mental problem. Lack of insight is a common feature in psychosis (Amador et al., 1993), schizophrenia (Amador, Flaum, & Andreasen, 1994; Amador, Strauss, Yale, & Gorman, 1991; Dickerson, Boronow, Ringel, & Parente, 1997), and mania (Swanson et al., 1995).

We are just beginning to understand the consequences of lack of insight (Ness & Ende, 1994) and its possible relationship to acute illness, violence, and legal questions. Husted (1999) has reviewed the literature on lack of insight as it pertains to the legal issue of treatment compliance and refusal. Others have focused on treatment refusal and civil commitment (McEvoy, Appelbaum, Apperson, Geller, & Freter, 1989) and other legal questions (Neumann, Walker, Weinstein, & Cutshaw, 1996).

The role of judgement.

A middle-aged man suffering from chronic schizophrenia spent most of his days walking around the urban and suburban areas of a large western US city. Late on a winter day he found himself 15 miles from home and very cold. He went to the nearest house and knocked on the door. No one was home and he broke in. He was arrested several hours later. At the time of his arrest he was in the kitchen making soup. When questioned about his motives he said that he broke into the house because he was cold and hungry.

Hales and Yudofsky (1999) define judgement as "the patient's capacity to make appropriate decisions and appropriately act on them in social situations." Although the offender in this case was taking his medication and was not floridly ill, one of the residual effects of his illness was impaired judgement. This is an important concept and its link to "crime" and violence is under-appreciated.

DISTAL ANTECEDENTS

In this section we will discuss treatment services and mental health law as important distal underpinnings to violence and criminality, and the ways in which factors associated with services and law might increase or decrease a person's chances of being "diverted" into criminal justice systems. The case below illustrates involvement in various aspects of the mental health and criminal justice systems—including the voluntary mental health system, civil commitment, probation, and a successful insanity defence and post-insanity defence commitment—that is typical for young chronic mentally ill patients in the US (Bloom, Williams, & Bigelow, 1992; Torrey, 1995).

More than 10 years ago, a 24-year-old single male was arrested and charged with bank robbery. At the time of his arrest he was living with his parents.

There were no reported problems during his early years, but in high school he began using drugs. Within several months of graduation he began to exhibit behaviour that caused his parents great concern. On two occasions he was seen in hospital emergency rooms because of social withdrawal, reversal of his sleep cycle, rapid mood swings, decrease in personal grooming habits, inability to secure employment, and hallucinatory experiences. The diagnosis was drug-induced psychosis secondary to use of hallucinogens and/or schizophrenia. Outpatient care with neuroleptic medication was instituted for a short period, but it produced no basic change. He was poorly motivated, apathetic, and uncooperative regarding treatment.

Two years later the patient was admitted to a state mental hospital on an emergency civil detention after a family altercation. Although the patient subsequently appeared for a civil commitment hearing, the judge ordered him discharged and he returned home. Several months later he was arrested, convicted of a property crime, and placed on probation (mandatory supervi-sion in the community). He complied poorly with the conditions of his pro-bation and the court held a hearing to review his probationary status. During the hearing he acted in a bizarre manner and the judge ordered an outpatient psychiatric evaluation. The evaluating psychiatrist found the patient to be hallucinating and unresponsive and recommended hospitalization. The judge ordered the patient hospitalized in a treatment unit for mentally disordered offenders at a state mental hospital. The patient was placed on neuroleptic medication and his response was rapid and positive.

Following the patient's discharge from hospital, the court modified the conditions of his probation to require mental health treatment and referred him to a local community mental health programme. Since he was resistant to treatment, he had to be maintained on intramuscular neuroleptic medica-tion for a year. Subsequently he refused his medication altogether. His men-tal condition deteriorated rapidly and 3 months later he was arrested for bank robbery.

In the week prior to the offence he was very disorganized. His descrip-tion of the robbery was vague and disconnected. He said he was riding a bus around the city when the bus passed a bank. He heard a voice that said, "Rob the bank." He got off the bus, went into the bank, and asked a teller for money, which the teller gave to him. He was unarmed at the time. He took the money and set off for his home. On the way home he placed the money in a postal box. Soon after he arrived home, he was arrested.

Mental status examination conducted as part of the court-ordered evalua-tion revealed a tall, dishevelled young man who related poorly during the interview. He showed a paucity of speech, long periods of silence, and dis-connected thought patterns and associations. At times he appeared to be hal-lucinating. His mood changed rapidly during the interview—from menacing, to fearful, to one of inappropriate hilarity. The examining psychiatrist diag-nosed him as having chronic undifferentiated schizophrenia and concluded that he met the criteria for an insanity defence because the severity of his mental illness significantly influenced his ability to appreciate the criminality of his conduct.

Following a trial before a judge he was found Not Guilty by Reason of Insanity and committed to the jurisdiction of the Psychiatric Security Review Board (PSRB) for a maximum term of 10 years. The judge determined that his initial placement under PSRB jurisdiction would be on conditional-release status. The patient remained in the community for the first 5 years of PSRB jurisdiction. However, he had to be re-hospitalized on several occa-sions during the second half of the term because of deteriorated mental con-dition. After 10 years, when the period of jurisdiction had expired, the PSRB discharged him.

Adequacy of treatment services

The adequacy of treatment services is one critical factor in the linkage between seri-ous illness and violence. In order to help the reader to understand the evolution of services in the US, we will briefly review the last 50 years of institutional and community treatment programmes.

Mental health services in the US. The large state mental hospital, a 19th-century institution, dominated mental health services in the US until after the middle of the 20th century. The *National Mental Health Act* of 1946 created the National Institutes of Mental Health. The NIMH focused initially on the development of mental health services. The report of the Joint Commission on Mental Illness and Health (1961) recommended supplanting the large, isolated state mental hospital with a national programme focused on the development of community mental health centres. Subsequent administrations attempted to implement these recommendations and, later, to slow down the development of the community centres. In 1981 the Reagan administration ended the federal effort in this area in favour of block grants to states and support of individuals through disability programmes. The federal role in mental health services is aptly described by Foley and Sharfstein (1983).

With the federal government essentially out of the business of direct funding of services, the last 20 years have been characterized by state initiatives, by the continuing decline of state hospital beds, by changes in mental health law (see below), by an increasing focus on the chronically ill in community-based care (see below), and most recently by the shift away from public programmes and towards corporately driven managed models of mental health care. The US is currently immersed in this latter phase of service delivery with all the problems attendant to the various types of managed-care programmes.

Institutional resources. In the early part of the history described above, community resources flowed from an institutional base. Outpatient clinics were initially supported by state hospitals and their outreach programmes. That situation is reversed today, with institutional resources flowing from the community. Given this change, there are questions about the adequacy of the number of institutional beds for the mentally ill and about the quality of inpatient services. One might safely assume that there is an inadequate supply of beds and/or appropriate community resources (see below), since so many mentally ill US residents are now housed in forensic units and jails.

Bloom, Williams, Land, McFarland, and Reichlin (1998) note a dramatic swing away, in the state of Oregon, from state hospitals to other inpatient settings, some associated with community hospitals and some with county-supported mental health institutions. Each setting has its own form of governance and oversight, which complicates issues related to adequacy and quality of care. This kind of diversification of setting is likely to increase as managed-care programmes gain greater control of public mental health programmes, making their evaluation and oversight more difficult.

Community treatment systems. The discovery of psychotropic medications, coupled with the deinstitutionalization movement in the US in the 1950s and 1960s, ushered in an era of optimism for the prospects of community treatment for severe mental illness. However, it soon became evident that community treatment as originally conceived was incapable of addressing the wide range of problems experienced by patients living in the community. Patients with severe psychiatric disorders either had difficulty accessing mental health treatment or were non-compliant, the result being high rates of relapse and re-hospitalization. Patients' families were often saddled with the responsibility of caring for them; however, they received little help from professionals and often developed negative feelings towards their mentally ill loved one, leading to a tense emotional climate in the family and increased vulnerability to psychiatric relapse.

In addition to the problem of accessing and coordinating outpatient treatment for severe mental illness, deinstitutionalization made the psychosocial deficits of severe mental illness more visible in the community. Typical problems included poor social relationships, rampant unemployment, and a lack of leisure and recreational activities. Other than studies that looked formally at depression, little has been done to estimate the influence of boredom, inactivity, and lack of productivity on symptom development and alcohol and drug abuse among the chronically mentally ill. The prominent social deficits of persons receiving optimal pharmacological treatment underscored the need for interventions to improve these areas of functioning.

A major consequence of deinstitutionalization was patients' ready access to alcohol and drugs. Rates of substance-use disorders among people with severe mental illness soared in the US as patients returned to the community, while many individuals with mental illness never entered state hospitals at all. Housing was also critical in this area. Many deinstitutionalized patients became homeless, and many lived in marginal circumstances in neighbourhoods where there was heavy drug traffic. Exposure to drug dealers and opportunity for victimization are important factors in the association between chronic illness and drug abuse.

The apparent dire needs of patients with severe mental illness living in the community spurred efforts to improve treatment and psychosocial outcomes. Some services for the chronically ill are based on traditional outpatient models that derive from psychotherapy, and some services are focused, intensive, and based on the assessment of specific deficits in the individual. It appears from the literature that it is the latter type of service that reduces the likelihood of violence (Dvoskin & Steadman, 1994); this type of service can fit quite well into the treatment components of mandated community treatment programmes for individuals who are involuntarily committed secondary to a civil or criminal court commitment (see below).

Effect of mental health laws on treatment
Laws affecting the mentally ill in the US are constantly evolving (Appelbaum, 1994; Bloom & Rogers, 1987). Over the past 25 years, several issues have been debated on the national level. These include changes in civil commitment such as the most recent focus on outpatient civil commitment, the insanity defence and post-insanity defence commitment procedures, the "right to treatment," the "right to refuse treatment," and the "duty to protect." The US Supreme Court has provided guidance on most of these areas, but to a large extent it is local politics, state legislatures, and local courts that have determined how each of these areas is approached in the various jurisdictions. Mental health law in a particular jurisdiction thus becomes an amalgam of how particular issues of national interest are or are not codified in that jurisdiction. We will briefly discuss several of these areas.

Although these issues have not been empirically explored, we believe such exploration is possible. Table 1 defines the major mental health and law interactions on a three-point scale of treatment orientation. We postulate that a jurisdiction's approach to mental health law will greatly influence the care and treatment of the mentally ill in that jurisdiction. A jurisdiction may, for example, develop more or less treatment-oriented solutions to each of the problems described above, and as a result its care of the mentally ill will be tilted towards either treatment within the mental health system or incarceration in the corrections system. Again, we hypothesize that jurisdictions whose laws are more treatment-oriented will experience less criminality and violence on the part of the mentally ill than jurisdictions whose laws are less treatment-oriented.

Table 1. Treatment orientation of mental health laws

	Most (1)	Intermediate (2)	Least (3)
Civil commitment standard	Gravely disabled Limited dangerousness	Dangerousness Limited gravely disabled	Dangerousness only
Outpatient commitment	Long-term commitment based on chronic illness	Short-term commitment based on chronic illness	No outpatient commitment
Treatment refusal procedures	No treatment refusal procedure	Administrative procedure	Judicial procedure
Insanity defence	American Law Institute	Modified McNaughten	No functional insanity defence
Post-insanity defence procedures	Post-insanity procedures with CR and defined commitment	Post-insanity procedures with limited CR and indefinite commitment	Hospitalization until no longer mentally ill and dangerous
Duty to protect	No statutory or case law	Statute	Tarasoff-like case

Civil commitment statutes are the cornerstone of law and mental health interactions, because they influence the lives of many people. These statutes have become a lightning rod for often intense disagreement among various interest groups: providers, consumers, families, and civil libertarians (Bloom & Williams, 1994b; Isaac & Armat, 1990; LaFond & Durham, 1992; Miller, 1987).

Outpatient commitment. As illustrated by the *New York Times* editorial in the introduction to this chapter, the controversy surrounding outpatient civil commitment has grown as the problems of under-treated chronically mentally ill persons in various communities have become more apparent and as very short hospital stays and revolving-door types of admissions become the norm (Appelbaum, 1986; Hiday & Scheid-Cook, 1987; Miller, 1992). Generally, those who favour the statutes believe they will enhance the treatment of the chronically mentally ill in the community, while those who oppose the statutes view them as a poor substitute for community mental health services and as an unfortunate extension of the coercion inherent in

civil commitment (Monahan et al., 1999). In addition to these philosophical dis-
agreements, the statutes pose procedural problems. These include the question of
how to handle medication refusal in the community setting (Appelbaum, 1988) and
the larger question of what to do with a patient who does not comply with the treatment plan, when criteria for revocation then become an issue. Even with these technical problems, outpatient civil commitment is potentially useful (Swanson et al.,
1997; Torrey & Kaplan, 1995), especially if combined with adequate community
treatment and a workable procedure for administration of medication.

The insanity defence and the treatment of insanity acquittees represent a small but
important component area of mental health law. The insanity defence is very controversial, with disagreement about the moral necessity for the defence itself (Bonnie,
1983) and about reasonable alternatives to the defence (Keilitz & Fulton, 1984).
There are two main models for the insanity defence in the US. Table 1 rates the
American Law Institute (ALI) test as the most treatment-oriented, the modified
McNaughten test in the middle, and experiments in which jurisdictions attempt to do
without an insanity defence as the least conducive to treatment.

   Following an insanity verdict, most acquittees are involuntarily committed to a
mental health facility, usually a state forensic hospital. Generally, release criteria are
based on a court finding of no longer mentally ill and/or no longer dangerous. In the
past several decades some jurisdictions have developed conditional release programmes for insanity acquittees (Bloom & Williams, 1994a; Bloom, Williams, &
Bigelow, 1991; Bluglass, 1993; Griffin, Steadman, & Heilbrun, 1991; Lamb, Weinberger, & Gross, 1988; McGreevy, Steadman, Dvoskin, & Dollard, 1991; Tellefsen,
Cohen, Silver, & Dougherty, 1992; Wiederanders, 1992; Wiederanders, Bromley, &
Choate, 1997). Many of these programmes are designed along the lines of assertive
case management (see below) and have demonstrated effectiveness in reducing the
number of arrests and dangerous behaviours.

   Table 1 describes a continuum of treatment orientation from programmes that
incorporate jurisdictional limits and conditional release to those that have no such
limits and are solely hospital-based.

Treatment refusal is another area of debate within the mental health community.
This issue is an offshoot of modern commitment statutes that separate civil commitment from civil competency, which opens the possibility for competent committed
patients to refuse treatment. The battle has been focused on psychotropic medication. Various administrative or judicial procedures have been developed in the US
(Appelbaum, 1988; Bloom, Williams, Land, Hornbrook, & Mahler, 1997). Table 1
assumes that no procedure at all is most conducive to mental health treatment and a
judicial type procedure is least conducive.

The duty to protect is less clearly related to the issues discussed, but it has been
a very important area of law and mental health interaction (Beck, 1985, 1990). The
"duty" relates to the Tarasoff decision (*Tarasoff v. Regents of University of California,* 1974, 1976) in the state of California and basically calls upon clinicians to
attempt to protect innocent third parties from potential violence at the hands of the

clinician's clients. The issue is important because it requires clinicians to strike a balance between protecting the longstanding privilege accorded confidential communications with patients and protecting the interests of third parties—which requires them to abrogate that privilege.

Some jurisdictions have tried Tarasoff-like cases, others have passed statutes that define the duty more precisely, and others, like Oregon, have neither tried any such cases nor passed any such statutes (Bloom & Rogers, 1988).

Discussion: Effective Treatment for the Mentally Ill

What are the implications of these proximal and distal factors for the effective treatment of persons with major mental disorders who are at risk of entering the criminal justice or forensic mental health systems or who are at risk for recidivism?

There is little scientific literature on the overall effectiveness of comprehensive, multidimensional treatment programmes for mentally ill offenders. However, three areas of study provide some empirical basis for the development of such programmes: (1) evaluations of treatments and services for persons with major mental disorders that have been shown to be effective in reducing symptoms and increasing the level of psychosocial functioning, (2) evaluations of rehabilitation programmes that have been shown to be effective in reducing recidivism among non-disordered offenders, and (3) specialized forensic psychiatric community treatment programmes. Each area will be discussed briefly.

Studies which demonstrate effective treatments for individuals with major mental disorders constitute the basic first approach to dealing with these people. Such programmes have been shown to reduce the number and severity of symptoms, improve the level of psychosocial functioning, and enhance quality of life. Two key areas will be discussed: medication and psychosocial treatment.

MEDICATION

Considerable research progress has been made in the pharmacological treatment of the primary symptoms of major mental disorders. Appropriate long-term medication is an essential component of treatment for persons with these disorders. The development of new medications has significantly improved treatment. However, it must be remembered that medication improves only one aspect of the problems presented by these individuals. Many patients resist taking medication, especially on a long-term basis. Additional components of treatment designed to ensure compliance are required. (For further details, see the chapters by Tiihonen and Volavka in this volume.)

PSYCHOSOCIAL TREATMENT FOR SEVERE MENTAL ILLNESS

Over the past 2 decades, a variety of interventions have been developed to improve the course of severe mental illness and to enhance social and vocational functioning. Ample empirical support is now available for six interventions: the assertive community treatment model of case management; family intervention; social skills training; supported employment; integrated dual diagnosis (mental illness and substance abuse) treatment; and cognitive therapy for persistent psychosis. We will briefly review each of these treatment approaches and summarize research supporting the interventions.

Assertive community treatment

The high utilization of inpatient treatment services and non-compliance with outpatient treatment led to the development of the assertive community treatment (ACT) model in the late 1970s (Stein & Santos, 1998; Stein & Test, 1980). The primary difference between this approach to case management and traditional clinical case management or brokered case management is that the ACT model shifts the locus of patient-staff contact from the mental health centre to the community. The defining characteristics of the ACT model are: lower caseloads (10:1 patient:staff ratio compared to greater than 25:1 for standard case management); most services provided out of the clinic and in the community; shared caseloads across clinicians; direct provision of services by the treatment team (rather than services being brokered to other treatment providers); and 24-hour availability for crisis intervention. In most treatment settings, ACT has been developed primarily for those persons with severe mental illness who have a history of high utilization of hospital services or whose survival in the community is heavily dependent on ongoing support from treatment providers.

ACT has been one of the most extensively studied treatment approaches for persons with severe mental illness. A recent comprehensive review of the research on ACT (or a similar model, intensive case management) summarizes the results of 30 controlled studies with several thousand patients (Mueser, Bond, Drake, & Resnick, 1998). The most consistent effects of ACT were found to be decreased time in hospital, improved housing stability, decreased symptom severity, and improved quality of life. Surprisingly, most ACT studies found no effect on social functioning.

Family intervention

The high level of contact between persons with severe mental illness and their family members, coupled with lack of information provided to relatives on the management of psychiatric disorders, had untoward effects on both patients and their families. Relatives often experienced a significant burden when attempting to cope with an illness they little understood (Lefley, 1996), and growing evidence documented the negative effects of family stress on the course of the illness (Butzlaff & Hooley, 1998). Beginning in the 1970s, interventions were aimed at educating families in the nature and treatment of severe mental illness, decreasing stress in the family, and improving patient adherence to treatments. In addition to a focus on education, stress reduction, and improved management of the psychiatric illness, successful family intervention programmes seek to establish a collaborative relationship between the family and treatment providers, tend to provide services over a longer term (e.g., more than 6 months), and employ behavioural strategies, such as training in communication and problem-solving skills, for reducing tension. Several models of family intervention have been developed. These include behavioural approaches (Barrowclough & Tarrier, 1992; Falloon, Boyd, & McGill, 1984; McFarlane, 1990; Mueser & Glynn, 1999), broad-based systems approaches (Anderson, Reiss, & Hogarty, 1986), and primarily psychoeducational treatments (Kuipers, Leff, & Lam, 1992).

Research has provided strong support for the effectiveness of family intervention in severe mental illness. The preponderance of research on family intervention has focused on schizophrenia. A review of 11 controlled family intervention studies, comparing family therapy for at least 9 months to standard treatment with follow-up assessments conducted for 18 to 24 months post-treatment initiation, showed strong effects for family treatment for schizophrenia (Baucom, Shoham, Mueser, Daiuto, & Stickle, 1998). The primary effect of family intervention has been reduced numbers of relapses and re-hospitalizations. Across the 11 controlled studies, the cumulative relapse or re-hospitalization rates over 18 to 24 months were reduced from 63.6% for routine treatment to between 25.5 and 28% for a single-family or multiple-family group intervention. In addition to the evidence supporting family intervention for schizophrenia, some research suggests that family treatment can improve the symptoms and course of bipolar disorder, major depression, and anxiety disorders (reviewed by Mueser & Glynn, 1999). Furthermore, there is an extensive body of research demonstrating that family intervention is an effective treatment for persons with severe mental illness, affecting symptoms, relapse, and re-hospitalization.

Supported employment
Unemployment is a common problem among persons with severe mental illness. Although many patients express an interest in working, traditional approaches to vocational rehabilitation (e.g., sheltered workshops) have failed (Bond et al., 1990). The past several years have seen an interest in a new model of vocational rehabilitation, supported employment, based on the success of similar programmes for developmentally disabled persons (Wehman, 1981, 1986).

A variety of supported employment programmes for persons with severe mental illness have been developed. The following principles of the Individual Placement and Support (IPS) model (Becker & Drake, 1993) are shared by other supported employment programmes: an emphasis on competitive jobs in integrated work settings; attention to client preferences such as type of job; integration of vocational service and clinical treatment; and provision of ongoing support after job placement, such as coaching, emotional support, problem-solving, and negotiating reasonable accommodations with the employer.

A review of six controlled studies comparing supported employment models with other approaches to vocational rehabilitation provides strong evidence for the effectiveness of supported programmes (Bond, Drake, Mueser, & Becker, 1997). Across the six studies, a mean of 58% of patients who received supported employment obtained competitive jobs, compared to 21% of patients who received the comparison programme. Furthermore, a seventh control study has reported similar benefits for the IPS model (Drake, McHugo, et al., 1999). In addition to the positive effects of supported employment on competitive work, none of the studies suggest negative effects of work on persons with severe metal illness, such as increased symptoms, re-hospitalizations, or other aspects of psychosocial functioning (Bond et al., 1997).

Thus supported employment models have been shown to be effective in improving the competitive work outcomes of persons with severe mental illness. Beneficial effects of supported programmes do not appear to be influenced by either psychiatric diagnosis or the severity of the psychiatric illness, and negative effects of work have not been observed.

Social skills training

Impaired social functioning is one of the defining characteristics of schizophrenia (American Psychiatric Association, 1994) and is common in the broad population of people with severe mental illness (Bellack, Morrison, Wixted, & Mueser, 1990). Despite the prominence of social deficits in people with severe mental illness, assertive community treatment, family intervention, and supported employment have minimal impact on social functioning. Social skills training (SST) has been developed with a primary focus on improving the quality of social relationships.

SST is a structured approach to teaching interpersonal skills based on the principles of social learning theory (Bandura, 1969; Liberman, DeRisi, & Mueser, 1989). SST involves the breaking down of complex interpersonal skills into small, component, steps and teaching those steps through repeated modelling, role play, positive and corrective feedback, and homework assignments to generalize the skill to the patient's natural setting (Bellack, Mueser, Gingerich, & Agresta, 1997). SST is most often conducted in a group, although it can be individually applied as well.

The last 25 years have seen extensive research on the effectiveness of SST for persons with severe mental illness. Early studies focused on the feasibility of teaching new skills, including the acquisition and maintenance of skills, and the generalization of skills to patients' natural environments. Subsequent research has examined the effects of SST on different areas of functioning in controlled studies. The consensus of several reviews of SST research (Dilk & Bond, 1996; Mueser, Wallace, & Liberman, 1995; Smith, Bellack, & Liberman, 1996) is that it improves social skills and social functioning but tends to have little effect on psychiatric symptoms, relapses, or hospitalizations. These findings are consistent with those of two recent controlled studies of long-term SST for schizophrenia, which reported that skills training was associated with significant improvements in social functioning over 2 years (Liberman et al., 1998; Marder et al., 1996).

Integrated dual diagnosis treatment

Substance abuse in severe mental illness has repeatedly been linked to a wide range of negative outcomes, including relapse and re-hospitalization, housing instability, violence, incarceration, and health-risk behaviours (Drake & Brunette, 1998). Efforts to treat individuals with comorbid mental illness and substance-use disorders (i.e., dually diagnosed patients) have shown the separate treatment of the two disorders, by different groups of clinicians, to be ineffective (Ridgely, Goldman, & Willenbring, 1990). Problems with non-integrated dual diagnosis treatment include lack of coordination between treatments, philosophical differences in treatment approaches, and difficulty accessing one or both treatments. In response to the limitations of traditional approaches to the treatment of dual disorders, integrated dual diagnosis treatment programmes have been developed and tested (Carey, 1996).

Integrated dual diagnosis treatment is defined as that in which one clinician (or team of clinicians) treats the mental illness and the substance-use disorder simultaneously and in which the treatment for the two disorders is integrated. In addition to simultaneous treatment by one professional, effective integrated dual diagnosis programmes share a number of other features (Mueser, Drake, & Noordsy, 1998): (1) They usually incorporate assertive outreach to engage treatment-non-compliant patients living in the community and to monitor the effectiveness of treatment. (2) They recognize the importance of stages of treatment (or stages of change), in order to tailor interventions to the patient's current motivational state. (3) They are long term: most patients require long-term programmes, as substance-use disorders in persons with severe mental illness remit at a slow but steady rate when services are integrated. (4) They recognize the importance to recovery of safe and protective living environments for persons with a dual diagnosis. When living environments are conducive to continued substance abuse, alternative living arrangements may be sought or family- or social network-based treatment may be considered. (5) They must be comprehensive, designed to address the wide range of patient needs: social relationships, work, housing, health, and the ability to manage persistent symptoms. Helping patients to improve their functioning in different domains is critical for sustained improvement in substance abuse.

A recent comprehensive review of research on integrated dual diagnosis treatment led to several conclusions (Drake, Mercer-McFadden, Mueser, McHugo, & Bond, 1998). Simply adding dual diagnosis groups to existing mental health services had negligible effects on substance-abuse outcomes. The effect of integrated dual diagnoses treatment on other outcomes is unclear from controlled studies, but longitudinal research indicates that remissions in substance abuse are accompanied by benefits in other areas, such as enhanced quality of life and decreased depression (Drake, Xie, et al., 1999).

Cognitive therapy for psychosis
Persistent psychotic symptoms are a problem for about one third of patients with schizophrenia (Carpenter & Buchanan, 1994; Kane & Marder, 1993). Psychotic symptoms are linked to problems in a variety of areas, including higher levels of distress, increased vulnerability to relapse, and potential for violence to self and others. Cognitive therapy, a psychotherapeutic intervention initially developed for the treatment of depression (Beck, Rush, Shaw, & Emery, 1979), has recently been successfully applied to individuals with persistent psychotic symptoms.

The premise of cognitive therapy is that cognitive styles and core beliefs form the basis of emotional reactions to external events. Some individuals may be prone to cognitive distortions or erroneous beliefs due to certain learning experiences or vulnerability during times of stress. Once distorted thinking or erroneous beliefs have been developed, they may be perpetuated by selective attention to relevant information, and may subsequently influence thoughts related to psychotic symptoms. The essence of cognitive therapy for psychosis is evaluation of the evidence supporting those beliefs, and, when the evidence does not support them, identification of alternative and more realistic thoughts.

Research on the effects of cognitive therapy is in its infancy. However, the available evidence provides strong encouragement for its use. In a meta-analysis of six controlled studies with 250 subjects with schizophrenia, the mean effect size for reduction in severity of psychiatric symptoms was 0.72, corresponding to a large effect size (Gould, Mueser, Bolton, Mays, & Goff, in press). While there is a need to evaluate the generalizability of the effects of cognitive therapy to other patients, and to determine whether it also impacts on areas such as hospitalization or aggression, these findings suggest that cognitive therapy may be an important adjunctive treatment for patients with persistent psychotic symptoms.

OFFENDER TREATMENT

The second source of knowledge relevant to the development of treatment programmes for mentally ill offenders is the large body of research on the rehabilitation of non-disordered offenders (for reviews, see Andrews & Bonta, 1994; Gendreau, 1996; Lösel, 1995). It appears likely that the individual characteristics associated with antisocial behaviour among non-disordered offenders also play a role in the offending of at least some individuals with severe mental disorders. Among non-disordered offenders, research has demonstrated that the most important risk factors are: pro-criminal attitudes, values, and beliefs; personal cognitive supports of crime; pro-criminal friends and associates; inadequate socialization; impulsivity; lack of self-control; restless aggressive energy; egocentrism; below-average verbal intelligence; sensation and/or novelty seeking; poor problem-solving skills; a history of antisocial behaviour from a young age, in a variety of settings and involving many different types of behaviour; criminality, mental disorder, and substance abuse in the family of origin; poor parenting in childhood, including little affection, caring, or family cohesiveness, inadequate supervision, harsh and inconsistent discipline, neglect, and abuse; and low levels of education and career success (Andrews, 1995). The design of a treatment programme intended to modify offending and/or violent behaviour and develop the skills necessary for mentally ill offenders to live in the community without re-offending must address these characteristics.

Since the mid-1980s several meta-analyses have consistently identified positive crime-prevention effects resulting from these interventions. The meta-analyses indicate that rehabilitation programmes lead to anywhere from "mild" to "moderate" reduction in recidivism. Taking into account the clinical appropriateness of a particular programme, the average correlation between the intervention and reduced recidivism was 0.30. This indicates that psychologically appropriate treatment leads, on average, to a 40% reduction in recidivism compared to control conditions (Andrews et al., 1990; Lipsey, 1995). The meta-analyses found that the effective programmes were those that were conducted in the community and that were characterized by a high degree of structure and a behavioural or cognitive-behavioural orientation. In addition, treatment integrity was maintained. The staff were enthusiastic and the clients were at high risk to recidivate. Further, the effective programmes were multi-modal, targeting the many skills deficits presented by the offenders.

The planning and delivery of effective offender rehabilitation take into account individual differences in risk, need, and responsivity. The risk principle suggests that intensive rehabilitation is best reserved for individuals at highest risk for criminal conduct. The crimogenic need principle suggests that the appropriate targets of treatment are those changeable characteristics of individuals and their circumstances that have been demonstrated to be related to criminal conduct.

Andrews et al. (1990) identify the following intermediate targets for rehabilitation programmes: (1) reducing antisocial attitudes, antisocial feelings, antisocial friends and associates, and chemical dependencies; (2) increasing affection for and communication with family members, monitoring and supervision by family members, identification with anti-criminal role models, self-control, self-management, and problem-solving skills; (3) replacing lying, stealing, and aggressive behaviours with prosocial alternatives; and (4) modifying the costs and rewards of criminal and non-criminal activities, so that non-criminal activities are preferred.

In addition, some offenders require undemanding, sheltered, supportive living arrangements. Finally, it is essential that the offender be taught to recognize risky situations and that a concrete plan for dealing with those situations be devised and rehearsed with the offender (Andrews, 1995).

The responsivity principle suggests that approaches to treatment be matched to the above-listed intermediate targets and to the learning styles of individual offenders. The most effective types of rehabilitation are based on learning theory, and they employ cognitive-behavioural and social learning techniques such as modelling, graduated practice, role play, reinforcement, extinction, resource provision, concrete verbal suggestions, and cognitive restructuring.

For these treatments to be effective, staff authority must be established and maintained. Staff must clearly and fairly distinguish between rules and requests, and must relate with the offenders in open, enthusiastic, and caring ways. They must reinforce compliance with the various aspects of the rehabilitation programme, as well as model and consistently reinforce anti-criminal thinking and behaviour and prosocial behaviours.

The offender literature also shows us what does *not* work in reducing violence and crime in offenders: punishment, traditional dynamic psychotherapy, client-centred casework, treatments based on sociological approaches of lower-class origin and labelling, and treatments that do not address dynamic risk factors empirically related to crime.

FORENSIC PSYCHIATRIC OUTPATIENT PROGRAMMES

The third body of evidence that is relevant for developing treatment programmes for mentally ill offenders comprises a small number of evaluations of specialized community programmes for this group. The results of studies from Canada (Wilson, Tien, & Eaves, 1995), Germany (Müller-Isberner, 1996), and the US (Bloom et al., 1991; Bloom & Williams, 1994; Heilbrun & Griffin, 1993; Wiederanders, 1992; Wiederanders et al., 1997) show that violence and crime can be prevented through the use of assertive forensic psychiatric community programmes (many designed along the lines described above), even among mentally ill offenders who are at high risk for re-offending.

Given the different legal and institutional frameworks in which these community programmes have been developed, it is encouraging to find that they share a number of features. These include: compulsory participation; recognition and acceptance by the mental health professionals who administer the programme that they have a dual mandate—to treat the mental disorder and to prevent offending; and the legal power of mental health professionals to rapidly re-hospitalize patients against their will if they believe they may offend and/or behave violently, or if the patient's mental health status is deteriorating. Effective community treatment programmes address the multiple problems presented by mentally ill offenders, and are staffed by people who accept responsibility for ensuring compliance with all aspects of the programme.

Conclusion

While there is still no specific, comprehensive, evidence-based literature on the treatment of mentally disordered offenders, the ingredients for a state-of-the-art approach have been identified. Three dimensions have to be considered:

Legal foundation of treatment: Laws that protect the rights of the mentally ill but that give clinicians the power to act (including providing treatment against the patient's will) when there is an acute or chronic risk of violence and crime.

Resources for treatment: (1) Funds to pay for treatment and for sheltered housing. The public and policy-makers should consider the enormous costs of violence and crime (including the cost of warehouse policies). (2) Non-compliant patients with co-occurring substance abuse and antisocial personality disorder are at highest risk. However, these clients can be reached only by intensive and therefore costly forms of case management; due to financial restrictions, the system tends to lose these neediest clients.

Components of treatment: Treatment must be based on empirical knowledge. Approaches to treating the mentally disordered offender should be multimodal and multidisciplinary, extracting and using knowledge from multiple sources.

The treatment of mentally disordered offenders should not be a self-promoting business. While overselling the idea of treatment should be strictly avoided, those working in the field should disseminate the idea that humane strategies for preventing violence and crime do exist, and are worth funding. Clinicians have a duty to provide effective treatment. Although they do not have to shoulder responsibility for inappropriate laws and insufficient funding, they do have a responsibility to promote the notion that reasonable legal and financial bases are required if we are to have crime-preventive programmes that are effective yet impose the fewest possible restrictions on clients.

Outpatient commitment, as proposed in the *New York Times* editorial that set the stage for this chapter, may be a means of getting forced access to those clients who are at risk of committing serious offences but whose illness prevents them from sensing the risk they pose to the public. However, outpatient commitment will not work if no service is delivered. It should be made clear that while outpatient commitment poses a burden on those mentally ill individuals who will be legally required to receive treatment, it also imposes a burden on the system to provide service.

Finally, it must be mentioned that any treatment approach must be accompanied by continuous assessment of risks and needs. Treatment efforts must be proportional to the risk, as assessed using structured actuarial devices (e.g., HCR-20: Webster, Douglas, Eaves, & Hart, 1997; Violence Prediction Scheme: Webster, Harris, Cormier, & Quinsey, 1994).

References

Abram, K.M., & Teplin, L.A. (1991). Co-occurring disorders among mentally ill jail detainees: Implications for public policy. *American Psychologist, 46,* 1036–1045.

Amador, X.F., Flaum, M., & Andreasen, N.C. (1994). Awareness of illness in schizophrenia and schizoaffective and mood disorders. *Archives of General Psychiatry, 51,* 826–836.

Amador, X.F., Strauss, D.H., Yale, Y.A., Flaum, M.M., Endicott, J., & Gorman, J.M. (1993). Assessment of insight in psychosis. *American Journal of Psychiatry, 150,* 873–879.

Amador, X.F., Strauss, D.H., Yale, S.A., & Gorman, J.M. (1991). Awareness of illness in schizophrenia. *Schizophrenia Bulletin, 17,* 113–132.

American Psychiatric Association. (1994). *Diagnostic and statistical manual of mental disorders (DSM-IV) (4th Rev. Ed.).* Washington: American Psychiatric Association.

Anderson, C.M., Reiss, D.J., & Hogarty, G.E. (1986). *Schizophrenia and the family.* New York: Guilford.

Andrews, D. (1995). The psychology of criminal conduct and clinical criminology. In L. Stewart, L. Stermac, & C. Webster (Eds.), *Clinical criminology: Toward effective correctional treatment* (pp. 130–150). Toronto: Correctional Service of Canada.

Andrews, D.A., & Bonta, J.L. (1994). *The psychology of criminal conduct.* Cincinnati: Anderson.

Andrews, D.A., Zinger, I., Hoge, R.D., Bonta, J., Gendreau, P., & Cullen, F.T. (1990). Does correctional treatment work? A clinically relevant and psychologically informed meta-analysis. *Criminology, 28,* 369–404.

Appelbaum, P.S. (1986). Outpatient commitment: The problems and the promise. *American Journal of Psychiatry, 143,* 1270–1272.

Appelbaum, P.S. (1988). The right to refuse treatment with antipsychotic medications: Retrospect and prospect. *American Journal of Psychiatry, 145,* 413–419.

Appelbaum, P.S. (1994). *Almost a revolution: Mental health law and the limits of change.* New York: Oxford University Press.

Bandura, A. (1969). *Principles of behavior modification.* New York: Holt, Rinehart & Winston.

Barrowclough, C., & Tarrier, N. (1992). *Families of schizophrenic patients: Cognitive behavioral intervention.* London: Chapman & Hall.

Baucom, D.H., Shoham, V., Mueser, K.T., Daiuto, A.D., & Stickle, T.R. (1998). Empirically supported couple and family interventions for adult mental health problems. *Journal of Consulting and Clinical Psychology, 66,* 53–88.

Beck, A.T., Rush, A.J., Shaw, B.F., & Emery, G. (1979). *Cognitive therapy of depression.* New York: Guilford.

Beck, J.C. (Ed.). (1985). *The potentially violent patient and the Tarasoff decision in psychiatric practice.* Washington: American Psychiatric Press.

Beck, J.C. (Ed.). (1990). *Confidentiality versus the duty to protect: Foreseeable harm in the practice of psychiatry.* Washington: American Psychiatric Press.

Beck, J.C., White, K.A., & Gage, B. (1991). Emergency psychiatric assessment of violence. *American Journal of Psychiatry, 148,* 1562–1565.

Becker, D.R., & Drake, R.E. (1993). *A working life: The Individual Placement and Support (IPS) program.* Concord, NH: New Hampshire–Dartmouth Psychiatric Research Center.

Bellack, A.S., Morrison, R.L., Wixted, J.T., & Mueser, K.T. (1990). An analysis of social competence in schizophrenia. *British Journal of Psychiatry, 156,* 809–818.

Bellack, A.S., Mueser, K.T., Gingerich, S., & Agresta, J. (1997). *Social skills training for schizophrenia.* New York: Guilford.

Bloom, J.D., & Rogers, J.L. (1987). The legal basis of forensic psychiatry: Statutorily mandated psychiatric diagnosis. *American Journal of Psychiatry, 144,* 847–853.

Bloom, J.D., & Rogers, J.L. (1988). The duty to protect others from your patients: *Tarasoff* spreads to the northwest. *Western Journal of Medicine, 148,* 231–234.

Bloom, J.D., & Williams, M.H. (1994a). *Management and treatment of insanity acquittees: A model for the 1990s.* Washington: American Psychiatric Press.

Bloom, J.D., & Williams, M.H. (1994b). Oregon's civil commitment law: 140 years of change. *Hospital and Community Psychiatry, 45,* 466–470.

Bloom, J.D., Williams, M.H., & Bigelow, D.A. (1991). Monitored conditional release of persons found Not Guilty by Reason of Insanity. *American Journal of Psychiatry, 148,* 444–449.

Bloom, J.D., Williams, M.H., & Bigelow, D.A. (1992). The involvement of schizophrenic insanity acquittees in the mental health and criminal justice systems. *Psychiatric Clinics of North America, 15,* 591–604.

Bloom, J.D., Williams, M.H., Land, C., Hornbrook, M.C., & Mahler, J. (1997). Treatment refusal procedures and service utilization: A comparison of involuntarily hospitalized populations. *Journal of the American Academy of Psychiatry and the Law, 25,* 349–357.

Bloom, J.D., Williams, M.H., Land, C., McFarland, B.H., & Reichlin, S. (1998). Changes in public psychiatric hospitalization in Oregon over the past two decades. *Psychiatric Services, 49,* 366–369.

Bluglass, R. (1993). Maintaining the treatment of mentally ill people in the community. *British Medical Journal, 306,* 159–160.

Bond, G., Witheridge, T., Dincin, J., Wasmer, D., Weff, J., & DeGraaf-Kaser, R. (1990). Assertive community treatment for frequent users of psychiatric hospitals in a large city: A controlled study. *American Journal of Community Psychology, 18*(6), 865–891.

Bond, G.R., Drake, R.E., Mueser, K.T., & Becker, D.R. (1997). An update on supported employment for people with severe mental illness. *Psychiatric Services, 48*(3), 335–346.

Bonnie, R.J. (1983). The moral basis of the insanity defense. *American Bar Association Journal, 69,* 194–197.

Borum, R., Swanson, J., Swartz, M., & Hiday, V. (1997). Substance abuse, violent behavior, and police encounters among persons with severe mental disorder. *Journal of Contemporary Criminal Justice, 13,* 236–249.

Butzlaff, R.L., & Hooley, J.M. (1998). Expressed emotion and psychiatric relapse. *Archives of General Psychiatry, 55,* 547–552.

Cain v. Rijken. (1985). 74 Or App 76,700 P.2d 1061.

Cain v. Rijken. (1986). 300 Or 706 717, P.2d 140.

Carey, K.B. (1996). Treatment of co-occurring substance abuse and major mental illness. In R.E. Drake & K.T. Mueser (Eds.), *Dual diagnosis of major mental illness and substance abuse. Vol. 2: Recent research and clinical implications* (pp. 19–31). San Francisco: Jossey-Bass.

Carpenter, W.T. Jr., & Buchanan, R.W. (1994). Schizophrenia. *New England Journal of Medicine, 330,* 681–690.

Cuffel, B.J., Shumway, M., Chouljian, T.L., & MacDonald, T. (1994). A longitudinal study of substance use and community violence in schizophrenia. *Journal of Nervous and Mental Disorders, 182*(12), 704–708.

Dickerson, F.B., Boronow, J.J., Ringel, N., & Parente, F. (1997). Lack of insight among outpatients with schizophrenia. *Psychiatric Services, 48,* 195–199.

Dilk, M.N., & Bond, G.R. (1996). Meta-analytic evaluation of skills training research for individuals with severe mental illness. *Journal of Consulting and Clinical Psychology, 64*(6), 1337–1346.

Dohrenwend, B.P., Shrout, P., Egri, G., & Mendelsohn, F. (1980). Measures of non-specific psychological distress and other dimensions of psychopathology in the general population. *Archives of General Psychiatry, 37,* 1229–1236.

Drake, R., Bartels, S., Teague, G., Noordsy, D., & Clark, R. (1993). Treatment of substance abuse in severely mentally ill patients. *Journal of Nervous and Mental Disorders, 181,* 606–611.

Drake, R.E., & Brunette, M.F. (1998). Complications of severe mental illness related to alcohol and other drug use disorders. In M. Galanter (Ed.), *Recent developments in alcoholism. Vol. 14: Consequences of alcoholism* (pp. 285–299). New York: Plenum.

Drake, R.E., McHugo, G.J., Bebout, R.R., Becker, D.R., Harris, M., Bond, G.R., & Quimby, E. (1999). A randomized clinical trial of supported employment for inner-city patients with severe mental illness. *Archives of General Psychiatry, 56,* 627–633.

Drake, R.E., Mercer-McFadden, C., Mueser, K.T., McHugo, G.J., & Bond, G.R. (1998). Review of integrated mental health and substance abuse treatment for patients with dual disorders. *Schizophrenia Bulletin, 24*(4), 589–608.

Drake, R.E., Mueser, K.T., Clark, R.E., & Wallach, M.E. (1996). The course, treatment, and outcome of substance disorder in persons with severe mental illness. *American Journal of Orthopsychiatry, 66,* 42–51.

Drake, R.E., Xie, H., McHugo, G.J., Teague, G.B., Mueser, K.T., Vaillant, G.E., & Wallach, M.A. (1999). *The five-year course of substance use disorder in patients with dual disorders.* Manuscript in preparation.

Dvoskin, J.A., & Steadman, H.J. (1994). Using intensive case management to reduce violence by mentally ill persons in the community. *Hospital and Community Psychiatry, 45,* 679–684.

Falloon, I.R.H., Boyd, J.L., & McGill, C.W. (1984). *Family care of schizophrenia: A problem-solving approach to the treatment of mental illness.* New York: Guilford.

Foley, H.A., & Sharfstein, H.A. (1983). *Madness and government: Who cares for the mentally ill?* Washington: American Psychiatric Press.

Gendreau, P. (1996). Offender rehabilitation: What we know and what needs to be done. *Criminal Justice and Behavior, 23,* 144–161.

Gould, R.A., Mueser, K.T., Bolton, E., Mays, V., & Goff, D. (1999). Cognitive therapy for psychosis in schizophrenia: A preliminary meta-analysis. Unpublished manuscript.

Griffin, P.A., Steadman, H.J., & Heilbrun, K. (1991). Designing conditional release systems for insanity acquittees. *Journal of Mental Health Administration, 18,* 231–241.

Hales, R.E., & Yudofsky, S.C. (1999). *Essentials of clinical psychiatry.* Washington: American Psychiatric Press.

Heilbrun, K., & Griffin, P. (1993). Community-based forensic treatment of insanity acquittees. *International Journal of Law and Psychiatry, 16,* 133–150.

Hiday, V.A., & Scheid-Cook, T.L. (1987). The North Carolina experience with outpatient commitment: A critical appraisal. *International Journal of Law and Psychiatry 10*, 215–232.

Hodgins, S. (1993). The criminality of mentally disordered persons. In S. Hodgins (Ed.), *Mental disorder and crime* (pp. 3–21). Newbury Park, CA: Sage.

Hodgins, S., Mednick, S.A., Brennan, P.A., Schulsinger, F., & Engberg, M. (1996). Mental disorder and crime. *Archives of General Psychiatry, 53,* 489–496.

Husted, J.R. (1999). Insight in severe mental illness: Implications for treatment decisions. *Journal of the American Academy of Psychiatry and the Law, 27,* 33–49.

Issac, R.J., & Armat, V.C. (1990). *Madness in the streets: How psychiatry and the law abandoned the mentally ill.* New York: Free Press.

Joint Commission on Mental Illness and Health. (1961). *Action for mental health.* New York: Basic.

Kane, J.M., & Marder, S.R. (1993). Psychopharmacologic treatment of schizophrenia. *Schizophrenia Bulletin, 19,* 287–302.

Keiltiz, I., & Fulton, J.P. (1984). *The insanity defense and its alternatives.* Washington: National Center for State Courts, R-085.

Kuipers, L., Leff, J., & Lam, D. (1992). *Family work for schizophrenia: A practical guide.* London: Gaskell.

LaFond, J.Q., & Durham, M.L. (1992). *Back to asylum: The future of mental health law and policy in the United States.* New York: Oxford University Press.

Lamb, H.R., Weinberger, L.E., & Gross, B.H. (1988). Court-mandated community outpatient treatment for persons found Not Guilty by Reason of Insanity: A five-year follow-up. *American Journal of Psychiatry, 145,* 450–456.

Lefley, H.P. (1996). *Family caregiving in mental illness.* Thousand Oaks, CA: Sage.

Liberman, R.P., DeRisi, W.J., & Mueser, K.T. (1989). *Social skills training for psychiatric patients.* Needham Heights, MA: Allyn & Bacon.

Liberman, R.P., Wallace, C.J., Blackwell, G., Kopelowicz, A., Vaccaro, J.V., & Mintz, J. (1998). Skills training versus psychosocial occupational therapy for persons with persistent schizophrenia. *American Journal of Psychiatry, 155,* 1087–1091.

Lindqvist, P., & Allebeck, P. (1990a). Schizophrenia and assaultive behavior: The role of alcohol and drug abuse. *Acta Psychiatrica Scandinavica, 82,* 191–195.

Lindqvist, P., & Allebeck, P. (1990b). Schizophrenia and crime: A longitudinal follow-up of 644 schizophrenics in Stockholm. *British Journal of Psychiatry, 157,* 345–350.

Link, B.G., & Stueve, A. (1994). Psychotic symptoms and the violent/illegal behavior of mental patients compared to community controls. In J. Monahan & H.J. Steadman (Eds.), *Violence and mental disorder* (pp. 137–159). Chicago: University of Chicago Press.

Lipsey, M.W. (1995). What do we learn from 400 research studies on the effectiveness of treatment with juvenile delinquents? In J. McGuire (Ed.), *What works: Reducing reoffending* (pp. 63–78). Chichester: Wiley.

Lösel, F. (1995). The efficacy of correctional treatment: A review and sythesis of meta-evaluations. In J. McGuire (Ed.), *What works: Reducing reoffending* (pp. 79–111). Chichester: Wiley.

Marder, S.R., Wirshing, W.C., Mintz, J., McKenzie, J., Johnston, K., Eckman, T.A., Lebell, M., Zimmerman, K., & Liberman, R.P. (1996). Two-year outcome for social skills training and group psychotherapy for outpatients with schizophrenia. *American Journal of Psychiatry, 153,* 1585–1592.

McEvoy, J.P., Appelbaum, P.S., Apperson, L.J., Geller, J.L., & Freter, S. (1989). Why must some schizophrenic patients be involuntarily committed? The role of insight. *Comprehensive Psychiatry, 30,* 13–17.

McFarlane, W.R. (1990). Multiple family groups and the treatment of schizophrenia. In M.I. Herz, S.J. Keith, & J.P. Docherty (Eds.), *Handbook of schizophrenia. Vol. 4: Psychosocial treatment of schizophrenia* (pp. 167–189). Amsterdam: Elsevier.

McGreevy, M.A., Steadman H.J., Dvoskin, J.A., & Dollard, N. (1991). New York State's system of managing insanity acquittees in the community. *Hospital and Community Psychiatry, 42,* 512–517.

McNiel, D.E. (1994). Hallucinations and violence. In J. Monahan & H.J. Steadman (Eds.), *Violence and mental disorder* (pp. 183–202). Chicago: University of Chicago Press.

McNiel, D.E., Binder, R.L., & Greenfield, T.K. (1988). Predictors of violence in civilly committed acute psychiatric patients. *American Journal of Psychiatry, 145,* 965–970.

Medicating the mentally ill. (1999, April 11). [Editorial.] *New York Times,* p. 16.

Miller, R.D. (1987). *Involuntary civil commitment of the mentally ill in the post-reform era.* Springfield, IL: Charles C. Thomas.

Miller, R.D. (1992). An update on involuntary civil commitment to outpatient treatment. *Hospital and Community Psychiatry, 43,* 79–82.

Monahan, J., Lidz, C.W., Hoge, S.K., Mulvey, E.P., Eisenberg, M.M., Roth, L.H., Gardner, W.P., & Bennett, N. (1999). Coercion in the provision of mental health services: The MacArthur studies. In J. Morrissey & J. Monahan (Eds.), *Research in community and mental health. Vol. 10: Coercion in mental health services* (pp. 13–20). Stamford, CT: JAI Press.

Mueser, K.T., Bond, G.R., Drake, R.E., & Resnick, S.G. (1998). Models of community care for severe mental illness: A review of research on case management. *Schizophrenia Bulletin, 24*(1), 37–74.

Mueser, K.T., Drake, R.E., Ackerson, T.H., Alterman, A.I., Miles, K.M., & Noordsy, D.L. (1997). Antisocial personality disorder, conduct disorder, and substance abuse in schizophrenia. *Journal of Abnormal Psychology, 106,* 473–477.

Mueser, K.T., Drake, R.E., & Noordsy, D.L. (1998). Integrated mental health and substance abuse treatment for severe psychiatric disorders. *Journal of Practical Psychiatry and Behavioral Health, 4*(3), 129–139.

Mueser, K.T., & Glynn, S.M. (1999). *Behavioral family therapy for psychiatric disorders,* 2nd ed. Oakland, CA: New Harbinger.

Mueser, K.T., Wallace, C.J., & Liberman, R.P. (1995). New developments in social skills training. *Behavior Change, 12,* 31–40.

Mueser K.T., Yarnold, P.R., Levinson D.R., Singh, H., Bellack, A.S., Kee, K., Morrison, R.L., & Yadalam, K.G. (1990). Prevalence of substance abuse in schizophrenia: Demographic and clinical correlates. *Schizophrenia Bulletin, 16,* 31–56.

Müller-Isberner, R. (1996). Forensic psychiatric aftercare following hospital order treatment. *International Journal of Law and Psychiatry, 19,* 81–86.

Ness, D.E., & Ende, J. (1994). Denial in the medical interview: Recognition and management. *Journal of the American Medical Association, 272,* 1777–1781.

Neumann, C.S., Walker E.F., Weinstein, J., & Cutshaw, M.A. (1996). Psychotic patients' awareness of mental illness: Implications for legal defense proceedings. *Journal of Psychiatry and Law,* Fall, 421–442.

Regier, D.A., Farmer, M.E., Rae, D.S., Locke, B.Z., Keith, S.J., Judd, L.L., & Goodwin, F.K. (1990). Comorbidity of mental disorders with alcohol and other drug abuse: Results from the Epidemiologic Catchment Area (ECA) study. *Journal of the American Medical Association, 264,* 2511–2518.

Ridgely, M.S., Goldman, H.H., & Willenbring, M. (1990). Barriers to the care of persons with dual diagnoses: Organizational and financing issues. *Schizophrenia Bulletin, 16,* 123–132.

Smith, T.E., Bellack, A.S., & Liberman, R.P. (1996). Social skills training for schizophrenia: Review and future directions. *Clinical Psychology Review, 16*(7), 599–617.

Steadman H.J., Mulvey, E.P., Monahan, J., Robbins, P.C., Appelbaum, P.S., Grisso, T., Roth, L.H., & Silver, E. (1998). Violence by people discharged from acute psychiatric inpatient facilities and by others in the same neighborhoods. *Archives of General Psychiatry, 55,* 393–412.

Stein, L.I., & Santos, A.B. (1998). *Assertive community treatment of persons with severe mental illness.* New York: Norton.

Stein, L.I., & Test, M.A. (1980). Alternatives to mental hospital treatment. I: Conceptual, model, treatment program and clinical evaluation. *Archives of General Psychiatry, 37,* 392–397.

Swanson, C.L., Freudenreich, O., McEvoy, J.P., Nelson, L., Kamaraju, L., & Wilson, W. (1995). Insight in schizophrenia and mania. *Journal of Nervous and Mental Disorders, 183,* 752–755.

Swanson, J.W., Swartz, M.S., George, L.K., Burns, B.J., Hiday, V.A., Borum, R., & Wagner, H.R. (1997). Interpreting the effectiveness of involuntary outpatient commitment: A conceptual model. *Journal of the American Academy of Psychiatry and the Law, 25,* 5–16.

Tarasoff v. Regents of University of California. (1974). 13 Cal 3d 177, 118 Cal Rptr 129, 529 P.2d 553.

Tarasoff v. Regents of University of California. (1976). 17 Cal 3d 425, 131 Cal Rptr 14, 551 P.2d 334.

Tardiff, K. (1989). *Assessment and management of violent patients.* Washington: American Psychiatric Press.

Tardiff, K., Marzuk, P.M., Leon, A.C., & Portera, B.A. (1997). A prospective study of violence by psychiatric patients after hospital discharge. *Psychiatric Services, 48,* 678–681.

Taylor, P.J. (1993). Schizophrenia and crime: Distinctive patterns in association. In S. Hodgins (Ed.), *Mental disorder and crime* (pp. 63–85). Newbury Park, CA: Sage.

Taylor, P.J., Garety, P., Buchanan, A., Reed, A., Wessley, S., Ray, K., Dunn, G., & Grubin, D. (1994). Delusions and violence. In J. Monahan & H.J. Steadman (Eds.), *Violence and mental disorder* (pp. 161–182). Chicago: University of Chicago Press.

Tellefsen, C., Cohen, M.I., Silver, S.B., & Dougherty, C. (1992). Predicting success on conditional release for insanity acquittees: Regionalized versus non-regionalized hospital patients. *Bulletin of the American Academy of Psychiatry and the Law, 20,* 87–100.

Torrey, E.F. (1995). [Editorial.] Jails and prisons: America's new mental hospital. *American Journal of Public Health, 85,* 1611–1613.

Torrey, E.F., & Kaplan, R.J. (1995). A national survey of the use of outpatient commitment. *Psychiatric Services, 46,* 778–784.

Webster, C.D., Douglas, K.S., Eaves, D., & Hart, S.D. (1997). *HCR-20: Assessing risk for violence, Version 2.* Burnaby, BC: Simon Fraser University.

Webster, C.D., Harris, G.T, Rice, M.E, Cormier, C., & Quinsey, V.L. (1994). *The violence prediction scheme: Assessing dangerousness in high risk men.* Toronto: Centre for Criminology, University of Toronto.

Wehman, P. (1981). *Competitive employment: New horizons for severely disabled individuals.* Baltimore: Brooks.

Wehman, P. (1986). Supportive competitive employment for persons with severe disabilities. *Journal of Applied Rehabilitation Counseling, 17,* 24–29.

Wiederanders, M.R. (1992). Recidivism of disordered offenders who were conditionally vs. unconditionally released. *Behavioral Sciences and the Law, 10,* 141–148.

Wiederanders, M.R., Bromley, D.L., & Choate, P.A. (1997). Forensic conditional release programs and outcomes in three states. *International Journal of Law and Psychiatry, 20,* 249–257.

Wilson, D., Tien, G., & Eaves, D. (1995). Increasing the community tenure of mentally disordered offenders: An assertive case management program. *International Journal of Law and Psychiatry, 18,* 61–69.

Joseph D. Bloom is Dean, School of Medicine, and Professor, Department of Psychiatry, Oregon Health Sciences University, Portland, Oregon, USA. Kim T. Mueser is Professor, Department of Psychiatry, Dartmouth Medical School and New Hampshire–Dartmouth Psychiatric Research Center, Concord, New Hampshire, USA. Rüdiger Müller-Isberner is Director, Haina Forensic Psychiatric Hospital, Haina, Germany.

Authors' Note

Comments or queries may be directed to Joseph Bloom, MD, School of Medicine, Oregon Health Sciences University, 3181 SW Sam Jackson Park Road (Mail code L 102), Portland OR 97201-3098 USA. Telephone: 503 494-6689. Fax: 503 494-3400. E-mail: <bloom@ohsu.edu>.

PHARMACOLOGICAL INTERVENTION FOR PREVENTING VIOLENCE AMONG THE MENTALLY ILL WITH SECONDARY ALCOHOL- AND DRUG-USE DISORDERS

JARI TIIHONEN
MARVIN S. SWARTZ

Introduction

Several studies have shown that both major mental disorders (MMD) and substance abuse are associated with increased risk of criminal, and, especially, violent offending (Eronen, Hakola, & Tiihonen, 1996a; Hodgins, 1992; Hodgins, Mednick, Brennan, Schulsinger, & Engberg, 1996; Tiihonen, Isohanni, Räsänen, Koiranen, & Moring, 1997). Since alcohol and drug abuse are more common among subjects with MMD (Regier et al., 1990; Ross, Glaser, & Germanson, 1988), it has been argued that the increased risk of offending among the mentally ill may be a consequence of frequent substance abuse in this population. However, several methodologically sound studies have suggested that MMD (odds ratios, or ORs, from 3.6 to 8.0) or substance abuse (ORs up to 10.7) alone increases the risk of violent offending (Eronen, Hakola, & Tiihonen, 1996a; Eronen, Tiihonen, & Hakola, 1996; Hodgins et al., 1996; Räsänen et al., 1998), although the greatest risk increase is seen among subjects with concurrent MMD and substance abuse (ORs from 17.2 to 25.2) (Eronen, Tiihonen, & Hakola, 1996; Räsänen et al., 1998) (see Table 1).

Table 1. Risk of violent behaviour among male index populations compared with the general male population

Diagnostic group/ Index population	Number of subjects obtained from studies/study design	Odds ratio	95% CI
Manic disorders (Eronen, Hakola, & Tiihonen, 1996a)	No males with manic disorders in 910 homicide offenders	—	—
Anxiety disorders (Eronen, Hakola, & Tiihonen, 1996a)	14 (1.5%) males with anxiety disorders in 910 homicide offenders	0.3	0.2–0.5
Dysthymia (Eronen, Hakola, & Tiihonen, 1996a)	13 (1.4%) males with dysthymia in 910 homicide offenders	0.6	0.3–1.0
General population		1	
Mental retardation (Eronen, Hakola, & Tiihonen, 1996a)	11 (1.2%) males with mental retardation in 910 homicide offenders	1.2	0.7–2.2

S. Hodgins (ed.), Violence among the Mentally Ill, 171–191.

Major depressive episode (Eronen, Hakola, & Tiihonen, 1996a)	27 (3.0%) males with major depressive episode in 910 homicide offenders	1.6	1.1–2.4
Non-compliance with substance abuse (Swartz et al., 1998a)	331 subjects with severe mental illness, risk of violent behaviour	2.29	1.01–5.21
Schizophrenia without alcoholism (Räsänen et al., 1998)	3 non-alcoholic schizophrenics convicted of violent crimes in a birth cohort ($n = 11,017$)	3.6	0.9–12.3
Men with major mental disorders (Hodgins, 1992)	82 in a birth cohort of 7,362 men suffered from a major mental disorder; their relative risk for violence was assessed	4.16	2.23–7.78
Major mental disorder (Hodgins et al., 1996)	Unselected birth cohort ($n = 324,401$), risk of violent offending	4.5	3.9–5.1
Schizophrenia (Tiihonen et al., 1997)	Unselected birth cohort ($n = 11,017$), risk of violent offending	7.0	3.1–15.9
Schizophrenia without alcoholism (estimate) (Eronen, Tiihonen, & Hakola, 1996)	48 non-alcoholic schizophrenics in 1,302 homicide offenders	7.25	4.7–5.4
Schizophrenia and schizophreniform psychoses (Eronen, Hakola, & Tiihonen, 1996a)	58 (6.4%) schizophrenics in 910 homicide offenders	8.0	6.1–10.4
Homicide offenders with one earlier homicide (Eronen, Tiihonen, & Hakola, 1996)	13-year sample of homicide recidivists ($n = 35$) among 1,584 homicide offenders	10.4	7.4–14.5
Alcoholism (Eronen, Hakola, & Tiihonen, 1996b)	357 (39.2%) alcoholic males in 910 homicide offenders	10.7	9.4–12.2
Antisocial personality disorder (Eronen, Hakola, & Tiihonen, 1996a)	103 (11.3%) males with antisocial personality disorder in 910 homicide offenders	11.7	9.5–14.4
Schizophrenia with alcoholism (estimate) (Eronen, Tiihonen, & Hakola, 1996)	38 (2.9%) alcoholic schizophrenic subjects in 1,302 homicide offenders	17.2	12.4–23.7
Schizophrenia with alcoholism (Räsänen et al., 1998)	4 alcoholic schizophrenics convicted of violent crimes in a birth cohort ($n = 11,017$)	25.2	6.1–97.2
Homicide offenders during first year after release from prison (Eronen, Hakola, & Tiihonen, 1996b)	13-year sample of homicide recidivists ($n = 35$) among 1,584 homicide offenders	253.8	145.8–441.9
Released forensic psychiatric patients during first year outside hospital (Tiihonen, Hakola, et al., 1996)	A follow-up study of released patients with mean follow-up period 7.8 years	293.9	119.2–724.7

The issue of preventing violent behaviour in forensic patients deserves special attention, because the highest risk for recurrent offending has been observed among individuals who have previously committed violent offences (Eronen, Tiihonen, &

Hakola, 1997). Studies on recidivistic violent offenders in Finland have found that about 70% of all homicide recidivists have early-onset alcoholism associated with severe antisocial or borderline personality disorder, and 15% have schizophrenia (Eronen, Hakola, & Tiihonen, 1996b). No reliable epidemiological data exist on milder recidivistic violent offences, or other crimes, as the detection and clearance rates for those offences are too low.

If one aims to develop specific anti-aggressive pharmacological treatments, it is essential that one understands the neurochemical mechanism underlying the violent behaviour. During the past decade, research on the neurochemistry of aggressive behaviour has focused quite strongly on the monoamines and, especially, serotonergic function in the brain. Several studies have consistently shown that low levels of cerebrospinal fluid (CSF) 5-hydroxyindoleacetic acid (5-HIAA) are associated with impulsive suicidal and aggressive behaviour among patients with personality disorder or substance abuse (Åsberg, Träskman, & Thoren, 1976; Linnoila et al., 1983; Virkkunen et al., 1994), but thus far such findings have not been confirmed among the mentally ill.

It has been suggested that both alcohol-induced euphoria and aggressive behaviour are associated with increased dopamine transmission in the brain. Since low-activity (L) allele of catechol-*O*-methyltransferase (COMT) gene results in a 3–4 times lower rate in the dopamine inactivation, it could be presumed that this polymorphism may have a role in the genetic background of substance abuse and aggressive behaviour. Indeed, recent studies have suggested that COMT polymorphism contributes to aggressive behaviour among schizophrenic patients and to the development of alcohol abuse (Lachman, Nolan, Mohr, Saito, & Volavka, 1998; Strous, Bark, Volavka, Parsia, & Lachman, 1997; Tiihonen et al., 1999). The results from these studies indicate that a low-activity allele (L) of the COMT gene is associated with aggressive or threatening behaviour among schizophrenics and an increased risk for alcoholism. These results are in line with findings that suggest dopamine activity is increased in paranoid (but not in catatonic) schizophrenia (Hietala et al., 1995), and with the findings that those drugs which increase aggression, such as ethanol, amphetamine, cocaine, and PCP, are associated with dopamine release in the brain (Rossetti, D'Aquila, Hmaidan, Gessa, & Serra, 1991; Sorensen, Jumphreys, Taylor, & Schmidt, 1992; Spanagel, Herz, Bals-Kubik, & Shippenberg, 1991; Yoshimoto, McBride, Lumeng, & Li, 1991). In addition, amphetamine results in greater dopamine release in the brains of schizophrenic patients than in healthy controls (Breier et al., 1997; Laruelle et al., 1996). These data can be used to rationalize why chemical substance abuse is especially detrimental to the mentally ill and their increased risk of violent behaviour.

Pharmacological Treatment of Mentally Ill Inpatients with MMD and Substance Abuse

The rule of thumb in the pharmacological treatment of aggressive behaviour among mentally disordered subjects is to treat the underlying disorder that contributes to violent behaviour. Those mentally ill patients who are hospitalized for their aggressive or dangerous behaviour have a high rate of comorbidity for personality disorders or substance abuse (Côté & Hodgins, 1990; Putkonen, Kotilainen, & Tiihonen, 2000; Taylor et al., 1998).

About one third of the homicides committed by the mentally ill in Finland were found to be a consequence of schizophrenic hallucinations or delusions; in the remaining cases it was not possible to establish a clear motive for the offence (Eronen, Räsänen, Hakola, & Tiihonen, 2000). Also, during hospital treatment some of the violent acts are caused by the psychotic symptoms, which can be prevented by efficient antipsychotic treatment. However, for the most part offences are a result of poor impulsive control, which can be treated pharmacologically with serotonergic drugs (such as lithium, anticonvulsants, antidepressants, beta-blockers, buspirone, and serenics). Among institutionalized mentally ill subjects (in hospitals and prisons), alcohol use is not a significant problem during incarceration, whereas the use of illicit drugs may be a significant problem, especially in prisons. However, substance abuse becomes a major problem when these subjects are discharged or released from the institutions.

ANTIPSYCHOTICS

There are several methodological difficulties in doing controlled clinical trials on the pharmacological treatment of violent behaviour; therefore, there are only a few well-controlled studies on the subject.

Among patients with a diagnosis of psychosis, standard neuroleptics having D_2-receptor-blocking properties such as haloperidol and zuclopenthixol are widely used and administered as intramuscular injections during the acute phase of aggressive behaviour. Although many patients respond well to the oral use of standard antipsychotics after the acute aggressive episode, the classic neuroleptics have several adverse effects, such as acathisia and irreversible tardive dyskinesia. Acathisia, in particular, may induce non-compliance and aggressive behaviour. So-called atypical antipsychotics, such as clozapine, risperidone, olanzapine, sertindol, quetiapine, ziprasidone, and zotepine, are weaker D_2-receptor blockers and therefore cause less extrapyramidal side effects. They also affect the serotonergic system—for example, by $5\text{-}HT_2$-receptor blockade. The suppression of aggressive behaviour by antipsychotic treatment in schizophrenic patients is apparently not fully explained by diminished delusions or by sedation, and recent studies suggest that clozapine (Chiles, Davidson, & McBride, 1994; Volavka, Zito, Vitrai, & Czobar, 1993), risperidone (Buckley et al., 1997; Czobor, Volavka, & Meibach, 1995; Marder, Davis, & Chouinard, 1997), and quetiapine (Cantillon, Arvanitis, Miller, & Kowalcyk, 1997) may have some selective effect on hostility and aggression. The studies by Czobor et al. and Marder et al. were double-blind controlled clinical trials demonstrating that risperidone has a greater selective effect on decreasing hostility than haloperidol. These data are described in detail in Jan Volavka's chapter in this book.

LITHIUM

Lithium is a mood stabilizer and therefore may reduce violent behaviour, especially among patients with bipolar disorder. However, it also affects the serotonergic system and may increase impulse control, leading to a decrease in impulsive aggressive behaviour among patients without bipolar disorder. The anti-aggressive effect of lithium has been demonstrated in one double-blind trial among mentally handicapped patients (Craft et al., 1987) and among violent prisoners without psychoses (Sheard, Marini, Bridges, & Wagner, 1976). The beneficial anti-aggressive effect of lithium among patients with schizophrenia and organic mental syndromes has been observed in an open trial (Tupin et al., 1973).

The results of the study by Sheard et al. (1976) indicate that lithium is effective in reducing violent behaviour, even at relatively low plasma levels (< 1.0 mmol/l). However, lithium may induce severe side effects, especially over the long term. Also, acute side effects may have a substantial impact on treatment compliance; for example, in the study by Sheard et al. about one third of the subjects stopped their medication because of adverse side effects such as hand tremor or shakiness, dryness of mouth, polyuria, or nausea. In long-term treatment, the most critical side effects are electrocardiogram (ECG) and electroencephalogram (EEG) abnormalities, dysfunction of the kidneys and subsequent increased creatinin levels, and hypoactivity of the thyroid gland resulting in decreased thyroxin (T4) levels. Because of the narrow therapeutic range of serum concentrations and the adverse effects, lithium levels and kidney, thyroid, and cardiac functions must be monitored with laboratory tests. During long-term treatment, laboratory tests should be carried out at 2- to 6-month intervals.

CARBAMAZEPINE

The beneficial anti-aggressive effect of carbamazepine among psychotic patients has been reported in several open trials since 1970 (Hakola & Laulumaa, 1982; Luchins, 1984; Shibahara, Hamada, & Uno, 1970). In a double-blind crossover study among patients with EEG abnormalities, most having a diagnosis of schizophrenia, a 50% reduction in the severity and a 30% reduction in the occurrence rate of aggressive incidents was observed during carbamazepine treatment when compared with a placebo (Neppe, 1983, 1988). A large double-blind study among patients with schizophrenia ($N = 127$) or schizoaffective disorder ($N = 35$) revealed a slightly better anti-aggressive effect for the carbamazepine group, in which the number of patients having marked or moderate improvement was 48%, vs. 30% for patients given a placebo ($p < 0.05$). There was no statistically significant change in the total BPRS scores, although the carbamazepine group showed more improvement in the areas of suspiciousness, uncooperativeness, and excitement (Okuma et al., 1989).

Carbamazepine has several potential side effects, such as liver dysfunction and agranulocytosis; therefore, liver and blood tests must be carried out before and during treatment. One must be careful when combining carbazepine with clozapine, since both these drugs increase the risk of agranulocytosis. It must be remembered that carbamazepine decreases the blood levels of several antipsychotics, and if carbamazepine treatment is terminated or switched to oxcarbazepine, for example, a 100% increase in the neuroleptic serum concentration may result if the neuroleptic dosage is not changed (Tiihonen, Vartiainen, & Hakola, 1995). Obviously, serum concentration increase may cause severe side effects, especially in patients receiving clozapine at the same time.

VALPROIC ACID

There have been no double-blind trials on the anti-aggressive effect of valproic acid. However, data obtained from an open-label study demonstrated that valproic acid reduced the number of hours spent in seclusion by patients with bipolar disorder or borderline personality disorder (Wilcox, 1994).

SSRIs

Selective serotonin re-uptake inhibitors (SSRIs), such as fluoxetine, increase central serotonergic transmission. Since habitual impulsive violent behaviour is associated with dysfunctions of the serotonergic system in the brain (Virkkunen et al., 1994; Virkkunen, DeJong, Bartko, Goodwin, & Linnoila, 1989; Virkkunen, Eggert, Rawlings, & Linnoila, 1996), it follows that these agents could enhance impulse control and suppress impulsive violent or criminal behaviour. The effectiveness of fluoxetine, the most widely used SSRI, has been demonstrated in two double-blind studies on the treatment of impulsive and aggressive behaviour among patients with personality disorders (Coccaro & Kavoussi, 1997; Saltzman et al., 1995). The anti-aggressive effect of SSRIs among patients with major mental disorders has been studied in only one double-blind placebo-controlled trial (Vartiainen et al., 1995). In this crossover study, 15 habitually aggressive patients in a high-security state mental hospital received citalopram or a placebo over 24 weeks. Citalopram was added to existing medication regimes, and many patients were also receiving clozapine. The results demonstrated a 27% lower rate of aggressive incidents with citalopram compared to placebo. Many of these patients had comorbid antisocial personality disorder and alcohol dependence, although it was not clear to what extent their aggressive and impulsive behaviour was actually attributable to the comorbid personality disorder rather than to psychotic illness.

Recent studies on pindolol augmentation during SSRI treatment suggest that pindolol enhances the antidepressant effect of SSRIs (Perez, Gilaberte, Faries, Alvarez, & Artigas, 1997; Räsänen, Hakko, & Tiihonen, 1999). Thus far, however, it is not known if pindolol also enhances the anti-aggressive effect of SSRIs.

BETA-BLOCKERS

Propranolol has been observed to decrease aggressive behaviour in schizophrenia in open studies (Sheppard, 1979; Sorgi, Ratey, & Polakoff, 1986). The anti-aggressive effect of nadolol among violent patients (most with schizophrenia) has been studied in two double-blind placebo-controlled studies (Albert et al., 1990; Ratey et al., 1992). Both studies revealed a reduction in either aggression or hostility.

Pindolol has a partial agonist effect on adrenergic receptors, which is the reason for its lower risk for cardiovascular side effects compared with some other beta-blockers. Thus far its efficacy has been examined only in a double-blind study of demented patients (Greendyke & Kanter, 1986). Pindolol is also a 5-HT$_{1A}$ antagonist. Presynaptic 5-HT$_{1A}$ autoreceptors detect increases of serotonin after SSRI treatment blocks presynaptic uptake sites of the serotonin re-uptake transporter (SERT). This leads to a negative feedback on serotonin release, and the delayed therapeutic effect of SSRIs (Figure 1). A recent study on the genetic polymorphism of the SERT allele revealed that those patients having short allele (S) benefited from pindolol augmentation during SSRI treatment, while those patients with long allele (L) did not (Smeraldi et al., 1998). A recent report suggests that habitually violent offenders with antisocial personality disorders and substance abuse have a higher S allele frequency than controls (Hallikainen et al., 1999). It is possible that S allele, or the SS genotype, may also contribute to violent behaviour among patients with MMD and both co-existing antisocial personality disorder and substance abuse. If so, pindolol augmentation during SSRI treatment might be beneficial, especially among those subjects having the S allele.

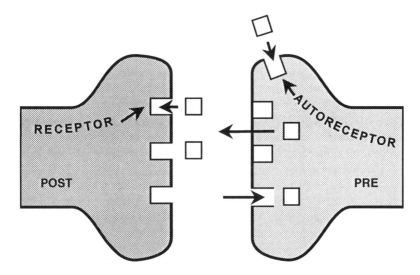

Figure 1. Increase of serotonin concentration (e.g., induced by SSRIs) in the synaptic cleft is detected by presynaptic 5-HT autoreceptor, which leads to negative feedback into the serotonin release

SERENICS

Eltoprazine is classified as belonging to the group of "serenics" that are 5-HT$_1$-receptor agonists. These agents have a selective anti-aggressive effect in animals (Rasmussen, Olivier, Raghoebar, & Mos, 1990). The role of 5-HT$_{1B}$-agonism has recently been demonstrated in a knockout gene study where mice lacking serotonin 5-HT$_{1B}$ receptors were shown to be very aggressive (Saudou et al., 1994).

The clinical efficacy of serenics in human aggression has been studied in mentally retarded (de Koning et al., 1994; Kohen, 1993; Tiihonen, Hakola, Paanila, & Turtiainen, 1993; Verhoeven, Tuinier, Sijben, van den Berg, & de Witte-van der Schoot, 1992) and schizophrenic (Tiihonen et al., 1993) patients. These studies have shown that eltoprazine may be effective in those patient groups. In the only double-blind study published to date, eltoprazine was found to be significantly more effective in treating hetero-aggressive or auto-aggressive behaviour, but only in the most aggressive mentally retarded patients (de Koning et al.). *L*-toperazine is another serenic compound being studied for its anti-aggressive effect. However, no results have been published thus far.

Pharmacological Treatment of Outpatients with MMD and Substance Abuse

At the moment, there are no published controlled studies on the efficacy of pharmacological treatment in preventing violence among outpatients with concurrent MMD and substance abuse, or even studies among patients with either MMD or substance abuse.

Data from a recent study indicate that outpatients treated in a forensic setting committed about 50% fewer new offences than a similar group of patients treated in a conventional setting (Müller-Isberner, 1996). The results of another recent study indicate that patients discharged from a forensic hospital commit fewer recidivist crimes than those discharged from an ordinary psychiatric hospital, and that patients who frequently visit their psychiatrist commit fewer new crimes (Hodgins, Lapalme, & Toupin, in press). These data strongly indicate that the crucial issue, in the long-term prevention of violent behaviour among patients with MMD and substance abuse, is effective compulsory outpatient treatment.

Long-term outpatient treatment that includes neuroleptic or mood-stabilizing medication is essential in preventing recidivistic violent behaviour among mentally ill patients after discharge from hospital (neuroleptic treatment should be used for at least 5 years continuously in patients with several relapses of psychosis [Kissling 1994]). In addition to frequent observation and follow-up with psychotherapeutic and sociobehavioural therapy, as well as neuroleptic or mood-stabilizing treatment, recidivistic violent behaviour among outpatients could be suppressed with other pharmacological treatments such as SSRIs and beta-blockers as described previously for inpatients. However, the compliance and side effects must be monitored carefully, which requires regular and relatively frequent visits by the patients. The main problem in treating and preventing (recidivistic) violent behaviour is the patient's poor compliance and attitude (Smith, 1989), especially when combined with substance abuse (Swartz et al., 1998a). This requires new approaches such as effective compulsory outpatient treatment, with supervised drug administration or use of depot-injection drugs, as an alternative to long-term incarceration.

Recidivistic violent behaviour in patients with a psychotic disorder is typically associated with cessation of voluntary treatment in outpatient care after discharge from hospital (i.e., seeing a doctor or nurse and using a neuroleptic medication), which results from an insufficient insight into their illness. In recent Finnish studies (which found about a 300-fold risk of committing a homicide during the first year outside the hospital), about 70% of all re-offenders and 100% of homicide re-offenders had stopped taking their medication and seeing their doctor (Tiihonen, Hakola, Eronen, Vartiainen, & Ryynänen, 1996; Vartiainen & Hakola, 1992). These studies, as well as studies on homicide recidivists by Eronen, Hakola, and Tiihonen (1996b) and a cohort study by Räsänen et al. (1998), suggest that co-existing alcohol or drug abuse among schizophrenic patients is an important factor in recidivist violent behaviour in this population; for example, most (88%) of the recidivist violent crimes were committed under the influence of alcohol (Vartiainen & Hakola). Therefore, any chemical substance abuse or dependence merits attention and should be treated as effectively and as vigourously as the psychotic illness. Dopamine-releasing agents such as ethanol, cocaine, and amphetamine can induce impulsive violent behaviour (Baggio & Ferrari, 1980; Barros & Miczek, 1996; Rossetti et al., 1991; Sorensen et al., 1992; Spanagel et al., 1991; Thor & Ghiselli, 1975), and substance abuse may make a substantial contribution to violent behaviour, even among mentally ill patients who are deliberately offensive due to their psychotic symptoms (e.g., delusions or hallucinations). During the last decade, several controlled trials have shown that there are efficacious pharmacological treatments for substance abuse. However, no such studies have been done among patients with comorbid major mental disorder. Intramuscular depot-neuroleptic treatment is effective in preventing relapse of psychotic illnesses, resulting in 50% lower relapse rates than treatment with oral medication (Kane, 1989; Kissling, 1994), but the low-dose neuroleptics typically used are associated with a significant risk of extrapyramidal side effects and tardive dyskinesia. Clozapine and new atypical neuroleptics possibly have some specific anti-aggressive effect (Citrome & Volavka, 1997), but at the present time none of these are available as depot injections (risperidone probably will be available in this form within the next year). However, the new antipsychotics risperidone, sertindole, and olanzapine have quite mild adverse effects, which results in better compliance.

SUBSTANCE ABUSE

Substance abuse is a major risk factor for violent behaviour among patients with MMD, especially in outpatient care (Steadman et al., 1998). Until approximately 10 years ago, the pharmacological treatment of alcohol dependence appeared to be quite ineffective. Disulfiram (Fuller et al., 1986; Fuller & Roth, 1979) and lithium (Dorus et al., 1989) have been studied in controlled clinical trials that have failed to demonstrate any significant differences in outcome for patients receiving the active medication and patients receiving placebo. Controlled studies by Naranjo and colleagues suggest that the SSRIs citalopram and zimelidine are effective in treating early stages of problem drinking (Naranjo et al., 1987; Naranjo & Sellers, 1989). Results from a recent study indicate that citalopram is significantly more effective than a placebo, even in the treatment of severe early-onset alcohol dependence

(Tiihonen, Ryynänen, Kauhanen, Hakola, & Salaspuro, 1996). However, some recent studies indicate that SSRIs may not have any significant effect in the reduction of craving and alcohol use (Agosti, 1995). Benzodiazepines are usually contraindicated in the treatment of outpatients with substance abuse (Uhde & Tancer, 1995).

Results from two double-blind placebo-controlled studies using naltrexone were published in 1992. Both demonstrated its efficacy in the treatment of alcohol dependence (O'Malley et al., 1992; Volpicelli, Alterman, Hayashida, & O'Brien, 1992). The results showed that patients receiving placebo had approximately twice the rate of relapse of those receiving naltrexone. A recent large clinical trial found that 43% of patients receiving acamprosate remained abstinent during a 1-year follow-up period, compared to 21% of patients receiving placebo (Sass, Soyka, Mann, & Zieglgänsberger, 1996). On the basis of this evidence from large clinical trials it can be concluded that both naltrexone and acamprosate are safe and effective agents for treating alcohol-dependent patients.

The pharmacological treatment of drug abuse has focused mainly on patients with opioid dependence. Pharmacological treatments for individuals abusing cocaine, amphetamines, and other drugs are still at a developmental stage, although some studies have shown lower rates of cocaine use in buprenorphine-maintained patients (Kosten, Kleber, & Morgan, 1989a, 1989b). Ibogaine, which is an *N*-methyl-*D*-aspartate (NMDA) antagonist, is regarded as a potential pharmacological treatment for cocaine and stimulant abuse (Popik et al., 1995). Studies on the treatment of opioid dependence have shown that although methadone-maintenance (Schottenfeld & Kleber, 1995) and buprenorphine-maintenance (Schottenfeld, Pakes, Oliveto, Ziedonis, & Kosten, 1997) treatments are quite successful, the use of illicit drugs, especially cocaine, persists in up to 40% of patients (Schottenfeld et al.). Methadone treatment is more likely to be effective when higher doses, longer durations of treatment, and more realistic goals are set (Wodak, 1994). Levo-α-acetylmethadol (LAAM) has similar properties to methadone but a longer half-life, which should result in clinical advantages. Naltrexone is used in the prevention of opiate relapse in detoxified patients (Tennant, Rawson, Cohen, & Mann, 1984), and clonidine has been used in opioid detoxification (Warner, Kosten, & O'Connor, 1997). The clinical treatment of cannabis and hallucinogen abuse has not been adequately described, perhaps because these categories of drugs are not markedly addictive and medical problems resulting from their use are not frequent (Callaway & M'Kenna, 1998).

In order to be effective, pharmacological treatments for alcohol abuse and other forms of drug abuse must be integrated into a programme that includes, for example, counselling and supportive or cognitive therapy. The results from studies on naltrexone treatment for alcohol dependence indicate that the cumulative rate of abstinence was highest for patients treated with naltrexone and supportive therapy, and that among the patients who relapsed, those who received both naltrexone and coping-skills therapy were the least likely to relapse (O'Malley et al., 1992). Methadone-maintenance treatment is an attractive option for the majority of opiate-dependent individuals, and is especially cost-effective for the society (Wodak 1994). Since many such patients are likely to combine methadone with illicit narcotics, they are typically not allowed to receive their methadone without supervision. Methadone is most successfully used in structured programmes that include other treatment components such as social-skills and job training, in conjunction with strict monitoring of use of methadone and other drugs by urine analysis.

Table 2. Preventing violence among the mentally ill with secondary alcohol- and drug-use disorders

Inpatients	Outpatients
Atypical neuroleptics	Regular and frequent monitoring of the mental
clozapine	state -> hospitalization if necessary
risperidone	Long-lasting (> 5 years) neuroleptic treatment
olanzapine?	Depot-neuroleptics: relapse risk ↓, compliance ↓
quetiapine?	Atypical neuroleptics: adverse effects ↓, compli-
SSRIs	ance ↑, no depot injections available at the mo-
Lithium	ment
Carbamazepine	Naltrexone?
Beta-blockers	Acamprosate?
	No benzodiazepines

Evaluating the Effectiveness of Pharmacologic Interventions

Substance-abuse comorbidity is a clearly potent risk factor for violence and other negative outcomes in mentally ill individuals (Bartels, Drake, & Wallach, 1995; Cuffel, Shumway, Chouljian, & MacDonald, 1994; Fulwiler, Grossman, Forbes, & Ruthazer, 1997; Osher & Drake, 1996; Swanson, 1994; Swanson, Borum, Swartz, & Monahan, 1996; Swartz et al., 1998a; Swofford, Kasckow, Schelley-Gilkey, & Inderbitzin, 1996). As discussed earlier, there are promising pharmacologic interventions for reducing violence in mentally ill individuals with comorbid substance-abuse disorders. New antipsychotic agents offering greater efficacy and tolerability, as well as other adjuvant agents, show promise in violence-prevention in limited naturalistic and controlled trials. However, there are no community-based, quasi-experimental, or randomized controlled trials examining the effectiveness of these pharmacologic agents in reducing violence in the community. Evidence to date is limited to highly selected clinical trials with limited generalizability. The paucity of such community-based evidence of the effectiveness of pharmacologic agents in reducing violence also highlights the challenges of evaluating community-based interventions for violence prevention. These challenges are briefly discussed below.

MEASURING SUBSTANCE-ABUSE COMORBIDITY

Accurate measurement of substance-abuse comorbidity, as well as medication adherence, is fraught with difficulties (Drake, Alterman, & Rosenberg, 1993; McPhillips et al., 1997). Patients are reluctant to admit to illicit substance use for fear of alienating providers or family members, or they may fear legal sanctions. As a result, clinician chart diagnoses identifying substance abuse often miss or underestimate it (Drake et al., 1993). In addition, even minor levels of substance use, below the threshold of a diagnosis, may well compromise the functioning and impulse control of mentally ill individuals (Drake, Rosenberg, & Mueser, 1996). As a result, measurement of substance use requires precision even at the threshold of occasional use. Unfortunately, self-report or family report of substance use is very unreliable and serum urine drug testing is limited to a short timeframe of detection for most substances. Drugs of abuse are also freely substituted on the street and individuals may not know the actual substances they are using. As a result, accurate reports of specific drugs of abuse and their relationship to violence are very limited. Analysis of illicit drug use by radioimmunoassay of hair (RIAH) demonstrates extensive under-reporting of illicit drug use by self-report and underestimates provided by urine drug testing (McPhillips et al.). RIAH may become a useful clinical tool for detecting illicit drug use. A small sample of hair, taken from the head, may be used to estimate illicit drug use in the preceding 30–90 days in the major illicit drug classes of opiates, barbiturates, PCP, cocaine, and marijuana (Kintz, 1996; Magura, Freeman, Siddiqi, & Lipton, 1992).

ASSESSING MEDICATION COMPLIANCE

Self-report of medication compliance is equally limited, because patients are frequently reluctant to acknowledge non-adherence (Fenton, Blyler, & Heinssen, 1997). Laboratory measures of compliance are limited as well. While serum levels can be used to detect the presence or absence of medications, quantification of the level of adherence is difficult or impractical for most antipsychotic regimens, although it is more feasible for mood-stabilizing agents. As a result, community-based trials of promising interventions are hampered by poor estimates of both treatment adherence and illicit drug use.

UNDERSTANDING THE ORDERING OF EFFECTS IN PATHWAYS TO VIOLENCE RISK

Comorbid substance abuse is clearly associated with violent behaviour in the community, but it is not clear how or what mechanisms underlie their association. Substance abuse is correlated with a number of adverse risk factors, which, singularly or in combination with substance abuse, raise the risk of violent behaviour. In addition, substance abuse may, in some cases, not be causative but a proxy measure for other risk factors for adverse outcomes. Several potential non-mutually exclusive hypotheses about the relationship of substance abuse, mental illness, and violence are plausible. In fact, several of these potential pathways to violence may act in concert. A number of these pathways are discussed below.

Substance abuse reduces impulse control
In this potential pathway, substance-abuse comorbidity lowers the threshold of impulse control in the mentally ill individual, in either an intoxicated or a withdrawal phase of use.

Substance abuse exacerbates psychotic and other symptoms
This pathway suggests that a general exacerbation or loss of control of psychotic symptoms, not an effect on impulse control per se, raises the risk of violence in mentally ill individuals with co-occurring substance abuse. Thus, the pathway to violent behaviour is through a general exacerbation of the illness.

Substance abuse is a proxy measure for personality disorder
This pathway argues that substance abuse is a relative epiphenomenon and serves as a proxy measure of personality disorder and/or poor impulse control. Because substance abuse and personality disorder are highly correlated, it is difficult to understand the relationship among substance abuse, personality disorder, and violence. Nonetheless, it is plausible that substance abuse merely identifies antisocial or impulsive mentally ill individuals already at high risk for violence.

Medication side effects lead to self-medication with illicit substances
This pathway suggests that mentally ill individuals use substances to ameliorate unwanted side effects of prescribed medications. For example, alcohol abuse could be an attempt to reduce akathisia from prescribed antipsychotics. This pathway would also suggest that reduction of side effects should be the most effective way to reduce substance use.

Medication non-compliance leads to substance use
Medication non-compliance is closely correlated with substance-abuse comorbidity in mentally ill individuals. Substance abuse may represent a substitution of one preferred drug for another (Swartz et al., 1998a, 1998b), thus the most direct means of reducing violence risk would be by enhanced medication compliance. This would also entail the optimization of prescribed drug regimens, the use of depot antipsychotic agents, or other psychosocial interventions designed to enhance compliance.

Psychotic and other symptoms lead to self-medication
Substance-abuse comorbidity can also relate to residual symptomatology. Attempts to ameliorate painful negative or positive symptoms are purported to lead to substance abuse. The downstream effects of substance abuse by disinhibition or other mechanisms would then increase the risk for violence. In this instance, improved pharmacologic management of the underlying psychiatric illness would be a key pathway to violence prevention.

Exposure to adverse social environments leads to substance use and aggressive behaviour
Many mentally ill individuals live in poor urban neighbourhoods with high levels of crime, violence, victimization, and substance use. A mentally ill person in such a neighbourhood may be particularly vulnerable to substance use due to lack of meaningful or structured activities, greater susceptibility to the influence of substance-abusing peers, or other community factors. Victimization and violent perpetration is often a part of these predatory environments (Hiday, Swartz, Swanson, Borum, &

Wagner, 1999). A reduction of violence risk in this instance would require broader environmental interventions to provide a safer residential environment.

Boredom and lack of structure lead to substance use
Despite the dissemination of new models of vocational rehabilitation, opportunities for competitive employment or meaningful work are limited for many mentally ill individuals. Many mentally ill people also lack opportunities for social and recreational engagement. As a result, boredom and lack of structure may lead to substance abuse and increased violence risk.

The potential diverse pathways to violence risk in the presence of mental illness and substance abuse suggest likely limits to the effectiveness of pharmacologic interventions to reduce violence risk. This poses a methodologic challenge in demonstrating effective community-based pharmacologic interventions and suggests that such interventions will likely need to be paired with key psychosocial interventions. The diversity of pathways also suggests limited points of leverage in reducing violence risk through pharmacologic means alone.

Pharmacologic interventions do show promise in reducing violence risk, by: (a) reducing psychiatric symptoms and improving functioning, (b) reducing unwarranted side effects such as akathisia, (c) improving impulse control, (d) improving adherence to medication regimens by improving efficacy and tolerability, and (e) providing sustained action through use of depot preparations where necessary. However, pathways to violence risk through the social environment—adverse neighbourhoods, lack of vocational and recreational resources, boredom—cannot be remedied by pharmacologic interventions alone. These social-environmental factors may well attenuate the effectiveness of pharmacologic agents in community trials. Depending on the degree of "noise" posed by environmental factors, it may be difficult to detect the "signal" of effective drug regimens.

Given the heterogeneity of violent behaviour in mentally ill individuals, multi-pronged pharmacologic interventions will be required. Pairing these medication regimens with psychosocial interventions that promote medication adherence, providing meaningful social engagement and structure, and enhancing residential safety will likely be key to demonstrating their effectiveness.

Conclusions

Several studies indicate that clozapine (and possibly other atypical neuroleptics as well), carbamazepine, lithium, beta-blockers, and SSRIs can be used to prevent violent behaviour among inpatients with MMD. The results indicate that effective, regular, and long-term compulsory outpatient care and supervised drug administration after discharge represent an absolute necessity in forensic patients having a psychotic disorder, substance abuse, previous offences, and insufficient insight into their mental illness. If the mental state of a patient with previous offences and psychotic disorder deteriorates significantly, he/she should be hospitalized immediately. Unfortunately, legislation does not allow compulsory long-term outpatient treatment and follow-up after discharge from hospital in all countries (e.g., in Finland the duration of compulsory outpatient follow-up and treatment is 6 months).

References

Agosti, V. (1995). The efficacy of treatments in reducing alcohol consumption: A meta-analysis. *International Journal of Addictions, 30*, 1067–1077.

Albert, M., Allan, E.R., Citrome, L., Laury, G., Sison, C., & Sudilovsky, A. (1990). A double-blind, placebo-controlled study of adjunctive nadolol in the management of violent psychiatric patients. *Psychopharmacology Bulletin, 26*, 367–371.

Åsberg, M., Träskman, L., & Thoren, P. (1976). 5-HIAA in the cerebrospinal fluid: A biochemical suicide predictor? *Archives of General Psychiatry, 33*, 1193–1197.

Baggio, G., & Ferrari, F. (1980). Role of brain dopaminergic mechanisms in rodent aggressive behavior: Influence of (+/-) N-n-propyl-norapomorphine on three experimental models. *Psychopharmacology, 70*, 63–68.

Barros, H.M.T., & Miczek, K.A. (1996). Neurobiological and behavioral characteristics of alcohol-heightened aggression. In D.M. Stoff & R.B. Cairns (Eds.), *Aggression and violence: Genetic, neurobiological, and biosocial perspectives* (pp. 237–264). Hillsdale, NJ: Erlbaum.

Bartels, S.J., Drake, R.E., & Wallach, M.A. (1995). Long-term course of substance use disorders among patients with severe mental illness. *Psychiatric Services, 46*(3), 248–251.

Breier, A., Su, T-P., Saunders, R., Carson, R.E., Kolachana, B.S., de Bartolomeis, A., Weinberger, D.R., Weisenfeld, N., Malhotra, A.K., Eckelman, W.C., & Pickar, D. (1997). Schizophrenia is associated with elevated amphetamine-induced synaptic dopamine concentrations: Evidence from a novel positron emission tomography method. *Proceedings of National Academy of Sciences of the United States of America, 94*, 2569–2574.

Buckley, P.F., Ibrahim, Z.Y., Singer, B., Orr, B., Donenwirth, K., & Brar, P.S. (1997). Aggression and schizophrenia: Efficacy of risperidone. *Journal of American Academy of Psychiatry and the Law, 25*, 173–181.

Callaway, J.C., & M'Kenna, D.J. (1998). Neurochemistry of psychedelic drugs. In S.T. Karch (Ed.), *Drug abuse handbook* (pp. 485–498). Boca Raton, FL: CRC Press LLC.

Cantillon, M., Arvanitis, L.A., Miller, B.G., & Kowalcyk, B.B. (1997, December). *"Seroquel" (quetiapine fumarate) reduces hostility and aggression in patients with acute schizophrenia* [Abstract], 36th Annual Meeting of the American College of Neuropsychopharmacology, 171.

Chiles, J.A., Davidson, P., & McBride, D. (1994). Effects of clozapine on use of seclusion and restraint at a state hospital. *Hospital and Community Psychiatry, 45*, 269–271.

Citrome, L., & Volavka, J. (1997). Psychopharmacology of violence. Part II: Beyond the acute episode. *Psychiatric Annals, 27*, 696–703.

Coccaro, E.F., & Kavoussi, R.J. (1997). Fluoxetine and impulsive aggressive behavior in personality-disordered subjects. *Archives of General Psychiatry, 54*, 1081–1088.

Côté, G., & Hodgins, S. (1990). Co-occurring mental disorders among criminal offenders. *Bulletin of the American Academy of Psychiatry and the Law, 18*, 271–281.

Craft, M., Ismail, A.I., Krishnamurti, D., Mathews, J., Regan, A., Seth, R.V., & North, P.M. (1987). Lithium in the treatment of aggression in mentally handicapped patients: A double-blind trial. *British Journal of Psychiatry, 150*, 685–689.

Cuffel, B.J., Shumway, M., Chouljian, T.L., & MacDonald, T. (1994). A longitudinal study of substance use and community violence in schizophrenia. *Journal of Nervous and Mental Diseases, 182,* 704–708.

Czobor, P., Volavka, J., & Meibach, R.C. (1995). Effect of risperidone on hostility in schizophrenia. *Journal of Clinical Psychopharmacology, 15,* 243–249.

De Koning, P., Mak, M., de Vries, M.H., Allsopp, L.F., Stevens, R.B., Verbruggen, R., van den Borre, R., van Peteghem, P., Kohen, D., Arumainayagam, M., Browne, R.V., Tyrer, S.P., Read, S.G., Jones, A., Sacks, B.I., Tokola, R., Kaski, M., Järvelin, M., Hagert, U., Claden, C., Doubliez, P., Pallegoix, M., & Gaussares, C. (1994). Eltoprazine in aggressive mentally handicapped patients: A douple-blind, placebo-controlled and baseline-controlled multi-centre study. The Eltoprazine Aggression Research Group. *International Clinical Psychopharmacology, 9,* 187–194.

Dorus, W., Ostrow, D.G., Anton, R., Cushman, P., Collins, J.F., Schaefer, M., Charles, H.L., Desai, P., Hayashida, M., Malkerneker, U., Willenbring, O., Fiscella, R., & Sather, M.R. (1989). Lithium treatment of depressed and nondepressed alcoholics. *Journal of the American Medical Association, 262,* 1646–1652.

Drake, R.E., Alterman, A.I., & Rosenberg, S.R. (1993). Detection of substance use disorders in severely mentally ill patients. *Community Mental Health Journal, 29,* 175–192; discussion 193–194.

Drake, R.E., Rosenberg, S.D., & Mueser, K.T. (1996). Assessing substance use disorder in persons with severe mental illness. *New Directions in Mental Health Services, 70,* 3–17.

Eronen, M., Hakola, P., & Tiihonen, J. (1996a). Mental disorders and homicidal behavior in Finland. *Archives of General Psychiatry, 53,* 497–501.

Eronen, M., Hakola, P., & Tiihonen, J. (1996b). Factors associated with homicide recidivism in a 13-year sample of homicide offenders in Finland. *Psychiatric Services, 47,* 403–406.

Eronen, M., Räsänen, P., Hakola, P., & Tiihonen, J. (2000). *Schizophrenic homicide offenders in Finland between 1984 and 1995.* Unpublished material.

Eronen, M., Tiihonen, J., & Hakola, P. (1996). Schizophrenia and homicidal behavior. *Schizophrenia Bulletin, 22,* 83–89.

Eronen, M., Tiihonen, J., & Hakola, P. (1997). Psychiatric disorders and violent behavior. *International Journal of Psychiatry in Clinical Practice, 1,* 179–188.

Fenton, W.S., Blyler, C.R., & Heinssen, R.K. (1997). Determinants of medication compliance in schizophrenia: Empirical and clinical findings. *Schizophrenia Bulletin, 23,* 637–651.

Fuller, R.K., Branchey, L., Brightwell, D.R., Derman, R.M., Emrick, C.D., Iber, F.L., James, K.E., Lacoursiere, R.B., Lee, K.K., Lowenstam, I., Manny, I., Neiderhiser, D., Nocks, S., & Show, J.J. (1986). Disulfiram treatment of alcoholism: A Veterans Administration co-operative study. *Journal of the American Medical Association, 256,* 1449–1455.

Fuller, R.K., & Roth, H.P. (1979). Disulfiram for the treatment of alcoholism: An evaluation in 128 men. *Annals of Internal Medicine, 90,* 901–904.

Fulwiler, C., Grossman, H., Forbes, C., & Ruthazer, R. (1997). Early-onset substance abuse and community violence by outpatients with chronic mental illness. *Psychiatric Services, 48,* 1181–1185.

Greendyke, R.M., & Kanter, D.R. (1986). Therapeutic effects of pindolol on behavioral disturbances associated with organic brain disease: A double-blind study. *Journal of Clinical Psychiatry, 47,* 423–426.

Hakola, H.P., & Laulumaa, V.A. (1982). Carbamazepine in treatment of violent schizophrenics. *Lancet, 1,* 1358.

Hallikainen, T., Saito, T., Lachman, H.M., Volavka, J., Pohjalainen, T., Ryynänen, O-R., Kauhanen, J., Syvälahti, E., Hietala, J., & Tiihonen, J. (1999). Association between low activity serotonin transporter promoter genotype and early onset alcoholism with habitual impulsive violent behavior. *Molecular Psychiatry, 4,* 285–388.

Hiday, V.A., Swartz, M.S., Swanson, J.W., Borum, R., & Wagner, H.R. (1999). Criminal victimization of persons with severe mental illness. *Psychiatric Services, 50,* 62–88.

Hietala, J., Syvälahti, E., Vuorio, K., Räkkolainen, V., Bergman, J., Haaparanta, M., Solin, O., Kuoppamäki, M., Kirvelä, O., Ruotsalainen, U., & Salokangas, K.R. (1995). Presynaptic dopamine function in striatum of neuroleptic-naive schizophrenic patients. *Lancet, 346,* 1130–1131.

Hodgins, S. (1992). Mental disorder, intellectual deficiency, and crime: Evidence from a birth cohort. *Archives of General Psychiatry, 49,* 476–483.

Hodgins, S., Lapalme, M., & Toupin, J. (in press). Criminal activities and substance use of patients with major affective disorders and schizophrenia: A two-year follow-up. *Journal of Affective Disorders.*

Hodgins, S., Mednick, S.A., Brennan, P.A., Schulsinger, F., & Engberg, M. (1996). Mental disorder and crime: Evidence from a Danish birth cohort. *Archives of General Psychiatry, 53,* 489–496.

Kane, J.M. (1989). Schizophrenia: Somatic treatment. In H.I. Kaplan & B.J. Sadock (Eds.), *Comprehensive textbook of psychiatry. Vol 1, 5th ed.* (pp. 777–792). Baltimore: Williams & Wilkins.

Kintz, P. (1996). Drug testing in addicts: A comparison between urine, sweat, and hair. *Therapeutic Drug Monitoring, 18,* 450–455.

Kissling, W. (1994). Compliance, quality assurance and standards for relapse prevention in schizophrenia. *Acta Psychiatrica Scandinavica, 89*(suppl 382), 16–24.

Kohen, D. (1993). Eltoprazine for aggression in mental handicap. *Lancet, 341,* 628–629.

Kosten, T.R., Kleber, H.D., & Morgan, C. (1989a). Role of opioid antagonists in treating intravenous cocaine abuse. *Life Science, 44,* 887–892.

Kosten, T.R., Kleber, H.D., & Morgan, C. (1989b). Treatment of cocaine abuse with buprenorphine. *Biological Psychiatry, 26,* 637–639.

Lachman, H.M., Nolan, K., Mohr, P., Saito, T., & Volavka, J. (1998). Association between COMT genotype and violence in schizophrenia and schizoaffective disorder. *American Journal of Psychiatry, 155,* 835–837.

Laruelle, M., Abi-Dargham, A., van Dyck, C.H., Gil, R., D'Souza, C.D., Erbos, J., McCance, E., Rosenblatt, W., Fingado, C., Zoghbi, S.S., Baldwin, R.M., Seibyl, J.P., Krystal, J.H., Charney, D.S., & Innis, R.B. (1996). Single photon emission computerized tomography imaging of amphetamine-induced dopamine release in drug-free schizophrenic subjects. *Proceedings of National Academy of Sciences of the United States of America, 93,* 9235–9240.

Linnoila, M., Virkkunen, M., Scheinin, M., Nuutila, A., Rimon, R., & Goodwin, R. (1983). Low cerebrospinal fluid 5-hydroxyindoleacetic acid concentration differentiates impulsive from nonimpulsive violent behaviour. *Life Science, 33,* 2609–2614.

Luchins, D.J. (1984). Carbamazepine in violent non-epileptic schizophrenics. *Psychopharmacology Bulletin, 20,* 569–571.

Magura, S.R., Freeman, C., Siddiqi, Q., & Lipton, D.S. (1992). The validity of hair analysis for detecting cocaine and heroin use among addicts. *International Journal of Addictions, 27,* 51–69.

Marder, S.R., Davis, J.M., & Chouinard, G. (1997). The effect of risperidone on the five dimensions of schizophrenia derived by factor analysis: Combined results of the North American trials. *Journal of Clinical Psychiatry, 58,* 538–546.

McPhillips, M.A., Kelly, F.J., Barnes, T.R., Duke, P.J., Gene-Cos, N., & Clark, K.F. (1997). Detecting comorbid substance misuse among people with schizophrenia in the community: A study comparing the results of questionnaires with analysis of hair and urine. *Schizophrenia Research, 25,* 141–148.

Müller-Isberner, J.R. (1996). Forensic psychiatric aftercare following hospital order treatment. *International Journal of Law and Psychiatry, 19,* 81–86.

Naranjo, C.A., & Sellers, E.M. (1989). Serotonin uptake inhibitors attenuate ethanol intake in problem drinkers. *Recent Developments in Alcoholism, 7,* 255–266.

Naranjo, C.A., Sellers, E.M., Sullivan, J.T., Woodley, D.V., Kadlec, K., & Sykora, K. (1987). The serotonin uptake inhibitor citralopram attenuates ethanol intake. *Clinical Pharmacology and Therapeutics, 41,* 266–274.

Neppe, V.M. (1983). Carbamazepine as adjunctive treatment in nonepileptic chronic inpatients with EEG temporal lobe abnormalities. *Journal of Clinical Psychiatry, 44,* 326–331.

Neppe, V.M. (1988). Carbamazepine in nonresponsive psychosis. *Journal of Clinical Psychiatry, 49*(suppl), 22–28.

Okuma, T., Yamashita, I., Takahashi, R., Itoh, H., Otsuki, S., Watanabe, S., Sarai, K., Hazama, H., & Inanaga. K. (1989). A double-blind study of adjunctive carbamazepine versus placebo on excited states of schizophrenic and schizoaffective disorders. *Acta Psychiatrica Scandinavica, 80,* 250–259.

O'Malley, S.S., Jaffe, A.J., Chang, G., Schottenfeld, R.S., Meyer, R.E., & Rounsaville, B. (1992). Naltrexone and coping skills therapy for alcohol dependence. *Archives of General Psychiatry 49,* 881–887.

Osher, F.C., & Drake, R.E. (1996). Reversing a history of unmet needs: Approaches to caring for persons with co-occurring addictive and mental disorders. *American Journal of Orthopsychiatry, 66*(1), 4–11.

Perez, V., Gilaberte, I., Faries, D., Alvarez, E., & Artigas, F. (1997). Randomized, double-blind placebo-controlled trial of pindolol in combination with fluoxetine antidepressant treatment. *Lancet, 349,* 1594–1597.

Popik, P., Layer, R.T., Fossom, L.H., Benveniste, M., Geter-Douglass, B., Witkin, J.M., & Skolnick, P. (1995). NMDA antagonist properties of the putative antiaddictive drug ibogaine. *Journal of Pharmacology and Experimental Therapeutics, 275,* 753–760.

Putkonen, A., Kotilainen, I., & Tiihonen, J. (2000). Personality disorders among psychotic homicide offenders. Unpublished manuscript.

Räsänen, P., Hakko, H., & Tiihonen, J. (1999). Pindolol and major affective disorders: A three-year followup study of 30,485 patients. *Journal of Clinical Psychopharmacology, 19,* 297–302..

Räsänen, P., Tiihonen, J., Isohanni, M., Rantakallio, P., Lehtonen, J., & Moring, J. (1998). Schizophrenia, alcohol abuse, and violent behavior: A 26-year followup study of an unselected birth cohort. *Schizophrenia Bulletin, 24,* 437–441.

Rasmussen, D.L., Olivier, B., Raghoebar, M., & Mos, J. (1990). Possible clinical application of serenics and some implications of their preclinical profile for their clinical use in psychiatric disorders. *Drug Metabolism and Drug Interactions, 8,* 159–186.

Ratey, J.J., Sorgi, P., O'Driscoll, G.A., Sands, S., Daehler, M.L., Fletcher, J.R., Kadish, W., Spruiell, G., Polakoff, S., & Lindem, K.J. (1992). Nadolol to treat aggression and psychiatric symptomatology in chronic psychiatric inpatients: A double-blind, placebo-controlled study. *Journal of Clinical Psychiatry, 53,* 41–46.

Regier, D.A., Farmer, M.E., Rae, D.S., Locke, B.Z., Keith, S.J., Judd, L.L., & Goodwin, F.K. (1990). Comorbidity of mental disorders with alcohol and other drug abuse: Results from the Epidemiologic Catchment Area (ECA) study. *Journal of the American Medical Association, 264,* 2511–2518.

Ross, H.E., Glaser, F.B., & Germanson, T. (1988). The prevalence of psychiatric disorders in patients with alcohol and other drug problems. *Archives of General Psychiatry, 45,* 1023–1031.

Rossetti, Z.L., D'Aquila, P.S., Hmaidan, Y., Gessa, G.L., & Serra, G. (1991). Repeated treatment with imipramine potentiates cocaine-induced dopamine release and motor stimulation. *European Journal of Pharmacology, 201,* 243–245.

Saltzman, C., Wolfson, A.N., Schatzberg, A., Looper, J., Henke, R., Albanese, M., Schwartz, J., & Miyawaki, E. (1995). Effect of fluoxetine on anger in symptomatic volunteers with borderline personality disorder. *Journal of Clinical Psychopharmacology, 15,* 23–29.

Sass, H., Soyka, M., Mann, K., & Zieglgänsberger, W. (1996). Relapse prevention by acamprosate. Results from a placebo-controlled study on alcohol dependence. *Archives of General Psychiatry, 53,* 673–680.

Saudou, F., Amara, D.A., Dietrich, A., LeMeur, M., Ramboz, S., Segu, L., Buhot, M.C., & Hen, R. (1994). Enhanced aggressive behavior in mice lacking 5-HT$_{1B}$ receptor. *Science, 265,* 1875–1878.

Schottenfeld, R.S., & Kleber, H.D. (1995). Methadone maintenance. In H.I. Kaplan & B.J. Sadock (Eds.), *Comprehensive textbook of psychiatry, Vol. 5* (pp. 2031–2038). Baltimore: Williams & Wilkins.

Schottenfeld, R.S., Pakes, J.R., Oliveto, A., Ziedonis, D., & Kosten, T.R. (1997). Buprenorphine vs. methadone maintenance treatment for concurrent opioid dependence and cocaine abuse. *Archives of General Psychiatry, 54,* 713–720.

Sheard, M.H., Marini, J.L., Bridges, C.I., & Wagner, E. (1976). The effect of lithium on impulsive aggressive behavior in man. *American Journal of Psychiatry, 133,* 1409–1413.

Sheppard, G.P. (1979). High-dose propranolol in schizophrenia. *British Journal of Psychiatry, 134,* 470–476.

Shibahara, T., Hamada, S., & Uno, K. (1970). Psychotropic effect of carbamazepine (Tegretol). *Journal of New Remedies and Clinics, 19,* 509–515.

Smeraldi, E., Zanardi, R., Benedetti, F., Di Bella, D., Perez, J., & Catalano, M. (1998). Polymorphism within the promoter of the serotonin transporter gene and antidepressant efficacy of fluvoxamine. *Molecular Psychiatry, 3,* 508–511.

Smith, L.D. (1989). Medication refusal and the rehospiralized mentally ill inmate. *Hospital and Community Psychiatry, 40,* 491–496.

Sorensen, S.M., Jumphreys, T.M., Taylor, V.L., & Schmidt, C.J. (1992). 5-HT$_2$ receptor antagonists reverse amphetamine-induced slowing of dopaminergic neurons by interfering with stimulated dopamine synthesis. *Journal of Pharmacology and Experimental Therapics, 260,* 872–878.

Sorgi, P.J., Ratey, J.J., & Polakoff, S. (1986). ß-adrenergic blockers for the control of aggressive behaviors in patients with chronic schizophrenia. *American Journal of Psychiatry, 143,* 775–776.

Spanagel, R., Herz, A., Bals-Kubik, R., & Shippenberg, T.S. (1991). β-endorphin-induced locomotor stimulation and reinforcement are associated with an increase in dopamine release in the nucleus accumbens. *Psychopharmacology* [Berlin], *104,* 51–56.

Steadman, H.J., Mulvey, E.P., Monahan, J., Robbins, P.C., Appelbaum, P.S., Grisso, T., Roth, L.H., & Silver, E. (1998). Violence by people discharged from acute psychiatric inpatient facilities and by others in the same neighborhoods. *Archives of General Psychiatry, 55,* 393–401.

Strous, R., Bark, N., Volavka, J., Parsia, S.S., & Lachman, H.M. (1997). Association of COMT codon 158 polymorphism aggressive and antisocial behavior in schizophrenia. *Psychiatry Research, 69,* 71–77.

Swanson, J.W. (1994). Mental disorder, substance abuse, and community violence: An epidemiological approach. In J. Monahan & H.J. Steadman (Eds.), *Violence and mental disorder: Developments in risk assessment*. Chicago: University of Chicago Press.

Swanson, J.W., Borum, R., Swartz, M.S., & Monahan, J. (1996). Psychotic symptoms and disorders and the risk of violent behavior in the community. *Criminal Behavior and Mental Health, 6,* 309–329.

Swartz, M.S., Swanson, J.W., Hiday, V.A., Borum, R., Wagner, H.R., & Burns, B.J. (1998a). Violence and severe mental illness: The effects of substance abuse and nonadherence to medication. *American Journal of Psychiatry, 155,* 226–231.

Swartz, M.S., Swanson, J.W., Hiday, V.A., Borum, R., Wagner, H.R., & Burns, B.J. (1998b). Taking the wrong drugs: The role of substance abuse and medication noncompliance in violence among severely mentally ill individuals. *Social Psychiatry and Psychiatric Epidemiology, 33*(suppl 1), S75–80.

Swofford, C.D., Kasckow, J.W., Scheller-Gilkey, G., & Inderbitzin, L.B. (1996). Substance use: A powerful predictor of relapse in schizophrenia. *Schizophrenia Research, 20,* 145–151.

Taylor, P.J., Leese, M., Williams, D., Butwell, M., Daly, R., & Larkin, E. (1998). Mental disorder and violence: A special (high security) hospital study. *British Journal of Psychiatry, 172,* 218–226.

Tennant, F.S. Jr., Rawson, R.A., Cohen, A.J., & Mann, A. (1984). Clinical experience with naltrexone in suburban opioid addicts. *Journal of Clinical Psychiatry, 45,* 42–45.

Thor, D.H., & Ghiselli, W.P. (1975). Suppression of mouse killing and apomorphine-induced social aggression in rats by local anesthesia of the mystacial vibrissae. *Journal of Comparative Physiology and Psychology, 88,* 40–46.

Tiihonen, J., Hakola, P., Eronen, M., Vartiainen, H., & Ryynänen, O-P. (1996). Risk of homicidal behavior among discharged forensic psychiatric patients. *Forensic Science International, 79,* 123–129.

Tiihonen, J., Hakola, P., Paanila, J., & Turtiainen, M. (1993). Eltoprazine for aggression in schizophrenia and mental retardation. *Lancet, 341,* 307.

Tiihonen, J., Hallikainen, H., Lachman, H., Saito, S., Volavka, J., Kauhanen, J., Salonen, J., Ryynänen, O-P., Koulu, M., Karvonen, M., Pohjalainen, T., Syvälahti, E., & Hietala, J. (1999). Association between the functional variant of the catechol-*O*-methyltransferase (COMT) gene and type 1 alcoholism. *Molecular Psychiatry, 4,* 286–289.

Tiihonen, J., Isohanni, M., Räsänen, P., Koiranen, M., & Moring, J. (1997). Specific major mental disorders and criminality: A 26-year prospective study of the 1966 northern Finland birth cohort. *American Journal of Psychiatry, 154,* 840–845.

Tiihonen, J., Ryynänen, O-P., Kauhanen, J., Hakola, H.P.A., & Salaspuro, M. (1996). Citalopram in the treatment of alcoholism: A double-blind placebo-controlled study. *Pharmacopsychiatry, 29,* 27–29.

Tiihonen, J., Vartiainen, H., & Hakola, P. (1995). Carbamazepine-induced changes in plasma levels of neuroleptics. *Pharmacopsychiatry, 28,* 26–28.

Tupin, J.P., Smith, D.B., Clanon, T.L., Kim, L.I., Nugent, A., & Groupe, A. (1973). The long-term use of lithium in aggressive prisoners. *Comprehensive Psychiatry, 14,* 311–317.

Uhde, T.W., & Tancer, M.E. (1995). Benzodiazepine receptor agonists and antagonists. In H.I. Kaplan & B.J. Sadock (Eds.), *Comprehensive textbook of psychiatry V, Vol. II, 6th ed.* (p. 1939). Baltimore: Williams & Wilkins.

Vartiainen, H., Tiihonen, J., Putkonen, A., Koponen, H., Virkkunen, M., Hakola, P., & Lehto, H. (1995). Citalopram, a selective serotonin reuptake inhibitor, in the treatment of aggression in schizophrenia. *Acta Psychiatrica Scandinavica, 91,* 348–351.

Vartiainen, H.T., & Hakola, H.P.A. (1992). How changes in mental health law adversely affect offenders discharged from security hospital. *Journal of Forensic Psychiatry, 3,* 563–570.

Verhoeven, W.M.A., Tuinier, S., Sijben, N.A.S., van den Berg, Y.W.H.M., & de Witte-van der Schoot, E.P.P.M. (1992). Eltoprazine in mentally retarded self-injuring patients. *Lancet, 340,* 1037–1038.

Virkkunen, M., DeJong, J., Bartko, J., Goodwin, F.K., & Linnoila, M. (1989). Relationship of psychobiological variables to recidivism in violent offenders and impulsive fire setters: A follow-up study. *Archives of General Psychiatry, 46,* 600–603.

Virkkunen, M., Eggert, M., Rawlings, R., & Linnoila, M.L. (1996). A prospective follow-up study of alcoholic violent offenders and fire setters. *Archives of General Psychiatry, 53,* 523–529.

Virkkunen, M., Rawlings, R., Tokola, R., Poland, R.E., Guidotti, A., Nemeroff, C., Bissette, G., Kalogeras, K., Karonen, S-L., & Linnoila, M. (1994). CSF biochemistries, glucose metabolism, and diurnal activity rhythms in alcoholic, violent offenders, fire setters, and healthy volunteers. *Archives of General Psychiatry, 51,* 20–27.

Volavka, J., Zito, J.M., Vitrai, J., & Czobar, P. (1993). Clozapine effects on hostility and aggression in schizophrenia. *Journal of Clinical Psychopharmacology, 13,* 287–289.

Volpicelli, J.R., Alterman, A.I., Hayashida, M., & O'Brien, C.P. (1992). Naltrexone in the treatment of alcohol dependence. *Archives of General Psychiatry, 49,* 876–880.

Warner, E.A., Kosten, T.R., & O'Connor, P.G. (1997). Pharmacotherapy for opioid and cocaine abuse. *Medical Clinics of North America, 8,* 909–925.

Wilcox, J. (1994). Divalproex sodium in the treatment of aggressive behavior. *Annals of Clinical Psychiatry, 6,* 17–20.

Wodak, A. (1994). Managing illicit drug use: A practical guide. *Drugs, 47,* 446–457.

Yoshimoto, K., McBride, W.J., Lumeng, L., & Li, T.K. (1991). Alcohol stimulates the release of dopamine and serotonin in the nucleus accumbens. *Alcohol, 9,* 17–22.

Jari Tiihonen is Professor and Medical Director, Department of Forensic Psychiatry, University of Kuopio and Niuvanniemi Hospital, Kuopio, Finland. Marvin S. Swartz is Professor and Head, Division of Social and Community Psychiatry, Duke University Medical Center, Durham, North Carolina, USA.

Authors' Note

Comments or queries may be directed to Jari Tiihonen, MD, PhD, Department of Forensic Psychiatry, University of Kuopio, Niuvanniemi Hospital, FIN-70240 Kuopio, Finland. Telephone: 358 17 203 202. Fax: 358 17 203 494. E-mail: <Jari. Tiihonen@uku.fi>.

PHARMACOLOGICAL INTERVENTIONS FOR PREVENTING VIOLENCE AMONG THE MENTALLY ILL WITH CO-OCCURRING PERSONALITY DISORDERS

JAN VOLAVKA
LESLIE CITROME

Antisocial Personality Disorder and Psychopathy

Antisocial personality disorder (APD) is partly defined by the history of violent behaviour (DSM-IV), and psychopathy is known to be associated with violent crime (Hare, 1996; Hare & McPherson, 1984). Psychopathy is a term that had been used rather loosely until Cleckley (1976) endowed it with specific content, conceptual framework, and clinical descriptions. Hare and his group have developed the concept and provided several versions of a diagnostic instrument—the Psychopathy Checklist. The version most frequently used in criminal offender populations is called the Hare Psychopathy Checklist-Revised (PCL-R); this is a 20-item rating scale. A cut-off score of 30 (or 25 by some authors) implies the diagnosis of psychopathy.

A 12-item version of the PCL-R was developed for use in the study of violence in the mentally disordered; it is called Psychopathy Checklist: Screening Version (PCL:SV) (Table 1) (Hart, Hare, & Forth, 1994). Each of the 12 items on the PCL:SV is scored on a 3-point scale: 0 = does not apply; 1 = applies to a certain extent; 2 = item applies. A cut-off score of 18 implies definite diagnosis of psychopathy; 13 implies possible psychopathy. The relative merits of the diagnosis of psychopathy (Hare, 1980) versus APD (DSM-IV) are a matter of continuing debate (Hare, 1996). APD is defined primarily in terms of behaviour (i.e., persistent violation of social norms), whereas psychopathy refers to characteristic affective and interpersonal styles (Factor 1) as well as to socially deviant behaviours (Factor 2) (Table 1).

Although most psychopaths also meet the criteria for APD, most subjects diagnosed with antisocial personality disorder do not meet the criteria for psychopathy: Psychopathy is a narrower concept.

S. Hodgins (ed.), Violence among the Mentally Ill, 193–209.
© 2000 *Kluwer Academic Publishers. Printed in the Netherlands.*

Table 1. The Hare Psychopathy Checklist: Screening Version (PCL:SV)

F1: Interpersonal/affective traits	F2: Social deviance
1. Superficial	7. Impulsive
2. Grandiose	8. Poor behavior controls
3. Manipulative	9. Lacks goals
4. Lacks remorse	10. Irresponsible
5. Lacks empathy	11. Adolescent antisocial behavior
6. Doesn't accept responsibility	12. Adult antisocial behavior

Source: Hart, Hare, and Forth (1994)

Comorbidity of Major Mental Disorders with Personality Disorders

There is general agreement that APD and schizophrenia may co-occur; for example, 63% of Canadian criminal offenders diagnosed with schizophrenia were also diagnosed with APD (Côté & Hodgins, 1990). Furthermore, when APD is diagnosed in combination with a major mental disorder (including schizophrenia), the patient's risk of crime is increased as compared to patients who have a major disorder without APD. Surprisingly, the patients with the combination of major disorder and APD were no more likely to behave violently than those with a major disorder without APD (Hodgins & Côté, 1993).

The possibility of co-occurrence of psychopathy and schizophrenia is less clear than the case for APD and schizophrenia. In administering the PCL-R to various groups of mentally disordered offenders, Hodgins, Côté, and Toupin (1998) observed a low rate of co-occurrence of psychopathy and major mental disorder. Similar results were reported by others who used the PCL in similar populations (Freese, Müller-Isberner, & Jockel, 1995; Nedopil, Hollweg, Hartmann, & Jaser, 1998; Owen, Tarantello, Jones, & Tennant, 1998). However, the PCL scores among schizophrenics hospitalized on a special unit for aggressive patients were significantly higher than those of comparison non-aggressive schizophrenia patients (Rasmussen, Levander, & Sletvold, 1995).

Using a strategy similar to that employed by Rasmussen et al. (1995), Nolan, Volavka, Mohr, and Czobor (1999) administered the PCL:SV to a set of persistently violent schizophrenic or schizoaffective patients ($N = 26$) and to non-violent schizophrenic or schizoaffective controls ($N = 25$). The results are displayed in Table 2. Mean psychopathy scores were higher for the violent than for the non-violent patients. Five (19%) of the violent patients had scores exceeding the cut-off for psychopathy, and 13 (50%) scored in the possible psychopathic range. All of the non-violent patients scored below the cut-off for possible psychopathy. The higher PCL scores in the violent group were not solely due to the assaultive acts by which that group was defined. If that were the case, the association between violence and psychopathy would have been tautological and trivial. As seen in Table 2, violent subjects scored higher on both Factor 1 (interpersonal and affective traits) and Factor 2 (antisocial behaviour). Thus, it appears that the comorbidity between psychopathy and major mental disorders is low in general forensic populations but high among persistently violent schizophrenic patients.

Table 2. Hare Psychopathy Checklist: Screening Version (mean ± standard deviation) as a function of history of violent behaviour

	Non-violent ($n = 25$)	Violent ($n = 26$)	Total ($n = 51$)	F (df)	p
Total	4.84 + 2.15	14.31 + 3.38	9.67 + 5.55	141.04 (1,49)	.000
Factor 1	2.08 + 1.58	5.89 + 2.20	4.02 + 2.70	50.08 (1,49)	.000
Factor 2	2.76 + 1.96	8.42 + 2.44	5.65 + 3.60	84.42 (1,49)	.000

These findings may imply that persistently violent schizophrenic patients can be classified into subtypes (depending on the presence or absence of comorbid psychopathy). We hypothesize that these subtypes differ in their pathogenesis. Possible implications of these findings for prevention and treatment strategies remain to be explored.

Comorbidity of Major Mental Disorders with Personality Disorders and Substance Use Disorders

Although another chapter of this volume is focused on substance use disorders and violence, it is impossible to separate this topic from our present discussion of major mental disorders comorbid with personality disorders. Among patients with major mental disorders (schizophrenia or schizoaffective disorder) and comorbid substance abuse, those diagnosed with APD demonstrated more severe forms of alcohol and drug abuse and more aggressive behaviour (Mueser et al., 1997). These findings suggest that patients with major mental disorders and comorbid APD represent a high-risk subgroup "by virtue of an additional risk of APD for aggressive and generally non-compliant behaviour and by virtue of the heightened risk for substance abuse" (Mueser et al., p. 476). These results have major implications for pharmacological interventions to prevent violence in patients with major mental disorders plus APD.

Poor compliance with pharmacological treatment in combination with substance use significantly elevates the risk for violent behaviour in patients with major mental disorders (Swartz et al., 1998). The well-established elevation of risk for violence in patients with major mental disorders by comorbid substance use (Scott et al., 1998; Steadman et al., 1998; Swanson, 1994) may be due in part to underlying APD and non-compliance with treatment. Whatever the relationships among comorbid personality disorders, comorbid substance use disorders, and treatment compliance, successful treatment of violent behaviour in major mental disorders requires attention to comorbid conditions and assurance of treatment compliance.

Treatment Compliance (Adherence)

Compliance with antipsychotic treatment is very important for the prevention of violent behaviour by patients with major mental disorders. In some patients, side effects are the reason for non-compliance. Switching such patients to an antipsychotic that causes fewer side effects and using the minimal effective dose levels may solve the problem. Other patients stop their medicine because they have difficulty remembering to take it or to keep their appointments. These patients may be managed using an intramuscular depot (slow-release) form of medication; these injections are given only once every 2 to 4 weeks. For various reasons, including poor insight into their illness, some violent schizophrenic patients resist, overtly or covertly, taking any form of medication. As long as they are in the hospital, this resistance can usually be overcome by clinical and legal methods that vary across hospitals and jurisdictions. However, the situation is more difficult when these patients are residing in the community. There are patients who become violent in the community after they stop their medication, the violence leads to a hospital admission, they respond well to medication in the hospital and are discharged, then stop taking the medicine, become violent, and the cycle starts again. The combination of non-adherence to treatment and the abuse of drugs and alcohol is particularly likely to result in violent behaviour (Swartz et al., 1998).

In order to break this cycle of violence, several US states have adopted or are experimenting with outpatient commitment programmes intended largely for psychotic patients with records of repeated violent behaviour and poor compliance with treatment. Under this system, a court orders the patient to follow a course of treatment (usually including antipsychotic medication) while living in the community. The patient is supervised; if he or she fails to comply, the police can be called and the patient involuntarily hospitalized. Proponents of this system argue that the outpatient commitment programmes will improve adherence to treatment, reduce violent behaviour by patients in the community, reduce the need for hospitalization, and result in shorter hospital stays for the involuntarily hospitalized patients committed through these programmes. While civil libertarians complain that the outpatient commitment violates patients' rights, its proponents argue that these programmes are needed to help schizophrenic patients who have no insight into their illness and to protect their potential victims. The effectiveness of outpatient commitment in the prevention of violence by patients with major mental disorders has not yet been formally demonstrated. A preliminary trial designed to test outpatient commitment in New York City has yielded some results that are interesting for outpatient care in general, but has provided no information about the effect of outpatient commitment on violence, since patients with a history of violence were not included (unpublished report). Another trial, by Swartz and colleagues, is in progress in North Carolina.

Transient or Persistent Violence

Most patients with major mental disorders do not exhibit violent behaviour. In those patients who do, violence subsides within several weeks after they start antipsychotic treatment and—if applicable—stop using alcohol and drugs. In these *transiently violent* patients, ensuring continued adherence to antipsychotic treatment (using typical or atypical medications) and abstinence from substance use will constitute long-term prevention of violent behaviour. However, there is a subgroup of schizophrenic patients who remain violent in spite of antipsychotic treatment and lack of access to alcohol and drugs. Such patients contribute disproportionate numbers of violent incidents recorded in psychiatric hospitals: In a US survey, 5% of inpatients were responsible for 53% of violent incidents (Convit, Isay, Otis, & Volavka, 1990). In an Australian study, 12% of inpatients accounted for 69% of violent incidents (Owen et al., 1998).

These *persistently violent* patients present a major challenge to long-term management. In many cases, these patients are best managed at specialized secure units with highly trained staff. Their illness (and its neurobiological underpinning) is apparently different from the more typical schizophrenia seen in the transiently violent and the non-violent patients (Krakowski, Convit, Jaeger, Lin, & Volavka, 1989a, 1989b; Volavka & Krakowski, 1989). These patients do not respond well to typical antipsychotics; nevertheless, they are sometimes treated with high doses of these agents (Krakowski, Kunz, Czobor, & Volavka, 1993).

Pharmacological Management

ATYPICAL ANTIPSYCHOTICS

The antiaggressive effects of these agents are under intensive investigation. The specificity of such antiaggressive effects is an important consideration. It can be understood in two ways: First, in order to be specific, the antiaggressive effect should not be mediated by sedation; the independence of antiaggressive and sedative effects of clozapine has been demonstrated (Chiles, Davidson, & McBride, 1994). Second, the specific antiaggressive effect should be relatively independent of general antipsychotic effects; this independence has also been demonstrated for clozapine (Volavka , Zito, Vitrai, & Czobor, 1993). This subtype of specificity is important for the consideration of an agent as a potential antiaggressive treatment in persons who are not psychotic.

Many reports support the long-term, perhaps specific, antiaggressive efficacy of clozapine in schizophrenic and schizoaffective patients. This evidence, however, is based on open, uncontrolled studies in which patients were assigned to clozapine treatment on a clinical basis (rather than being randomized) and the data were collected in a retrospective record review; these studies are summarized in Table 3.

In spite of the methodological weaknesses of individual studies, the cumulative evidence for the antiaggressive effects of clozapine appears to be relatively strong. The antiaggressive effects of clozapine are not limited to patients with the diagnoses of schizophrenia or schizoaffective disorder (Volavka & Citrome, 1999).

Other atypical antipsychotics may also have antiaggressive effects that may be similar to those of clozapine, but not much data are available yet (Table 3). There is some evidence that risperidone may reduce hostility (Czobor, Volavka, & Meibach, 1995) and aggression (Buckley et al., 1997) in schizophrenic patients. Analogous data for olanzapine and quetiapine are being analyzed and prepared for publication. In general, the literature on antiaggressive effects of antipsychotics is plagued by serious methodological problems that are reviewed and analyzed elsewhere (Volavka & Citrome, 1999).

Table 3. Studies of the effects of atypical antipsychotics on hostile and aggressive behaviour in patients with major mental disorders

Author, year	Drug	N	Diagnosis	Study type	Control group	Patient assign- ment	Measure of effect
Michals et al., 1993	CLO[*]	9	Brain injury	Open; retro- spective rec- ord review	None	Clinical	Clinical response documented in the medical record
Maier, 1992	CLO	25	Schizo- phrenia, schizoaf- fective	Open; retro- spective rec- ord review	None	Clinical	Security Level, discharge
Mallya et al., 1992	CLO	107	"chronic" patients	Open; retro- spective rec- ord review	None	Clinical	Seclusion and restraint
Ratey et al., 1993	CLO	5	Schizo- phrenia	Open; retro- spective rec- ord review	None	Clinical	Seclusion and re- straint, aggressive incidents, BPRS
Volavka et al., 1993	CLO	223	Schizo- phrenia	Open; retro- spective rec- ord review	None	Clinical	BPRS Hostility item
Ebrahim et al., 1994	CLO	27	Schizo- phrenia, schizoaf- fective	Open; retro- spective rec- ord review	None	Clinical	Seclusion and restraint, BPRS, Level of Privileges
Chiles et al., 1994	CLO	139	Schizo- phrenia, schizoaf- fective	Open; retro- spective rec- ord review	None	Clinical	Seclusion and restraint, NOSIE
Buckley et al., 1995	CLO	30	Schizo- phrenia	Open; retro- spective rec- ord review	None	Clinical	Seclusion and restraint, BPRS
Wilson & Claussen, 1995[+]	CLO	100	Chronic psychosis	Open; retro- spective rec- ord review	None	Clinical	Episodes of aggression
Czobor et al., 1995	RIS[#]	139	Schizo- phrenia	Randomized clinical trial	Haloperidol, placebo	Random	PANSS Hostility item
Rabi- nowitz et al., 1996	CLO	75	Schizo- phrenia	Open; retro- spective rec- ord review	None	Clinical	Incidents of physical or verbal aggression, BPRS Hostility item
Buckley et al., 1997	RIS	27	Schizo- phrenia, schizoaf- fective	Open; case- control study	Conven- tional anti- psychotics	Clinical	Seclusion and restraint
Cantillon et al., 1997	QUE[&]	351	Schizo- phrenia	Randomized clinical trial	Haloperidol, placebo	Random	BPRS Hostility item

Author, year	Drug	N	Diagnosis	Study type	Control group	Patient assign-ment	Measure of effect
Marder et al., 1997 $	RIS	513	Schizo-phrenia	Randomized clinical trial	Haloperidol, placebo	Random	BPRS Factor 4 (uncontrolled hos-tility/excitement)

Legend
* CLO Clozapine
# RIS Risperidone
& QUE Quetiapine
+ Includes data from an earlier publication (Wilson, 1992)
$ Uses same database as Czobor et al., 1995
BPRS: Brief Psychiatric Rating Scale (Guy, 1986)
PANSS: Positive and Negative Symptom Scale (Kay, Fiszbein, & Opler, 1987)
NOSIE: Nurses' Observation Scale for Inpatient Evaluation (Honigfeld & Klett, 1965)

ADJUNCTIVE TREATMENTS

Many patients with major mental disorders who are persistently violent are treated with a combination of an antipsychotic and an adjunctive medication.

Mood stabilizers

These substances are widely used in the management of mood disorders. Although the antiaggressive effect of mood stabilizers in schizophrenic patients is generally not mentioned in psychopharmacology textbooks, these compounds are apparently used quite widely for this indication. An expert consensus statement recommends mood stabilizers as adjunctive treatment for "persistent excitement" in schizophrenic patients receiving typical antipsychotics (Frances, Docherty, & Kahn, 1996). Persistent excitement may include persistent aggressive behaviour (but aggression is not explicitly addressed in the consensus statement).

Lithium. The number of infractions involving violent behaviour was reduced by lithium treatment of recurrently violent prisoners in open trials (Sheard, 1971; Tupin et al., 1973) as well as in a double-blind, placebo-controlled study (Sheard, Marini, Bridges, & Wagner, 1976). Lithium plasma levels in these trials were mostly below 1.0 Meq/L; such relatively low levels are not generally associated with lethargy or general suppression of motor activity in adult patients. Most prisoners in the open trial (Tupin et al.) had various organic mental syndromes or schizophrenia, whereas the subjects in the controlled trial were described as having "nonpsychotic personality disorders" (Sheard et al.).

The effectiveness of lithium therapy in schizophrenia is not established. Active affective symptoms, previous affective episodes, and a family history of affective disorder may predict a favourable response to lithium (Atre-Vaidya & Taylor, 1989), but also provide clues that the diagnosis may be something other than schizophrenia (Citrome, 1989). A double-blind placebo-controlled, parallel-design clinical trial, involving seriously ill state hospital patients with schizophrenia who had not responded to prior trials of typical neuroleptics, demonstrated no advantage of lithium combined with haloperidol over haloperidol alone (Wilson, 1993). When lithium was added to neuroleptics for the treatment of resistant schizophrenic patients classified as "dangerous, violent, or criminal," no benefits were seen after 4 weeks of adjunctive lithium therapy (Collins, Larkin, & Shubsachs, 1991). However, there are case reports of patients with paranoid schizophrenia with aggressive or disorderly behaviours who responded to the addition of lithium to their neuroleptic treatment, then deteriorated after the lithium was discontinued, but subsequently improved when it was reinstituted (Prakash, 1985).

Carbamazepine. The antiaggressive effects of carbamazepine as an adjunctive treatment in schizophrenic and schizoaffective patients has been suggested by two placebo-controlled studies. The first study (Neppe, 1983) was small and included patients with other diagnoses. The second study (Okuma et al., 1989) involved 162 schizophrenic or schizoaffective patients receiving various antipsychotics (open-label) who were randomized to one of two adjunctive treatments: carbamazepine or placebo (double-blind). The study demonstrated a significantly better effect of carbamazepine on agitation and aggression. Unfortunately, these two behaviours were commingled in data analysis; thus, the report does not permit an assessment of antiaggressive effects per se. In addition to these placebo-controlled studies, observations suggest antiaggressive effects of carbamazepine in schizophrenic and schizoaffective patients (Hakola & Laulumaa, 1982; Luchins, 1984; Yassa & Dupont, 1983). Thus, adjunctive carbamazepine may indeed cause antiaggressive effects in such patients. However, definitive studies demonstrating such effects are lacking.

Valproate. In a survey of 12,444 inpatients in New York State psychiatric hospitals, 28% of all patients diagnosed with schizophrenia received valproate (valproic acid or divalproex sodium) in 1996 (Citrome, Levine, & Allingham, 1998). This percentage increased to 35% in 1998 (Citrome et al., unpublished data). A previous survey of a smaller subset of the same inpatient population suggested that the intended effects of this treatment were improvements in impulse control and reduction in aggressive behaviour (Citrome, 1995).

Valproate may have antiaggressive effects, but the evidence for its efficacy is based only on uncontrolled studies and case reports describing mostly patients with dementia, mental retardation, and brain injuries (Donovan et al., 1997; Geracioti, 1994; Giakas, Seibyl, & Mazure, 1990; Hollander, Grossman, Stein, & Kwon, 1996; Horne & Lindley, 1995; Lott, McElroy, & Keys, 1995; Mattes, 1992; Mazure, Druss, & Cellar, 1992; Mellow, Solano-Lopez, & Davis, 1993; Wilcox, 1994; Wroblewski, Joseph, Kupfer, & Kalliel, 1997). Very little is known about the antiaggressive efficacy of valproate in patients with schizophrenia. The widespread use of valproate for the control of aggressive behaviour in schizophrenic patients does not appear to be based on evidence of effectiveness. This is troubling, particularly in view of its potential for hepatotoxicity, as well as its effect on the cost of long-term treatment of schizophrenic patients.

Gabapentin. Another anticonvulsant, gabapentin has been used as a new treatment for bipolar disorder (Schaffer & Schaffer, 1997), and suggestions have been made that this agent may be useful in the management of behaviour dyscontrol (Ryback & Ryback, 1995). Similar to valproate, gabapentin has also been used as an adjunctive agent in the treatment of schizophrenia. In 1998, the prescription rate for gabapentin in New York State psychiatric hospital patients diagnosed with schizophrenia exceeded that for carbamazepine (3.7% vs. 3.5%) (Citrome et al., unpublished data).

Selective serotonin reuptake inhibitors (SSRIs)
Since reduced central serotonin turnover is associated with impulsive aggression (Coccaro, Kavoussi, Cooper, & Hauger, 1997), SSRIs would be expected to inhibit aggression. Indeed, fluoxetine has been shown to have antiaggressive effects in persons with personality disorders (Coccaro & Kavoussi, 1997) and perhaps—as an adjunctive treatment—in schizophrenic patients (Goldman & Janecek, 1990). In a double-blind crossover study, citalopram showed convincing antiaggressive effects as an adjunctive treatment in forensic patients diagnosed with schizophrenia (Vartiainen et al., 1995).

Benzodiazepines
For a long time, benzodiazepines as needed (p.r.n.) have been commonly used in the short-term management of aggression (see above). More recently, however, these compounds are increasingly used on a continuous basis (i.e., not merely p.r.n.) for the long-term management of persistently violent patients. Thus, some of these patients are, over many months, receiving regular daily doses of benzodiazepines for the control of aggressive behaviour. The effectiveness of such long-term treatment has not been demonstrated; indeed, one might expect development of tolerance (and attendant loss of efficacy) after several weeks of continued administration of benzodiazepines.

In several psychiatric facilities in New York State, clonazepam is prescribed routinely to control aggression in schizophrenic patients. There are several case reports suggesting the antiaggressive effects of clonazepam in various disorders other than schizophrenia. However, in a double-blind, placebo-controlled trial, adjunctive clonazepam had no beneficial effect in schizophrenic patients, and some of the patients showed an *increase* in violent behaviour after administration of clonazepam (Karson, Weinberger, Bigelow, & Wyatt, 1982). Thus, continuous benzodiazepine treatment of persistent aggressive behaviour in schizophrenia does not appear to be based on evidence of effectiveness. The use of clonazepam to control aggression in schizophrenic patients who do not have concomitant seizure disorder seems particularly questionable.

Beta-adrenergic blocking agents
These compounds have been used to treat persistent aggressive behaviour in a variety of conditions (Volavka, 1995, pp. 279–283). Isolated cases of successful treatment of aggression with propranolol in particularly assaultive schizophrenic patients have been reported (Sorgi, Ratey, & Polakoff, 1986; Whitman, Maier, & Eichelman, 1987). A retrospective chart review demonstrated antiaggressive effects of nadolol

in six patients with chronic schizophrenia (Sorgi et al.). A double-blind, placebo-controlled parallel-group trial of nadolol in aggressive, mostly schizophrenic patients ($N = 41$) demonstrated the superiority of nadolol in reducing incidents of overt aggression (Ratey et al., 1992). Unfortunately, there appeared to be a considerable difference in the level of aggression between the two treatment groups at baseline; it is not clear whether this difference affected the outcome.

Interestingly, nadolol is a relatively lipophobic compound that is accordingly believed not to cross the blood-brain barrier to any great extent (although this belief is not universal; see Whitman et al., 1987). Thus, these encouraging results with a lipophobic drug suggest that at least some of the antiaggressive action of beta-blocking agents may have a peripheral mechanism of action. A peripheral component of akathisia, tension, or anxiety might be improved by nadolol, and the antiaggressive effect may be mediated by these improvements. Akathisia may increase the propensity for aggressive behaviour (Crowner et al., 1990; Keckich, 1978).

Thus, although rigorously designed studies have not yet been done, adjunctive beta-adrenergic blocking agents may have antiaggressive effects in persistently violent schizophrenic patients. The mechanism of this effect is unclear. As mentioned above, the effects may be peripheral. It is also possible that the mechanism involves central antiadrenergic activity; this would be compatible with the recently reported association between persistent violence and the low-activity allele in the catechol-*O*-methyltransferase gene (Lachman, Nolan, Mohr, Saito, & Volavka, 1998; Strous, Bark, Parsia, Volavka, & Lachman, 1997). Finally, there may be pharmacokinetic interactions between beta-blockers and antipsychotics (Silver, Yudofsky, Kogan, & Katz, 1986). The beta-blocker treatment of aggression does not seem particularly popular; this may due be in part to the dose-limiting side effects (such as hypotension and bradycardia) of these compounds. The use of beta-blockers for the treatment of aggression in major mental disorders may have been supplanted by atypical antipsychotics, notably clozapine.

Future Directions

Pharmacological interventions with the explicit or implicit aim of preventing violence in patients with major mental disorders and comorbid personality disorders are implemented daily by thousands of practitioners. Nevertheless, the rationale for such interventions is not based on strong evidence. Providing such evidence should be the focus of future systematic research. We will outline the directions for such research.

COMORBID PERSONALITY DISORDERS

At this point, perceptive readers might have noticed that we did not explain how this comorbidity with major mental disorders affects pharmacological treatment decisions. Notwithstanding the ambitious title of our chapter, we regret to admit that we do not know the answer. Research addressing this problem has yet to be done. Such research will need to include studies of heterogeneity of violent behaviour.

CROSS-SECTIONAL HETEROGENEITY OF VIOLENT BEHAVIOUR

Violent behaviour is notoriously heterogeneous (Volavka, 1995). Some of the violent behaviour in psychotic patients is attributable directly to psychotic symptoms (e.g., delusions). At the other end of the spectrum, patients diagnosed with major mental disorders may commit predatory violent crimes. Such crimes may occur while the patients are showing no overt psychotic symptoms and while their psychosis is being treated (Volavka et al., 1995). It seems plausible that these two subtypes of violent behaviour will have different responses to pharmacological treatments. Future research should address this question.

Along similar lines, there are neurobiological differences between impulsive and premeditated violent behaviour (Bergeman & Seroczynski, 1998). It seems logical that pharmacological approaches to these two subtypes should be different. Research should elucidate this issue.

TEMPORAL HETEROGENEITY OF VIOLENT BEHAVIOUR AND THE DEVELOPMENT OF MENTAL ILLNESS

The history of violent patients with major mental disorders shows that their contact with psychiatric service agencies started earlier than it did for non-violent patients. This is particularly true for patients showing persistent violence and comorbidity with personality and substance use disorders. In these cases, it appears that the first psychiatric symptoms are those compatible with the diagnosis of conduct disorder. It is likely that optimal preventative and therapeutic efforts to help these patients will differ depending on their age and the stage of development of their illness. These issues would be best addressed by longitudinal prospective studies of relatively symptom-free high-risk subjects, as well as first-episode patients.

GENETIC HETEROGENEITY OF VIOLENT BEHAVIOUR AND ITS POSSIBLE PHARMACOGENETIC CONSEQUENCES

Violent behaviour in schizophrenic and schizoaffective male patients is associated with a polymorphism of the gene that codes for catechol-O-methyltransferase, one of the two enzymes responsible for the biotransformation of catecholamines (Lachman et al., 1998; Strous et al., 1997). It seems logical that this polymorphism might explain in some part the variability in antiaggressive clinical response to beta-adrenergic blockers such as propranolol. Along similar lines, low-activity serotonin transporter promoter genotype is found in Type 2 alcoholics (these patients are prone to violent behaviour) (Hallikainen et al., in press). Would the SSRI have particularly pronounced antiaggressive effect in patients who exhibit this genotype?

HETEROGENEITY DUE TO THE TYPE OF MAJOR MENTAL DISORDER (AXIS I)

Most of the research cited in this chapter has been concerned with schizophrenia and schizoaffective disorder. Much less is known about aggressive behaviour and its treatment in major mood disorders, delusional disorder, and atypical psychoses.

PSYCHOPATHY OR APD?

Research in the area of psychopharmacology of aggression in patients who have major mental disorder plus comorbid personality disorder should use a standard measure of personality disorder. We recommend that the PCL:SV be that standard measure. The reasons for this recommendation are as follows:

- The APD definition (DSM-IV) relies too heavily on violent behaviour, making it difficult to avoid a tautological error when using this concept in research on violence.
- Psychopathy has been redefined by Hare and his associates so that the important aspects of personality traits (such as affective and interpersonal components) are assessed separately from violent behaviour.
- Samples of persons diagnosed with APD are more heterogeneous than samples of persons diagnosed with psychopathy, with respect to personality, attitudes, and motivation for violent behaviour.
- Unlike the APD diagnosis, the PCL:SV has been developed specifically for use with persons with major mental disorders.
- Unlike the APD, the PCL:SV has psychometric properties (such as reliability) that have been extensively tested in samples of patients with major mental disorders. These results have been published. Training sessions for future PCL:SV raters are available.

References

Atre-Vaidya, N., & Taylor, M.A. (1989). Effectiveness of lithium in schizophrenia: Do we really have an answer? *Journal of Clinical Psychiatry, 50,* 170–173.

Bergeman, C.S., & Seroczynski, A.D. (1998). Genetic and environmental influences on aggression and impulsivity. In M. Maes & E.F. Coccaro (Eds.), *Neurobiology and clinical views on aggression and impulsivity* (pp. 63–80). Chichester: Wiley.

Buckley, P., Bartell, J., Donenwirth, K., Lee, S., Torigoe, F., & Schulz, S.C. (1995). Violence and schizophrenia: Clozapine as a specific antiaggressive agent. *Bulletin of the American Academy of Psychiatry and the Law, 23,* 607–611.

Buckley, P.F., Ibrahim, Z.Y., Singer, B., Orr, B., Donenwirth, K., & Brar, P.S. (1997). Aggression and schizophrenia: Efficacy of risperidone. *Journal of the American Academy of Psychiatry and the Law, 25,* 173–181.

Cantillon, M., Arvanitis, L.A., Miller, B.G., & Kowalcyk, B.B. (1997, December). *"Seroquel" (quetiapine fumarate) reduces hostility and aggression in patients with acute schizophrenia* [Abstract]. Paper presented at the 36th annual meeting of the American College of Neuropsychopharmacology, 171.

Chiles, J.A., Davidson, P., & McBride, D. (1994). Effects of clozapine on use of seclusion and restraint at a state hospital. *Hospital and Community Psychiatry, 45,* 269–271.

Citrome, L. (1989). Differential diagnosis of psychosis: A brief guide for the primary care physician. *Postgraduate Medicine, 85,* 273–274.

Citrome, L. (1995). Use of lithium, carbamazepine, and valproic acid in a state-operated psychiatric hospital. *Journal of Pharmacy Technology, 11,* 55–59.

Citrome, L., Levine, J., & Allingham, B. (1998). Utilization of valproate: Extent of inpatient use in the New York State Office of Mental Health. *Psychiatric Quarterly, 69,* 283–300.

Citrome, L., & Volavka, J. (1997). Psychopharmacology of violence. Part II: Beyond the acute episode. *Psychiatric Annals, 27,* 696–703.

Citrome, L., & Volavka, J. (1998). The efficacy of pharmacological treatments in preventing crime and violence among persons with psychotic disorders. In S. Hodgins & R. Müller-Isberner (Eds.), *Violence, crime, and mentally disordered offenders: Concepts and methods for effective treatment and prevention.* New York: Wiley.

Citrome, L., & Volavka, J. (1999). Schizophrenia: Violence and comorbidity. *Current Opinion in Psychiatry, 12,* 47–51.

Cleckley, H. (1976). *The mask of sanity (5th ed.).* St. Louis: Mosby.

Coccaro, E.F., & Kavoussi, R.J. (1997). Fluoxetine and impulsive aggressive behavior in personality-disordered subjects. *Archives of General Psychiatry, 54,* 1081–1088.

Coccaro, E.F., Kavoussi, R.J., Cooper, T.B., & Hauger, R.L. (1997). Central serotonin activity and aggression: Inverse relationship with prolactin response to D-fenfluramine, but not CSF 5-HIAA concentration, in human subjects. *American Journal of Psychiatry, 154,* 1430–1435.

Collins, P.J., Larkin, E.P., & Shubsachs, A.P.W. (1991). Lithium carbonate in chronic schizophrenia: A brief trial of lithium carbonate added to neuroleptics for treatment of resistant schizophrenic patients. *Acta Psychiatrica Scandinavica, 84,* 150–154.

Convit, A., Isay, D., Otis, D., & Volavka, J. (1990). Characteristics of repeatedly assaultive psychiatric inpatients. *Hospital and Community Psychiatry, 41,* 1112–1115.

Côté, G., & Hodgins, S. (1990). Co-occurring mental disorders among criminal offenders. *Bulletin of the American Academy of Psychiatry and the Law, 18,* 271–281.

Crowner, M.L., Douyon, R., Convit, A., Gaztanaga, P., Volavka, J., & Bakall, R. (1990). Akathisia and violence. *Psychopharmacology Bulletin, 26,* 115–117.

Czobor, P., Volavka, J., & Meibach, R.C. (1995). Effect of risperidone on hostility in schizophrenia. *Journal of Clinical Psychopharmacology, 15,* 243–249.

Donovan, S.J., Susser, E.S., Nunes, E.V., Stewart, J.W., Quitkin, F.M., & Klein, D.F. (1997). Divalproex treatment of disruptive adolescents: A report of 10 cases. *Journal of Clinical Psychiatry, 58,* 12–15.

Ebrahim, G.M., Gibler, B., Gacono, C.B., & Hayes, G. (1994). Patient response to clozapine in a forensic psychiatric hospital. *Hospital and Community Psychiatry, 45,* 271–273.

Frances, A., Docherty, J.P., & Kahn, D.A. (1996). The expert consensus guideline series. Treatment of schizophrenia. *Journal of Clinical Psychiatry, 57*(Suppl 12B), 1–58.

Freese, A., Müller-Isberner, R., & Jockel, D. (1995). Psychopathy and co-morbidity in a German hospital order population [Abstract]. *Issues in Criminological and Legal Psychology, 24,* 45–46.

Geracioti, T.D. Jr. (1994). Valproic acid treatment of episodic explosiveness related to brain injury [letter]. *Journal of Clinical Psychiatry, 55,* 416–417.

Giakas, W.J., Seibyl, J.P., & Mazure, C.M. (1990). Valproate in the treatment of temper outbursts [letter]. *Journal of Clinical Psychiatry, 51,* 525.

Goldman, M.B., & Janecek, H.M. (1990). Adjunctive fluoxetine improves global function in chronic schizophrenia. *Journal of Neuropsychiatry and Clinical Neurosciences, 2,* 429–431.

Guy, W. (1986). *ECDEU assessment manual for psychopharmacology.* Rockville, MD: National Institute of Mental Health.

Hakola, H.P.A., & Laulumaa, V.A. (1982). Carbamazepine in treatment of violent schizophrenics [letter]. *Lancet, 1,* 1358.

Hallikainen, T., Saito, T., Lachman, H.M., Volavka, J., Pohjalainen, T., Ryynänen, O.-P., Kauhanen, J., Syvalahti, E., Hietala, J., & Tiihonen, J. (in press). Association between low activity serotonin transporter promoter genotype with habitual impulsive behavior among antisocial early onset alcoholics. *Molecular Psychiatry.*

Hare, R.D. (1980). A research scale for the assessment of psychopathy in criminal populations. *Personality and Individual Differences, 1,* 111–119.

Hare, R.D. (1996). Psychopathy and antisocial personality disorder: A case of diagnostic confusion. *Psychiatric Times, February,* 39–40.

Hare, R.D., & McPherson, L.M. (1984). Violent and aggressive behavior by criminal psychopaths. *International Journal of Law and Psychiatry, 7,* 35–50.

Hart, S.D., Hare, R.D., & Forth, A.E. (1994). Psychopathy as a risk marker for violence: Development and validation of a screening version of the revised psychopathy checklist. In J. Monahan & H.J. Steadman (Eds.), *Violence and mental disorder: Developments in risk assessment* (pp. 81–98). Chicago: University of Chicago Press.

Hodgins, S., & Côté, G. (1993). Major mental disorder and antisocial personality disorder: A criminal combination. *Bulletin of the American Academy of Psychiatry and the Law, 21,* 155–160.

Hodgins, S., Côté, G., & Toupin, J. (1998). Major mental disorders and crime: An etiological hypothesis. In D. Cooke, A. Forth, & R.D. Hare (Eds.), *Psychopathy: Theory, research and implications for society* (pp. 231–256). Dordrecht: Kluwer.

Hollander, E., Grossman, R., Stein, D.J., & Kwon, J. (1996). Borderline personality disorder and impulsive-aggression: The role for divalproex sodium treatment. *Psychiatric Annals* (Suppl 26), S464–S469.

Honigfeld, G., & Klett, G. (1965). The nurses' observation scale for inpatient evaluation: A new scale for measuring improvement in chronic schizophrenia. *Journal of Clinical Psychology, 21,* 65–71.

Horne, M., & Lindley, S.E. (1995). Divalproex sodium in the treatment of aggressive behavior and dysphoria in patients with organic brain syndromes [letter]. *Journal of Clinical Psychiatry, 56,* 430–431.

Karson, C.N., Weinberger, D.R., Bigelow, L., & Wyatt, R.J. (1982). Clonazepam treatment of chronic schizophrenia: Negative results in a double-blind, placebo-controlled trial. *American Journal of Psychiatry, 139,* 1627–1628.

Kay, S.R., Fiszbein, A., & Opler, L.A. (1987). The positive and negative syndrome scale (PANSS) for schizophrenia. *Schizophrenia Bulletin, 13,* 261–276.

Keckich, W.A. (1978). Neuroleptics: Violence as a manifestation of akathisia. *Journal of the American Medical Association, 240,* 2185–2185.

Krakowski, M.I., Convit, A., Jaeger, J., Lin, S., & Volavka, J. (1989a). Neurological impairment in violent schizophrenic inpatients. *American Journal of Psychiatry, 146,* 849–853.

Krakowski, M.I., Convit, A., Jaeger, J., Lin, S., & Volavka, J. (1989b). Inpatient violence: Trait and state. *Journal of Psychiatric Research, 23,* 57–64.

Krakowski, M.I., Kunz, M., Czobor, P., & Volavka, J. (1993). Long-term high-dose neuroleptic treatment: Who gets it and why? *Hospital and Community Psychiatry, 44,* 640–644.

Lachman, H.M., Nolan, K.A., Mohr, P., Saito, T., & Volavka, J. (1998). Association between catechol-*O*-methyltransferase genotype and violence in schizophrenia and schizoaffective disorder. *American Journal of Psychiatry, 155,* 835–837.

Lott, A.D., McElroy, S.L., & Keys, M.A. (1995). Valproate in the treatment of behavioral agitation in elderly patients with dementia. *Journal of Neuropsychiatry and Clinical Neurosciences, 7,* 314–319.

Luchins, D.J. (1984). Carbamazepine in violent non-epileptic schizophrenics. *Psychopharmacology Bulletin, 20,* 569–571.

Maier, G.J. (1992). The impact of clozapine on 25 forensic patients. *Bulletin of the American Academy of Psychiatry and the Law, 20,* 297–307.

Mallya, A.R., Roos, P.D., & Roebuck-Colgan, K. (1992). Restraint, seclusion, and clozapine. *Journal of Clinical Psychiatry, 53,* 395–397.

Marder, S.R., Davis, J.M., & Chouinard, G. (1997). The effects of risperidone on the five dimensions of schizophrenia derived by factor analysis: Combined results of the North American trials. *Journal of Clinical Psychiatry, 58,* 538–546.

Mattes, J.A. (1992). Valproic acid for nonaffective aggression in the mentally retarded. *Journal of Nervous and Mental Diseases, 180,* 601–602.

Mazure, C.M., Druss, B.G., & Cellar, J.S. (1992). Valproate treatment of older psychotic patients with organic mental syndromes and behavioral dyscontrol. *Journal of the American Geriatrics Society, 40,* 914–916.

Mellow, A.M., Solano-Lopez, C., & Davis, S. (1993). Sodium valproate in the treatment of behavioral disturbance in dementia. *Journal of Geriatric Psychiatry and Neurology, 6,* 205–209.

Michals, M.L., Crismon, M.L., Roberts, S., & Childs, A. (1993). Clozapine response and adverse effects in nine brain-injured patients. *Journal of Clinical Psychopharmacology, 13,* 198–203.

Mueser, K.T., Drake, R.E., Ackerson, T.H., Alterman, A.I., Miles, K.M., & Noordsy, D.L. (1997). Antisocial personality disorder, conduct disorder, and substance abuse in schizophrenia. *Journal of Abnormal Psychology, 106,* 473–477.

Nedopil, N., Hollweg, M., Hartmann, J., & Jaser, R. (1998). Comorbidity of psychopathy with major mental disorders. In D.J. Cooke, A. Forth, & R.D. Hare (Eds.), *Psychopathy: Theory, research and implications for society* (pp. 257–268). Dordrecht: Kluwer.

Neppe, V.M. (1983). Carbamazepine as adjunctive treatment in nonepileptic chronic inpatients with EEG temporal lobe abnormalities. *Journal of Clinical Psychiatry, 44,* 326–331.

Nolan, K.A., Volavka, J., Mohr, P., & Czobor, P. (1999). Psychopathy and violent behavior among patients with schizophrenia or schizoaffective disorder. *Psychiatric Services, 50,* 787–792.

Okuma, T., Yamashita, I., Takahashi, R., Itoh, H., Otsuki, S., Watanabe, S., Sarai, K., Hazama, H., & Inanaga, K. (1989). A double-blind study of adjunctive carbamazepine versus placebo on excited states of schizophrenic and schizoaffective disorders. *Acta Psychiatrica Scandinavica, 80,* 250–259.

Owen, C., Tarantello, C., Jones, M., & Tennant, C. (1998). Repetitively violent patients in psychiatric units. *Psychiatric Services, 49,* 1458–1461.

Prakash, R. (1985). Lithium-responsive schizophrenia: Case reports. *Journal of Clinical Psychiatry, 46,* 141–142.

Rabinowitz, J., Avnon, M., & Rosenberg, V. (1996). Effect of clozapine on physical and verbal aggression. *Schizophrenia Research, 22,* 249–255.

Rasmussen, K., Levander, S., & Sletvold, H. (1995). Aggressive and non-aggressive schizophrenics: Symptom profile and neuropsychological differences. *Psychology, Crime and Law, 2,* 119–129.

Ratey, J.J., Leveroni, C., Kilmer, D., Gutheil, C., & Swartz, B. (1993). The effects of clozapine on severely aggressive psychiatric inpatients in a state hospital. *Journal of Clinical Psychiatry, 54,* 219–223.

Ratey, J.J., Sorgi, P., O'Driscoll, G.A., Sands, S., Daehler, M.L., Fletcher, J.R., Kadish, W., Spruiell, G., Polakoff, S., Lindem, K.J., Bemporad, J.R., Richardson, L., & Rosenfeld, B. (1992). Nadolol to treat aggression and psychiatric symptomatology in chronic psychiatric inpatients: A double-blind, placebo-controlled study. *Journal of Clinical Psychiatry, 53,* 41–46.

Ryback, R., & Ryback, L. (1995). Gabapentin for behavioral dyscontrol [Letter]. *American Journal of Psychiatry, 152,* 1399.

Schaffer, C.B., & Schaffer, L.C. (1997). Gabapentin in the treatment of bipolar disorder [Letter]. *American Journal of Psychiatry, 154,* 291–292.

Scott, H., Johnson, S., Menezes, P., Thornicroft, G., Marshall, J., Bindman, J., Bebbington, P., & Kuipers, E. (1998). Substance misuse and risk of aggression and offending among the severely mentally ill. *British Journal of Psychiatry, 172,* 345–350.

Sheard, M.H. (1971). Effect of lithium on human aggression. *Nature, 230,* 113–114.

Sheard, M.H., Marini, J.L., Bridges, C.I., & Wagner, E. (1976). The effect of lithium on impulsive aggressive behavior in man. *American Journal of Psychiatry, 133,* 1409–1413.

Silver, J.M., Yudofsky, S.C., Kogan, M., & Katz, B.L. (1986). Elevation of thioridazine plasma levels by propranolol. *American Journal of Psychiatry, 143,* 1290–1292.

Sorgi, P.J., Ratey, J.J., & Polakoff, S. (1986). Beta-adrenergic blockers for the control of aggressive behaviors in patients with chronic schizophrenia. *American Journal of Psychiatry, 143,* 775–776.

Steadman, H.J., Mulvey, E.P., Monahan, J., Robbins, P.C., Appelbaum, P.S., Grisso, T., Roth, L.H., & Silver, E. (1998). Violence by people discharged from acute psychiatric inpatient facilities and by others in the same neighborhoods. *Archives of General Psychiatry, 55,* 393–401.

Strous, R.D., Bark, N., Parsia, S.S., Volavka, J., & Lachman, H.M. (1997). Analysis of a functional catechol-*O*-methyltransferase gene polymorphism in schizophrenia: Evidence for association with aggressive and antisocial behavior. *Psychiatry Research, 69,* 71–77.

Swanson, J.W. (1994). Mental disorder, substance abuse, and community violence: An epidemiological approach. In J. Monahan & H.J. Steadman (Eds.), *Violence and mental disorder: Developments in risk assessment* (pp. 101–136). Chicago: University of Chicago Press.

Swartz, M.S., Swanson, J.W., Hiday, V.A., Borum, R., Wagner, H.R., & Burns, B.J. (1998). Violence and severe mental illness: The effects of substance abuse and nonadherence to medication. *American Journal of Psychiatry, 155,* 226–231.

Tupin, J.P., Smith, D.B., Clanon, T.L., Kim, L.I., Nugent, A., & Groupe, A. (1973). The long-term use of lithium in aggressive prisoners. *Comprehensive Psychiatry, 14,* 311–317.

Vartiainen, H., Tiihonen, J., Putkonen, A., Koponen, H., Virkkunen, M., Hakola, P., & Lehto, H. (1995). Citalopram, a selective serotonin reuptake inhibitor, in the treatment of aggression in schizophrenia. *Acta Psychiatrica Scandinavica, 91,* 348–351.

Volavka, J. (1995). *Neurobiology of violence.* Washington: American Psychiatric Press.

Volavka, J., & Citrome, L. (1999). Atypical antipsychotics in the treatment of the persistently aggressive psychotic patient: Methodological concerns. *Schizophrenia Research, 35,* S23–S33.

Volavka, J., & Krakowski, M. (1989). Schizophrenia and violence. *Psychological Medicine, 19,* 559–562.

Volavka, J., Mohammad, Y., Vitrai, J., Connolly, M., Stefanovic, M., & Ford, M. (1995). Characteristics of state hospital patients arrested for offenses committed during hospitalization. *Psychiatric Services, 46,* 796–800.

Volavka, J., Zito, J.M., Vitrai, J., & Czobor, P. (1993). Clozapine effects on hostility and aggression in schizophrenia. *Journal of Clinical Psychopharmacology, 13,* 287–289.

Whitman, J.R., Maier, G.J., & Eichelman, B. (1987). Beta-adrenergic blockers for aggressive behavior in schizophrenia [letter]. *American Journal of Psychiatry, 144,* 538–539.

Wilcox, J. (1994). Divalproex sodium in the treatment of aggressive behavior. *Annals of Clinical Psychiatry, 6,* 17–20.

Wilson, W.H. (1992). Clinical review of clozapine treatment in a state hospital. *Hospital and Community Psychiatry, 43,* 700–703.

Wilson, W.H. (1993). Addition of lithium to haloperidol in non-affective, antipsychotic non-responsive schizophrenia: A double blind, placebo controlled, parallel design clinical trial. *Psychopharmacology, 111,* 359–366.

Wilson, W.H., & Claussen, A.M. (1995). 18-month outcome of clozapine treatment for 100 patients in a state psychiatric hospital. *Psychiatric Services, 46,* 386–389.

Wroblewski, B.A., Joseph, A.B., Kupfer, J., & Kalliel, K. (1997). Effectiveness of valproic acid on destructive and aggressive behaviours in patients with acquired brain injury. *Brain Injury, 11,* 37–47.

Yassa, R., & Dupont, D. (1983). Carbamazepine in the treatment of aggressive behavior in schizophrenic patients: A case report. *Canadian Journal of Psychiatry, 28,* 566–568.

Jan Volavka is Chief, Clinical Research Division, Nathan S. Kline Institute for Psychiatric Research, Orangeburg, New York, USA, and Professor of Psychiatry, New York University, New York, New York, USA. Leslie Citrome is Director, Clinical Research and Evaluation Facility, Nathan S. Kline Institute for Psychiatric Research, Orangeburg, New York, USA, and Clinical Associate Professor of Psychiatry, New York University, New York, New York, USA.

Authors' Note

Portions of this chapter draw on the following publications: Citrome and Volavka, 1997, 1998, 1999; Nolan, Volavka, Mohr, and Czobor, 1999; Volavka, 1995; Volavka and Citrome, 1995.

Comments or queries may be directed to Jan Volavka, MD, PhD, Clinical Research Division, Nathan S. Kline Institute for Psychiatric Research, 140 Old Orangeburg Road, Building 37, Orangeburg NY 10962-1167 USA. Telephone: 914 398-6567. Fax: 914 398-6566. E-mail: <Volavka@NKI.RFMH.ORG>.

Section III

PREVENTING VIOLENCE IN HOSPITALS

INSTITUTIONAL VIOLENCE AMONG THE MENTALLY ILL

V.L. QUINSEY

During the mid-1960s I worked as an attendant on the admission ward of a psychiatric hospital. An Ojibway boy about my age was admitted from a local jail where he had been held following an arrest for drunkenness. After admission, he was started on a standard detoxification routine. However, his behaviour grew increasingly bizarre. He assumed a crucified posture in front of the ward door, reported that he saw the devil in the darkness, and became afraid to go to sleep at night. He was also very intelligent, challenging my assertion that his hallucinations had no basis in external reality using sophisticated arguments fashioned with his limited English vocabulary. He was also very sad to be missing the wild rice harvest on the Indian reserve.

One day this patient walked down the long corridor and, without a word, attacked me. He punched and I blocked while being forced slowly backwards down the corridor. We passed a laundry room where two of my colleagues were folding clothes. These surprised attendants came to my aid, and, after great difficulty, we subdued the patient. This event drew attention to the fact that this acutely psychotic schizophrenic was being treated with vitamins instead of antipsychotic drugs. The patient responded very well to appropriate medication and, while he missed the wild rice harvest, was soon discharged.

The aggression of this patient appeared to be related to acute psychosis, not antisocial personality disorder or criminality, and it disappeared with the psychotic symptoms when he received antipsychotic medication. His attack appeared to arise literally out of the blue, with no possible recent provocation by me.

Was this a typical aggressive act committed by a psychiatric patient? Is aggression closely associated with the intensity of psychiatric symptoms, or is it tied more closely to antisocial personality? How well does aggressive behaviour respond to various medications? Are assaults by psychiatric patients generally unprovoked, and are they directed towards particular individuals or are they random? Before dealing with these and related questions, we must concern ourselves with the measurement of the phenomenon we hope to explain and control, together with some preliminary methodological issues.

Methodological Issues

There is a large literature on institutional violence. Sources for the older literature include Lion and Reid (1983), Rice, Harris, Varney, and Quinsey (1989), and Tar-

S. Hodgins (ed.), Violence among the Mentally Ill, 213–235.
© 2000 *Kluwer Academic Publishers. Printed in the Netherlands.*

diff (1989), for the more recent literature, Bjørkly (1995). Unfortunately, most of the literature, even the most recent (e.g., Day, Franklin, & Marshall, 1998; Raja, Azzoni, & Lubich, 1997), is descriptive; very few studies examine either the prediction or the reduction of violence. Moreover, the conclusions that can be drawn from the descriptive literature are limited in scope, because the study of violence among the institutionalized mentally ill is bedevilled with methodological problems. Haller and Deluty (1988) identified some of those commonly occurring in the earlier literature: under-reporting of assaults; incomplete operational definitions of aggression and predictor variables; and lack of distinction between major and minor assaults, verbal and physical aggression, and victim types.

However, selection effects are involved in the less tractable methodological difficulties. Because violent acts frequently lead to psychiatric hospital admission, hospitalized patients are more likely to have a history of violent behaviour and to be more violent than an unselected sample of the mentally ill. Because discharge is associated with improvement in clinical symptoms, including a reduction in aggressive behaviour (e.g., Steinert, Hermer, & Faust, 1996), the tragedy of the psychiatric hospitals comes into play. The tragedy is that length of psychiatric hospitalization is directly correlated with patient refractoriness to available treatments. Thus, psychiatric hospitals always end up caring for the untreatable unless they can transfer their intractable cases to other hospitals, such as security or "special" hospitals.

These selection processes cause violence to be associated with different patient characteristics according to length of stay. For example, Noble (1997) concluded, on the basis of a literature review, that on acute wards violence is associated with acute schizophrenia, substance abuse, and personality disorder, whereas on chronic wards it is associated with chronic refractory schizophrenia and mental impairment and organic syndromes.

Differential admission and discharge of psychiatric patients means that the generalizability of results from inpatient studies is difficult to characterize. This problem is worsened by the relationship of dual diagnosis to institutional placement. Both developmental handicap and mental illness have some relationship with aggressive behaviour. Jurisdictions vary in their policies regarding the disposition of persons with dual diagnoses; they may be placed in psychiatric facilities, institutions for the developmentally handicapped, or both, to varying degrees (Quinsey, Skilling, & Rougier-Chapman, 1997). Finally, jurisdictions vary in the liberality with which they use the insanity defence and thus in the proportion of mentally ill individuals in prison or in hospital.

Psychiatric units are thus analogous to the "islands" beloved of biogeographers. The analogy to species is diagnostic group. The proportion of patients in various diagnostic groups is determined by rates of immigration (admission) and extinction (discharge). These rates in turn are determined by the bureaucratic closeness of other islands (psychiatric units) or continents (the correctional system and the developmentally handicapped system) and the mutation rate (changes in the legal policies governing admission to the various geographical entities). To mix the metaphor, because immigration and extinction are both related to assaultiveness in a manner that varies over islands, the correlation of assaultiveness and diagnosis can be expected to vary in substantively uninteresting ways.

Measurement

There has been significant progress over the past 20 years in the measurement of institutional assaults. Researchers more often establish inter-observer reliability in the measurement of assaults now than in the past, and there is an increasing tendency to use the same measures in different studies (for a critical review of "aggression" in psychiatric patients, see Gothelf, Apter, & Van-Praag, 1997). Nevertheless, there are problems in measuring assault frequency. The most important difficulty is the failure to control for opportunity. Confinements or lengthy time outs are often contingent upon serious assaults, and frequency estimates that do not control for confinement-related curtailed opportunity will be too low, and very likely differentially too low, with more serious assaults and assaulters.

The most widely used instrument, the Overt Aggression Scale (Silver & Yudofsky, 1987; Yudofsky, Silver, Jackson, Endicott, & Williams, 1986), measures verbal aggression, physical aggression against objects, physical aggression against self, and physical aggression against others. A rating scale of severity is provided within each of the four categories. A fifth category deals with interventions and has a severity scale ranging from talking to the patient to using restraints. A Total Aggression Score is obtained by adding the weighted score for the most severe degree of aggression within each category to the weighted score for the most restrictive intervention. Because the Total Aggression Score completely confounds staff and patient behaviour, I strongly recommend not calculating it. In a study of the Overt Aggression Scale on three wards at each of two psychiatric hospitals, the scale documented more aggressive incidents than did official hospital documents. It is not clear whether this discrepancy was caused by staff filling out the scale (i.e., preferring the rating scale to the regular documentation).

Less commonly employed measures include a modification of the Overt Aggression Scale (Kay, Wolkenfeld, & Murrill, 1988a, 1988b) and the Scale for the Assessment of Aggressive and Agitated Behaviors (Brizer, Convit, Krakowski, & Volavka, 1987). Hallsteinsen, Kristensen, Dahl, and Eilertsen (1998) have developed an extended form of the Staff Observation Aggression Scale, the SOAS-E. This instrument is designed to record violent and non-violent aggressive behaviours of psychiatric inpatients together with the warning signals and provocations that may precede them.

The nature of the outcome measure deserves more attention that it receives. Rating scales that incorporate severity ratings may or may not be what investigators want to interpret. Scales like the Overt Aggression Scale conflate severity and frequency. This approach sensibly weights more serious assaults more than less serious ones but at the cost of asserting that, say, 20 verbal threats are equivalent to one physical assault.

A more labour-intensive system for measuring a more restricted but more easily interpreted domain was developed by Quinsey and Varney (1977) for recording physical assaults. In this method, a researcher visited each ward daily and identified potential incidents by talking to ward staff and patients and reviewing the ward log. Each likely incident involving actual or attempted forceful physical contact was recorded by interviewing each of the staff and patient participants and, where possible, a witness. A description of the antecedents to and consequences of the assault were recorded together with what happened during the incident. Informants were also asked why the assault occurred. Good inter-rater agreement was found in the original and subsequent studies (Rice et al., 1989).

An even more laborious method of recording assaults has been developed by Brizer, Crowner, Convit, and Volavka (1988), in which assaults are identified through continuous videotaping, for subsequent analysis. This method has many advantages, chief among them the ability to recode assault data from videotaped archives. This relatively unobtrusive method of recording assaults, unencumbered by the vagaries of recall and reporting practices, allows for a number of questions to be resolved more clearly than by using trained observers or relying on front-line staff to record incidents. For example, in both the original study and a subsequent investigation (Crowner, Peric, Stepcic, & Van-Oss, 1994), incident reports were found to underestimate actual assaults. The 1994 investigation demonstrated that the more serious the physical assaults, the more likely they were to be included in incident reports.

The following review deals primarily with aggression as defined by physical assaults. Where other, more general, measures of aggression are discussed, the nature of the measure is described.

Characteristics of Assaulters

A small minority of patients are involved in the majority of assaults (e.g., Bjørkly, 1999; Cheung, Schweitzer, Tuckwell, & Crowley, 1997; Convit, Isay, Otis, & Volavka, 1990; Harris & Varney, 1986; Noble, 1997; Quinsey & Varney, 1977; Rasmussen & Levander, 1996a). Assaultive patients are more likely to be younger (e.g., Convit et al., 1990), to have prior histories of intra-institutional assaults, and to be lower-functioning than non-assaultive patients (Harris & Varney[1]; Quinsey & Varney).

Rasmussen and Levander (1996b) studied physical aggression in a maximum security psychiatric institution. Over 6.5 years, 55% of the 94 patients were involved in at least one of 1,945 incidents. However, 87% of the incidents were caused by six patients. More females than males were assaultive, including one woman who contributed 58% of the assaults. Assaults were more frequent on weekdays but no other temporal patterns emerged. The most common precipitating event was attempting to calm an upset patient. Patients who attacked less often caused less harm than those who attacked more often, although serious injury was very rare. Positive psychiatric symptoms, borderline symptoms, and assistance in daily care were positively related to assault frequency in a regression equation, while age, modified PCL-R score, and depressive symptoms were negatively related.

Krakowski, Jaeger, and Volavka (1988) followed 44 consecutive admissions to a unit for the treatment of violent patients. Psychopathology, as measured by the Brief Psychiatric Rating Scale (BPRS) (Overall & Gorham, 1962), was positively related, both cross-sectionally and longitudinally, to unfocused violence (primarily against property) but not as strongly as activity therapists' ratings of social dysfunction (level of functioning). Although BPRS ratings were not related to verbal aggression or physical assault, social dysfunction was correlated with physical assault among patients with functional psychiatric disorders during the first week post-admission. Patients with diagnoses of personality disorder or mental retardation and those with younger ages at first hospitalization were more persistently violent than those with a diagnosis of schizophrenia or major affective disorder.

In a subsequent study, Krakowski, Convit, Jaeger, Lin, and Volavka (1989a) compared 77 admissions to a unit for the treatment of violent patients, divided into a transiently and a persistently violent group, with a comparison group of 44 non-violent patients. The comparison group was matched on age, race, chronicity, and diagnosis (except that no non-assaultive personality disorder patients could be found for the comparison group). Violent behaviours included physical assaultiveness, verbal threat, and destruction of property. Logistic regressions indicated that persis-tently violent patients were more neurologically impaired and had experienced greater overall family disturbance than either of the other two groups. Both violent groups had more frequently been convicted for a violent crime than comparison subjects. EEG recordings did not differentiate among the groups.

The relationship of diagnosis and sex of patient to aggression has been mixed (Rasmussen & Levander, 1996b), probably because of the selection effects described earlier. For example, the relationship of psychopathy to institutional assaultiveness can be expected to vary because of selection. Some of the items that contribute to a psychopathy score, such as failure on prior conditional release, criminal versatility, juvenile delinquency, glibness, and so forth, are primarily relevant to patients who have had opportunities to commit crimes in the community and have a minimum degree of verbal skills. In unit populations where there is a substantial proportion of highly assaultive but very low-functioning individuals, psychopathy may be found to correlate negatively with institutional violence.

Despite the negative findings reviewed above for the BPRS, there is some evi-dence that acute psychotic symptoms are related to assaultiveness (Junginger, 1996). In a series of studies of a matched group of 31 aggressive and 31 non-aggressive schizophrenics (Cheung, Schweitzer, Crowley, & Tuckwell, 1997a, 1997b, 1997c; Cheung, Schweitzer, Crowley, Yastrubetskaya, & Tuckwell, 1996), it was found that assaultiveness was associated with both positive and negative symptoms and with general psychopathology. Cheung et al. (1997a) interpreted their results as indicat-ing that three sets of symptoms were related to assaults: symptoms with verbal or physical aggression being part of their definition, symptoms reflecting frontal lobe impairment, and excitement. General psychopathology, personality traits, and his-tory of aggression were related to assaultiveness but not so highly as negative affec-tive responses to delusions or hallucinations. Assaultive patients tended to have per-secutory delusions and non-aggressive patients tended to have grandiose delusions. Neuroleptic side effects and command hallucinations were not significantly corre-lated with assaults. Command hallucinations were also found to be unrelated to as-saultiveness by Hellerstein, Frosch, and Koenigsberg (1987).

Further findings supporting the idea that acute symptoms bear a stronger relation to assaultiveness than diagnosis come from a longitudinal study of 34 patients diag-nosed as schizophrenic or schizoaffective (Harrow, Rattenbury, & Stoll, 1988). In focused interviews, the researchers studied patients' belief-conviction about their delusions, perspective about whether other people would regard their ideas as aberrant or unrealistic, and emotional commitment (immediacy, importance, urgency) to their delusions. The same themes were evident from the premorbid period, through hospitalization, to the post-hospital phase. There was a relatively high level of belief-conviction throughout, but somewhat more (although poor) awareness of others' likely perceptions. The acute phase was marked primarily by increased emotional commitment that was in turn related to the likelihood of aggressive behaviour (cf. Buchanan, 1997).

A limited amount of data suggests that symptoms associated with antipsychotic medication are related to assaults. Using videotape technology, patients and victims (but not bystanders) in a unit for chronically violent psychiatric patients were found to have higher akasthisia scores in the 5-minute period preceding nine physical assaults (Crowner et al., 1990).

Suicidal and self-injurious behaviour has been linked to assaultiveness. Hillbrand (1995) compared Overt Aggression Scale scores of 103 male forensic patients assigned to one of four groups defined by their history of suicidal behaviour and their current level of self-injurious behaviour. Patients who had both characteristics were more assaultive than both patients who had neither and patients who exhibited previous suicidality but no current self-injurious behaviour. These group differences remained after controlling for age, diagnosis, length of hospitalization, and amount of medication.

Characteristics of Assaults

Staff are usually more likely than co-patients to be assaulted (Benjaminsen, Gotzsche-Larsen, Norrie, & Harder, 1996; Cheung, Schweitzer, Tuckwell, & Crowley, 1997; Harris & Varney, 1986; Quinsey & Varney, 1977). Those assaulted are usually nursing or attendant staff (Bjørkly, 1999; Carmel & Hunter, 1993; Lanza, 1992; Tam, Engelsmann, & Fugere, 1996) and are assaulted in the context of setting limits on patients or requesting activity from them (Benjaminsen et al.; Harris & Varney; Quinsey & Varney). Increasing proportions of inexperienced nursing staff have been associated with increases in assaults (James, Fineberg, Shah, & Priest, 1990); similarly, Rasmussen and Levander (1996b) found that untrained staff and female staff were differentially likely to be assaulted.

Staff and patients often give very different reasons for assaults. Staff often state that there was no reason for the assault or that the assault was a result of the patient's psychopathology. Patients, on the other hand, cite teasing by patients or staff, staff provocation in the form of giving them orders, and so forth (Harris & Varney, 1986; Quinsey & Varney, 1977). Crowner, Peric, Stepcic, and Ventura (1995) found very similar results in a study of 134 videotaped physical assaults committed by 40 psychiatric patients. Most patients refused to be interviewed, but those who did cooperate often claimed to have been playing with the victim, complained of verbal abuse, or said they wanted to stop objectionable behaviours by the victim. Taken together, these studies suggest that patients frequently perceive victim behaviours as provocative.

The injuries associated with assaults tend to be minor (Bjørkly, 1999; Harris & Rice, 1986; Noble, 1997; Reid, Bollinger, & Edwards, 1989). However, more serious injuries are associated with restraining patients, sprains, and the effects of falling (Harris & Rice, 1986).

Assaults often occur when patients are engaged in unstructured activity (Deitz & Rada, 1983; Harris & Varney, 1986; Quinsey & Varney, 1977). Silver and Yudofsky (1987) found that aggression increased at medication time and during shift changes and decreased at lunchtime.

Crichton (1997) summarizes the findings of British studies, most of which echo the rest of the literature. Minor violence is very common, particularly in low-security institutions where violence is a criterion for admission; serious violence is rarer but is more common in special security hospitals. Active psychotic symptoms, but not diagnoses, are associated with assault frequency. Female patients in secure facilities are more assaultive than male patients. A few patients cause the majority of assaults. Poor staffing levels and temporary staff are associated with assaults, as is patient idleness.

Neurobiology

Neurobiological correlates and potential causes of aggression have been investigated for decades (for a general review, see Stoff & Cairns, 1996). Part of the motivation for these investigations is the obvious: The proximal causes of all behaviours reside in the brain. Past experience and current environmental events also cause behaviours but do so through a neural route, not directly. A more specific and powerful impetus for this line of investigation has been the success of the dopamine hypothesis in schizophrenia with the associated psychopharmacological interventions. The literature on neurobiological correlates is vast. Some recent studies on institutional violence are reviewed below.

Balaban, Alper, and Kasamon (1996) conducted a meta-analysis of 39 studies examining the relationship of the serotonin metabolite 5-hydroxyindoleacetic acid (5-HIAA) to human aggression. Psychiatric patients were lower in 5-HIAA than non-psychiatric groups, but there was not a significant correlation between 5-HIAA and aggression. Maguire et al. (1997) likewise found no difference on serotonin function measured by ^{3}HT-Paroxetine binding to platelet membranes between aggressive and non-aggressive schizophrenic patients matched on age, sex, and duration of illness.

Convit, Czobor, and Volavka (1991) recorded the EEGs of 21 men treated on a unit for the management of violent behaviour. Both the number of instances of violence (including verbal and physical violence towards staff and assaults against property) and the number of staff interventions were related to increased delta and decreased alpha band activity in the parieto-occipital and temporal areas, independently of medication or length of stay on the unit. Increased levels of violence were associated with relatively greater power of delta band activity in the left hemisphere.

In a large study of neurobiological correlates of assaultiveness, Krakowski et al. (1997) followed 102 hospital admissions for 4 weeks. Of these, 33 had been arrested for a violent crime. Sixty-nine patients who were physically assaultive in the hospital were matched on age, race, sex, diagnosis, and length of hospitalization with 33 who were not. Patients who exhibited multiple assaults were divided into the persistently violent ($N = 9$), the transiently violent (those whose frequency of inpatient assaults markedly declined, $N = 20$), and the sporadically violent (those with one assault, $N = 13$). Patients with a history of community violence (but not crime in general) did not differ from other patients on the WAIS-R but were more impaired on indices of frontal lobe impairment, the Wisconsin Card Sorting Test, the Finger Tapping Test, and the Purdue Pegboard Test. Patients were more likely to be sporadically or persistently violent (i.e., not show clear post-admission deceleration) if they had a history of community violence and showed frontal lobe impairment. Transient post-admission violence appears to reflect an acute psychotic episode with different neurobiological correlates than persistent violence.

Prediction of Assaults

Hillbrand, Spitz, Foster, Krystal, and Young (1998) examined the relationship between serum creatine kinase elevations (caused by muscle activity) and Overt Aggression Scale scores of 164 consecutive male admissions to a forensic hospital. Among patients who received neuroleptic medication, high creatine kinase on admission was positively related to subsequent physical aggression, even when prior assaultiveness and restraint were controlled. Creatine kinase was a better predictor of assaultiveness than prior assaultiveness. It was of interest that creatine kinase functioned well as a static but not a dynamic predictor; changes in it were unrelated to temporal variations in assaultiveness.

Convit, Jaeger, Lin, Meisner, and Volavka (1988) developed a model based on neurological (EEG) abnormalities, history of violent crime, history of violent suicide attempts, and deviant-family childhood environment that significantly predicted which psychiatric patients would be physically assaultive during the first 3 months after their admission. In the prospective study, 79 male schizophrenics under 36 years of age were followed. Fifty-two of the 79 subjects were correctly classified by the model.

Heilbrun et al. (1998) correlated the Psychopathy Checklist (PCL) with physical aggression during the first and last 2 months of hospitalization among 218, mostly male, mentally disordered offenders. Twelve percent of the patients exhibited physical aggression in the first 2 months and 7% in the last 2 months. The PCL correlated significantly with physical aggression in the first period, although the magnitude of the correlation was very small ($r = .12$), but not in the second period.

From a previous study, McNiel and Binder (1994) selected five predictors of inpatient aggression to calculate a unit-weighted actuarial score: history of physical attacks and/or fear-inducing behaviour within 2 weeks prior to admission, absence of suicidal behaviour within 2 weeks prior to admission, schizophrenic or manic diagnosis, male sex, and—surprisingly, given the direction of its usual relation with aggression—currently married or living with a partner. The validation sample consisted of 338 patients of a locked, university-based inpatient unit. The Overt Aggression Scale was completed retrospectively from file data. Twenty-four percent of the sample physically attacked someone. The checklist resulted in a 25% relative improvement over chance in predicting which patients would exhibit physical aggression. This is an important demonstration of the power and utility of actuarial methods, particularly inasmuch as the predictors employed are customarily available to clinicians at the time of patient admission. The Violence Risk Appraisal Guide, a more difficult-to-complete instrument designed to predict post-release violent recidivism, also predicts violent re-offending of supervised mentally disordered offenders (Quinsey, Coleman, Jones, & Altrows, 1997) and institutional misconduct among prison inmates (Kroner & Mills, 1997).

DYNAMIC RISK INDICATORS

Dynamic risk indicators can be categorized according to whether they can be employed to estimate the long-term likelihood of violent acts. Temporally fixable dynamic predictors are those that can change or be made to change, such as the provision of treatment or the response to treatment, but that end at an identifiable point in time. These predictors become historical when they occur and can be used to predict a behaviour of interest over subsequent follow-up periods of any desired length. Temporally fixable dynamic predictors thus compete with static predictors for outcome variance.

In contrast, fluctuating dynamic predictors are those that change continuously in time, such as mood and sobriety. In particular, these predictors can change in the course of a follow-up period. The practical use of these predictors, therefore, is quite different from that of static or historical predictors. Because they change continuously, they are not appropriately used to forecast the likelihood of violent behaviour over long follow-up periods and do not compete for outcome variance with static or historical predictors; rather, they are best used to indicate imminence. In brief, static and historical predictors are suitable for indicating how much risk a person presents over the long term, and fluctuating dynamic predictors for indicating when risk changes within an individual over a short period. The shortness of the period is determined by the speed with which the predictor changes and the frequency of measurement.

Few studies have investigated fluctuating dynamic predictors of violence. In order to do so, it must be demonstrated that a *change* in the predictor is contemporaneously associated with violent acts. In an explicit investigation of dynamic prediction of serious violence, Quinsey, Coleman, et al. (1997) examined the aggression of institutionalized psychiatric patients directed at members of the community at large. They compared 60 mentally disordered male offenders who had eloped from hospital or re-offended while under supervision with 51 male offenders who had done neither. Re-offenders or elopers were identified by asking staff in forensic units at all 10 Ontario provincial psychiatric hospitals to provide the name of any forensic patient who had eloped or re-offended outside of the hospital in the previous 10 years, together with the date and nature of the incident. All identified re-offenders ($n = 33$) were included. Every re-offender had committed an offence off the ward where he resided that was serious enough that criminal charges were or could have been laid. Every eloper had been absent without leave and the incident was serious enough to warrant informing the police.

Of the 111 mentally disordered male offenders included, 60 had eloped or re-offended outside their hospital unit while living under supervision and 51 were comparison subjects. Re-offenders were categorized as violent ($n = 19$) or non-violent ($n = 14$) based on the most severe offence they had committed during the incident. In terms of the most serious re-offence among the 19 violent re-offenders, three committed murder, five attempted murder, one wounding, two assault causing bodily harm, three common assault, four rape, and one indecent assault.

Because there were many more elopers than re-offenders, 27 elopers were chosen randomly to bring the total number of elopers/re-offenders up to 60. If a subject had been involved in more than one incident of interest, the most serious was chosen as the *index event*. If there was more than one event in the same category, the earliest was chosen. Thus, if several violent, non-violent, and simple elopement incidents occurred for a given individual, the earliest violent incident was chosen as the index event.

Comparison subjects were matched with eloper/re-offender subjects on diagnosis (psychotic, not-psychotic), age (within 10 years), and level of supervision (secure custody, direct staff supervision, or indirect supervision). In addition to an actuarially based estimate of risk of violent re-offending, the Violence Risk Appraisal Guide (Quinsey, Harris, Rice, & Cormier, 1998) proximal dynamic variables were coded from clinical file information recorded either in the month before the elopement/re-offence or the control date for all subjects as well as from a control period (usually a year earlier) for the elopers/re-offenders. Seven dynamic variables statistically differentiated elopers/re-offenders from other patients after controlling for actuarial risk level, and also differentiated the period preceding elopement or re-offence from an earlier period among elopers/re-offenders. These robust predictors of eloping/re-offending involved primarily two kinds of items: those involving non-compliance with supervision and antisocial attitudes and those pertaining to emotional dysphoria and psychiatric symptoms.

Violent re-offenders were best differentiated from their controls by a proximal factor labelled "Dynamic Antisociality." Dynamic Antisociality included items concerning lack of remorse and empathy, procriminal sentiments, and unrealistic discharge plans. The finding that Dynamic Antisociality is a dynamic predictor may at first appear paradoxical because it contains some items that are very similar to those on the Psychopathy Checklist–Revised, or PCL-R (Hare, 1991), a well-known *static* predictor. The PCL-R, however, is scored on the basis of a person's lifetime history by searching for exemplars of the items. Thus, once an item is scored "certainly present" it can no longer change during that person's lifetime, and, in practice, the PCL-R is extremely stable over time when scored according to the manual. Dynamic Antisociality is potentially a dynamic indicator because it is scored for a month-long observation period, not a lifetime. The robust within-patient effect found in this study demonstrates that Dynamic Antisociality is dynamic within a limited time period. Its dynamic nature is compatible with the observations that procriminal sentiment is related to criminal recidivism and is modifiable by supervisory staff (Andrews, 1980).

The third factor, Poor Compliance, comprised only three items: escape attempts, exhibiting few positive coping skills, and poor compliance with rules. In contrast to Dynamic Antisociality, it was not related to violent or non-violent recidivism but was related to elopement.

Psychiatric Symptoms contained items reflecting both positive and negative schizophrenic symptoms. Psychiatric Symptoms was not significantly correlated with violent re-offending and was inconsistently correlated with nonviolent re-offending, but was strongly related to eloping. The finding that Psychiatric Symptoms failed to predict violent re-offending is consistent with the finding that a diagnosis of schizophrenia is associated with lower risk of violent re-offending (Gardner, Lidz, Mulvey, & Shaw, 1996; Quinsey et al., 1998; Villeneuve & Quinsey, 1995) because schizophrenic diagnosis is a static variable. In the present study, schizophrenic symptoms were treated as a dynamic variable. The question being addressed was conditional: "Given a schizophrenic patient, does the exacerbation of symptoms relate to eloping or re-offending?" The answer was positive with respect to elopement and negative with respect to very serious violent re-offending, suggesting that early intervention in response to psychotic symptoms and non-compliance with medication may reduce the likelihood of elopement. Violent re-offenders were more likely to be personality disordered and elopers more likely to be psychotic.

Somewhat similar findings are reported by Beauford, McNiel, and Binder (1997), who investigated situational risk factors associated with violence among 328 patients hospitalized on a locked ward. Information from physicians' admitting notes was coded on the Therapeutic Alliance Scale (Clarkin, Hurt, & Crilly, 1987). The scale was coded from 1 (patient is actively involved in therapy, explores problems, etc.) to 6 (patient sees no need for hospitalization and is constantly demanding discharge...totally denies emotional problems, etc.). The BPRS was filled out on admission as well, yielding scores for thinking disturbance, agitation-excitement, hostile-suspiciousness, anxious-depression, and withdrawal-retardation. Outcome data for the week following admission were gathered with the Overt Aggression Scale scored for no aggression, fear-inducing behaviour, and physical attacks.

Twelve percent of the patients physically attacked someone and 21% engaged in fear-inducing behaviour during the first week of admission. In descending order of their predictive value, the predictors were: pre-admission violence, initial Therapeutic Alliance score, age, and BPRS Agitation-Excitement. Therapeutic Alliance remained significantly associated with outcome after the effects of pre-admission violence were controlled. Recalling the classification of predictors presented earlier, pre-admission violence and age on admission are historical or static variables. Therapeutic Alliance and Agitation-Excitement are surely fluctuating and dynamic, although no prediction was made from the change in either of these variables in this study. Therefore, based only on this study, we cannot estimate the extent to which the predictive power of these two variables resulted from some static feature. For example, it could be that psychopaths are litigious and form a poor Therapeutic Alliance, so that Therapeutic Alliance, although in principle dynamic, serves in this instance as a proxy for a static variable, psychopathy. However, the similarity of the Therapeutic Alliance items with some items from the Dynamic Antisociality Scale, such as *complains about staff* and *has unrealistic discharge,* inspires confidence that changes in Therapeutic Alliance are related to violence.[2]

As noted earlier, psychotic symptoms have sometimes been associated with inpatient assaultiveness. In contrast to the findings of the Quinsey, Coleman, et al. (1997) investigation, these associations have been found in on-ward contexts where the assaults seldom cause serious injury. For example, Ross, Hart, and Webster (1998) studied 82 male and 49 female consecutive admissions to a 10-bed unit. The Overt Aggression Scale was completed biweekly. There were 234 incidents over 47 weeks. Thirty percent of the patients were physically assaultive. Correlations with physical aggression were .21 for the Psychopathy Checklist-Short Version, Part 2, and .20 for the clinical items of the HCR-20. The Psychosis Factor of the BPRS correlated .36 with physical aggression.

Management and Treatment

This section will deal only with studies employing measures of assault frequency or staff injury, not with descriptions of unevaluated programmes (e.g., Thackrey, 1987) or studies employing only patient self-report or clinician ratings (e.g., Renwick, Black, Ramm, & Novaco, 1997; Stermac, 1987). Neither will reports of single cases or small series of patients be reviewed. The literature on the management and treatment of aggressive mentally ill patients remains primitive. Despite the variety of interventions that have been tried, there are no meta-analytic reviews that permit the effect sizes of various treatments to be quantitatively compared. Of necessity, the review that follows is qualitative in nature, with all of the interpretative problems that entails.

DRUG TREATMENT

There exist many narrative reviews of the pharmacological literature. Most of these agree that the treatment of aggression in psychiatric patients should not rely on the sedative effects of antipsychotic medication. For example, Yudofsky, Silver, and Schneider (1987) conclude:

> A review of the literature reporting anticonvulsant, lithium, and propranolol treatment of aggression in over 300 patients reveals that most of these patients had been treated unsuccessfully with antipsychotic medications. While antispsychotic agents are certainly appropriate and effective when aggression is related to active psychosis, the use of neuroleptic agents to treat chronic aggression—especially that due to organic brain injury—is often ineffective and entails significant risks of serious complications. (p. 400)

One of these complications is the distraction of clinical staff from non-pharmacological interventions by the continual adjustments of antipsychotic medications. As documented by Harris (1989), these adjustments generally do not affect patient progress because patients tend to respond to medication either quickly or not at all.

Reviewers of this literature come to different conclusions about the most promising drugs for reducing aggression. Yudofsky et al. (1987) favour beta-blockers such as propanolol for organic brain diseases or injuries and other patients whose aggression is not tied directly to psychotic ideation, lithium for aggression related to mania, carbamazepine for aggression related to complex partial seizure disorder, and antipsychotics for aggression related to psychotic ideation and for the acute management of violence. Hughes (1998) is much more sanguine than Yudofsky et al. (1987) about the use of lithium for aggressive persons who are not manic.

Glazer and Dickson (1998) favourably review the evidence for the effectiveness of clozapine in reducing persistent aggression in schizophrenia. Menditto et al. (1996), for example, found evidence that the substitution of clozapine for standard antipsychotic medication among chronic schizophrenics who responded slowly to a rigorous social learning programme reduced the frequency of assaults and threatened assaults.

There is also a literature on specialty drugs related to various neurotransmitters. For example, Volavka et al. (1990) tested the effectiveness of tryptophan in the treatment of 20 aggressive psychiatric inpatients. Injections of antipsychotics and sedatives were administered as needed to control agitated or violent behaviour. In comparison to placebo, TRP treatment had no effect on the number of violent incidents nor on the hostility-suspiciousness factor of the BPRS, although it significantly reduced injections of antipsychotics and sedatives.

BEHAVIOURAL TREATMENT

The most impressive reductions in assaults among very seriously schizophrenic patients using any treatment type were achieved by Paul and Lentz (1977), who employed a 48-hour time-out contingency imbedded in a sophisticated token economy programme. The same time-out[3] procedure was less effective in a milieu therapy programme, where it did not totally eliminate assaults. This impressive reduction in assaultiveness produced by the behavioural social learning programme was not related to antipsychotic medication. Similar dramatic reductions in assaultiveness were achieved by Beck, Menditto, Baldwin, Angelone, and Maddox (1991), who implemented a social learning programme with a 24-hour time-out period for aggressive psychotic patients held in a maximum security psychiatric facility.

Unfortunately, the demonstration of complete programme control of staff behaviour in the Paul and Lentz (1977) social learning programme is unique in the literature. Behavioural treatment is usually not nearly as well implemented as it was in Paul and Lentz's programme and is, therefore, not as effective. For example, a behavioural programme developed at the maximum security Oak Ridge psychiatric facility awarded points for off-ward and on-ward work, room care and self-care, and ratings of mood and cooperation. These points were accumulated weekly, and the weekly net totals determined patients' privilege levels for the next week. Points were subtracted for misbehaviours according to a fixed fine schedule from the accumulating total as well as the current total, so they could, if large enough, result in an immediate drop in privilege level and an increase in staff surveillance. This programme has been described in several sources (Harris, 1989; Quinsey, 1981).

The programme appeared to increase the fairness and consistency with which privileges were awarded and taken away by staff. There was also evidence that the programme was a good assessment instrument because assaults were unlikely in locations in which the patients had to have exhibited success in the programme in order to obtain access and most likely in situations that patients were eligible to be in regardless of their privilege level (Harris & Varney, 1986; Quinsey & Varney, 1977; Rice et al., 1989).

An evaluation of this programme was conducted by examining predictors of high point earnings in weeks 7 through 12 after admission ($N = 113$) and the prediction of violent and general recidivism over a 6.5-year average follow-up period ($N = 92$) (Rice, Quinsey, & Houghton, 1990).

Intercorrelations among mood, cooperation, room care, self-care, work scores, and point earnings for the second week of treatment were all very high. Number of days confined was also highly negatively correlated with other programme variable predictors. Point earnings significantly increased over the 12-week period. Points earned in weeks 7 through 12 were predicted by point earnings in week 2, less confinement in the first 2 weeks, having criminal charges leading to admission, and having been found unfit for trial or Not Guilty by Reason of Insanity. Considering only those patients who started off poorly in the programme, those who improved were less likely to have been referred from another psychiatric hospital and less likely to have been married.

Length of stay in Oak Ridge (mean of 11 months and median of 4 months) was predicted by having charges leading to admission, being referred from another psychiatric hospital, having been confined more frequently in weeks 7 through 12, and having been more assaultive in the first 12 weeks in the programme. Following release, 51% of the patients were arrested and/or re-admitted to Oak Ridge. This form of failure was predicted by number of previous months in institutions, youthfulness, not having been found unfit for trial or Not Guilty by Reason of Insanity, and having been referred from another psychiatric hospital. Twenty-four percent of the patients were arrested or returned to Oak Ridge for committing a violent offence against persons. Violent re-offenders had spent more total previous months in institutions, were less likely to be psychotic, were less likely to have been employed prior to admission, and were more likely to have been confined during weeks 7 through 12.

The best predictor of future point earnings was past point earnings. At least half of the patients started off very well in the programme and continued to do well. Patients who did not improve were most often referrals from other hospitals who were assaultive and posed a management problem. Months until discharge was related to programme variables but added little to pre-admission predictors. Men found Not Guilty by Reason of Insanity or unfit for trial did better in the programme but were held for longer periods of time. Programme variables were very weakly related to general or violent recidivism.

There are a variety of explanations for these troubling but instructive results. First, there were issues of treatment design: The programme seldom involved immediate tangible reinforcements; the programme was neither individualized nor focused on the risk factors or "criminogenic needs" of the patients, and, in fact, the contingencies did not even make contact with the behaviour of almost half of the patients (who were performing well from the outset).

Similar difficulties were found in an earlier evaluation. Quinsey and Sarbit (1975) showed that patients were responsive to small alterations in the point system that allowed patients to buy commissary items or rent certain privileges with their points (in the form of tokens). Increases were found in points earned for on-ward work, mood and cooperation ratings, and total points earned, but no significant differences were observed in room care and self-care ratings or in fines incurred. Although the group data were quite consistent in showing orderly improvements in point earnings over a 4-month period, individual data indicated that only some patients were responsive to this change in contingency. There is very good reason to believe that patients in these programmes were not actually *learning* new behaviours. A large number of unpublished observations indicate that when additional contingencies were arranged for individual patients using the method ordinarily used for awarding points in this programme (e.g., tokens for particular behaviours), these behaviours increased in a step function. These all-or-none increases in what were often complex behaviours suggest strongly that the programme functioned primarily as a motivational system. The fact that modelling, shaping, and chaining were seldom used in the programme increase the plausibility of this interpretation.

Second, there were problems concerning programme intensity, integrity, and fidelity of implementation (Rice, Quinsey, & Houghton, 1990). Although inter-rater reliabilities were quite acceptable for most of the rated behaviours, their high inter-correlations indicate that they all reflected either a halo phenomenon or a measure of general psychiatric disturbance. Inter-rater reliabilities on the mood and cooperation ratings were variable. These data speak to the lack of specificity of measurement and, thus, reward. Although the programme was in effect continuously, it was targeted at only a small proportion of the patients' behaviours, particularly those involving compliance and security issues.

In a subsequent study, Harris and Rice (1992) documented ever-increasing fines and increasing numbers of punishable acts specified by this programme over a 15-year period, despite strenuous efforts of psychology staff to resist this punitive trend. The increasing punitiveness of the programme was correlated with increasing assaultiveness of the patients. In general, it appeared that whatever clinical utility the programme may have had was eroded over time by drift from behavioural principles of treatment.

STAFF TRAINING

Training programmes have to be either compatible with staff attitudes towards assaultive patients and their management or designed to modify them. An old literature on the "aide culture" amply documents punitive and moralistic attitudes among nursing staff (Ellsworth, 1968). Crichton (1997) used videotape vignettes to show that nursing staff tend to perceive patient assaults in moral terms. More specifically, Harris, Rice, and Preston (1989) examined the perceptions of staff and patients in a maximum security psychiatric institution concerning the least restrictive alternatives for the short-term control of disturbed behaviour. Staff and patients ranked the interventions in the same order of intrusiveness: mechanical restraint with constant observation, seclusion, sedative injection, loss of clothing, a sedative pill, and manual restraint. Experienced staff and patients rated the interventions as less aversive than inexperienced staff and patients. Staff, especially inexperienced staff, expected that the heavier techniques would prevent future occurrences but nevertheless had a greater preference than the patients for the heavier techniques. There was a large discrepancy between staff and patients in the relative frequency with which the various techniques were employed: patients reported that staff more frequently used heavy techniques, and staff reported that they more frequently used light techniques (though preferring to use heavier ones).

Careful documentation provides evidence that the aggression of mentally ill patients does not emanate solely from their psychopathology. Rather, aggressive incidents arise out of interactions among patients and between patients and staff. Some studies have found that staff are the recipients of patient aggression more frequently than patients, despite their smaller numbers. In a 10-year study of assaults in a maximum security psychiatric hospital, Rice et al. (1989) found that staff were the victims of assaults about half the time. These observations and a review of the literature on police-civilian disputes led Rice et al. (1989) to develop a 5-day course designed to train front-line staff in assault prevention as well as effective management of assaults when they occurred. The course covered the prevention of violence through security measures and calming interventions, dealing with explosive situations through defusing techniques, manual restraint, seclusion, and self-defence, and follow-up interventions including interviewing and conflict-resolution techniques. Training methods relied heavily on practice in simulated situations.

Restraint and self-defence techniques were chosen not only because of their effectiveness but also on the basis of their "learnability." A careful examination of trainees' spontaneous responses to simulated physical situations sometimes led to the identification of effective techniques that were easy to learn because they required only slight modfications to spontaneous reactions; in other instances, such an examination identified ineffective habits that could be corrected with practice (Quinsey, Marion, Upfold, & Popple, 1986; Rice et al., 1989). Practice in these techniques was designed not only to teach their mechanics but also to demonstrate the conditions (such as weight disparities between trainee and simulated patient) that influenced their effectiveness.

Evaluation of this programme focused on four sets of measures: (1) measures of knowledge and skills obtained from simulated crises, (2) measures of programme acceptance, including a 15-month post-course questionnaire, (3) measures of patient affect and morale, and (4) incidents of violence and injury (Rice, Helzel, Varney, & Quinsey, 1985). Eighty-nine staff who received the training improved more than control staff on tests of crisis-related skills and knowledge. Measures of programme acceptance indicated strongly favourable responses, and patient affect and morale increased relative to control wards. Assault frequency declined immediately after implementation of the course, and staff injuries were reduced.

Most, but not all, evaluations of staff training programmes have been positive. Infantino and Musingo (1985) evaluated a 3-day training programme in aggression-control techniques. The curriculum was based on criterion-referenced performance standards pertaining to verbal defusing and non-offensive physical action. Ninety-six attendant staff were followed for between 9 and 24 months. Thirty-seven percent of the 65 untrained staff were assaulted, of whom 19 were injured, and one of the 31 trained staff was assaulted and not injured. Contrary results were obtained by Parkes (1996) in an evaluation of training in control and restraint techniques in a medium security facility. Staff were more likely to be injured during restraint after training than before, possibly because the training programme taught staff to approach a patient from in front rather than from behind.

Taken together, these studies indicate that staff training can be effective in reducing staff injury if the training focuses on verbal interventions and sound physical techniques, has ethological validity, and ensures that staff acquire the techniques being taught. Future course development can benefit from Crowner, Douyon, Convit, and Volavka's (1991) videotape method of observation (especially if supplemented by audiotape recording). For example, Crowner, Stepcic, Peric, and Czobor (1994) found that 25 of 35 videotaped assaults were preceded by a warning, a provocation, or both. Of the 16 that were preceded by warnings, the nature of the warning was, in descending order of frequency: threatening gestures, approaching the victim and standing before him/her, pacing in front of the victim, intrusive gestures, and yelling at the victim. This kind of videotape can be profitably employed in staff training using methods developed by Rice et al. (1989).

Lastly, Flannery et al. (1998) report declines in assault frequency in three state hospitals following implementation of the Assaulted Staff Action Program previously shown to reduce assaults in a single institution. The programme involves peer support for staff who have been involved in an assault. Similarly, Quinsey (1977) report a reduction of assaults against staff in a maximum security psychiatric institution following the introduction of a peer and management staff debriefing and support task force that met with attendant staff after they had been involved in assaultive incidents.

Conclusions and Future Research

I last reviewed the literature on institutional violence in the mid-1980s, and it is apparent that we know quite a bit more now than we did then. For example: (1) Actuarial methods can estimate the long-term likelihood that individuals will be assaultive. (2) Dynamic variables signal the imminence of very serious assaults. (3) Certain medications can reduce assaults among patients with particular diagnoses. (4) Behavioural methods can eliminate or markedly reduce assaults among chronic schizophrenics. (5) Staff training in interviewing, security, and physical management can reduce assaults and staff injury.

Nevertheless, our understanding of institutional violence remains unsatisfactory. In the large literature on institutional violence among the mentally ill, only a few studies rise above simple description. Even some of the intervention research has a "medication of the month" flavour. Further improvement in our understanding will require theory. To date, much of the theory that has been applied to understanding institutional violence pertains strictly to proximal causal mechanisms. Proximal mechanisms, however, are best identified and understood in a functional context (for a discussion of these issues see McGuire & Troisi, 1998). Such a context could be provided by an ethological analysis of human aggression buttressed by a theory of ultimate cause. For example, a good portion of institutional assaults appear to result from dominance or status disputes of the type commonly seen among young men (e.g., Daly & Wilson, 1988). This interpretation is supported by assaulters' reports that their aggression resulted from teasing or provocation and by the success of staff training programmes that emphasize "face saving" verbal interventions. Of course, not all institutional aggression results from inter-male status competition with its link to the ultimate cause of intrasexual selection; there are undoubtedly other, functionally different, forms of institutional violence. It is also likely that aggression that may have been motivated originally by status competition comes to be controlled by reinforcement contingencies (as implied by the findings of Paul & Lentz, 1977). The point of this is that we require a functional typology of aggressive behaviour rooted in theories of ultimate causation that can inform our search for proximal causal mechanisms. The videotape technology developed by Crowner and associates appears admirably suited for an ethological analysis of institutional violence.

So, how about my Ojibway friend? From the literature, he appears to be among those patients whose assaultiveness was directly related to psychotic symptomatology and, therefore, one whose aggression could be controlled with antipsychotic medication. He would not be expected to be a persistently assaultive individual. Patients with character disorder and lower-functioning individuals are more likely to be chronically assaultive, with the former exhibiting markedly more serious assaults. The lack of some provocation to this assault was unusual, but the provocation may simply have not been observed.

Notes

1. The abstract of the Harris and Varney paper incorrectly states that psychotic patients were more likely to be assaultive than non-psychotic patients. In fact psychotic patients were *less* likely to be assaultive than non-psychotic patients.
2. Another item that has similar content to the Therapeutic Alliance Scale is *denies all problems* from the Management Problem Scale of the Problem Behavior Checklist (Quinsey et al., 1998). This item is related to static risk and number of clinical problems as rated by staff. It is also closely related to a known dynamic predictor of violence, the Inappropriate and Procriminal Social Behaviors Scale, a file version of the staff-rated Management Problem Scale (Quinsey, Coleman, et al., 1997).
3. For a review of the early behavioural literature on aversive techniques, see Harris and Ersner-Hershfield (1978).

References

Andrews, D.A. (1980). Some experimental investigations of the principles of differential association through deliberate manipulations of the structure of service systems. *American Sociological Review, 45,* 448–462.

Balaban, E., Alper, J.S., & Kasamon, Y.L. (1996). Mean genes and the biology of aggression: A critical review of recent animal and human research. *Journal of Neurogenetics, 11,* 1–43.

Beauford, J.E., McNiel, D.E., & Binder, R.L. (1997). Utility of the initial therapeutic alliance in evaluating psychiatric patients' risk of violence. *American Journal of Psychiatry, 154,* 1272–1276.

Beck, N.C., Menditto, A.A., Baldwin, L.J., Angelone, E., & Maddox, M. (1991). Reduced frequency of aggressive behavior in forensic patients in a social learning program. *Hospital and Community Psychiatry, 42,* 750–752.

Benjaminsen, S., Gotzsche-Larsen, K., Norrie, B., & Harder, L. (1996). Patient violence in a psychiatric hospital in Denmark: Rate of violence and relation to diagnosis. *Nordic Journal of Psychiatry, 50,* 233–242.

Bjørkly, S. (1995). Prediction of aggression in psychiatric patients: A review of prospective prediction studies. *Clinical Psychology Review, 15,* 475–502.

Bjørkly, S. (1999). A ten-year study of aggression in a special secure unit for dangerous patients. *Scandinavian Journal of Psychology, 40,* 57–63.

Brizer, D.A., Convit, A., Krakowski, M., & Volavka, J. (1987). A rating scale for reporting violence on psychiatric wards. *Hospital and Community Psychiatry, 38,* 769–770.

Brizer, D.A., Crowner, M.L., Convit, A., & Volavka, J. (1988). Videotape recording of inpatient assaults: A pilot study. *American Journal of Psychiatry, 145,* 751–752.

Buchanan, A. (1997). The investigation of acting on delusions as a tool for risk assessment in the mentally disordered. *British Journal of Psychiatry, 170,* 12–16.

Carmel, H., & Hunter, M. (1993). Staff injuries from patient attack: Five years' data. *Bulletin of the American Academy of Psychiatry and Law, 21,* 485–493.

Cheung, P., Schweitzer, I., Crowley, K., & Tuckwell, V. (1997a). Aggressive behaviour in schizophrenia: The role of psychopathology. *Australian and New Zealand Journal of Psychiatry, 31,* 62–67.

Cheung, P., Schweitzer, I., Crowley, K., & Tuckwell, V. (1997b). Aggressive behaviour in schizophrenia: Role of state versus trait factors. *Psychiatry Research, 72,* 41–50.

Cheung, P., Schweitzer, I., Crowley, K., & Tuckwell, V. (1997c). Violence in schizophrenia: Role of hallucinations and delusions. *Schizophrenia Research, 26,* 181–190.

Cheung, P., Schweitzer, I., Crowley, K., Yastrubetskaya, O., & Tuckwell, V. (1996). Aggressive behaviour and extrapyramidal side effects of neuroleptics in schizophrenia. *International Clinical Psychopharmacology, 11,* 237–240.

Cheung, P., Schweitzer, I., Tuckwell, V., & Crowley, K.C. (1997). A prospective study of assaults on staff by psychiatric in-patients. *Medicine, Science, and the Law, 37,* 46–52.

Clarkin, J.F., Hurt, S.W., & Crilly, J.L. (1987). Therapeutic alliance and hospital treatment outcome. *Hospital and Community Psychiatry, 38,* 871–875.

Convit, A., Czobor, P., & Volavka, J. (1991). Lateralized abnormality in the EEG of persistently violent psychiatric inpatients. *Society of Biological Psychiatry, 30,* 363–370.

Convit, A., Isay, D., Otis, D., & Volavka, J. (1990). Characteristics of repeatedly assaultive psychiatric inpatients. *Hospital and Community Psychiatry, 41,* 1112–1115.

Convit, A., Jaeger, J., Lin, S.P., Meisner, M., & Volavka, J. (1988). Predicting assaultiveness in psychiatric inpatients: A pilot study. *Hospital and Community Psychiatry, 39,* 429–434.

Crichton, J. (1997). The response of nursing staff to psychiatric inpatient misdemeanour. *Journal of Forensic Psychiatry, 8,* 36–61.

Crowner, M.L., Douyon, R., Convit, A., Gaztanaga, P., Volavka, J., & Bakall, R. (1990). Akathisia and violence. *Psychopharmacology Bulletin, 26,* 115–117.

Crowner, M.L., Douyon, R., Convit, A., & Volavka, J. (1991). Videotape recording of assaults on a state hospital inpatient ward. *Journal of Neuropsychiatry and Clinical Neurosciences, 3,* S9–S14.

Crowner, M.L., Peric, G., Stepcic, F., & Van-Oss, E. (1994). A comparison of videocameras and official incident reports in detecting inpatient assaults. *Hospital and Community Psychiatry, 45,* 1144–1145.

Crowner, M.L., Peric, G., Stepcic, F., & Ventura, F. (1995). Psychiatric patients' explanations for assaults. *Psychiatric Services, 46,* 614–615.

Crowner, M.L., Stepcic, F., Peric, G., & Czobor, P. (1994). Typology of patient-patient assaults detected by videocameras. *American Journal of Psychiatry, 151,* 1669–1672.

Daly, M., & Wilson, M. (1988). *Homicide.* New York: Aldine de Gruyter.

Day, H.D., Franklin, J.M., & Marshall, D.D. (1998). Predictors of aggression in hospitalized adolescents. *Journal of Psychology, 132,* 427–434.

Dietz, P.E., & Rada, R.T. (1983). Interpersonal violence in forensic facilities. In J.R. Lion & W.H. Reid (Eds.), *Assaults within psychiatric facilities* (pp. 47–59). New York: Grune & Stratton.

Ellsworth, R.B. (1968). *Nonprofessionals in psychiatric rehabilitation: The psychiatric aide and the schizophrenic patient.* New York: Appleton-Century-Crofts.

Flannery, R.B., Hanson, M.A., Penk, W.E., Goldfinger, S., Pastva, G.J., & Navon, M.A. (1998). Replicated declines in assault rates after implementation of the Assaulted Staff Action Program. *Psychiatric Services, 49,* 241–243.

Gardner, W., Lidz, C.W., Mulvey, E.P., & Shaw, E.C. (1996). Clinical versus actuarial predictions of violence by patients with mental illnesses. *Journal of Consulting and Clinical Psychology, 64,* 602–609.

Glazer, W.M., & Dickson, R.A. (1998). Clozapine reduces violence and persistent aggression in schizophrenia. *Journal of Clinical Psychiatry, 59*(suppl 3), 8–14.

Gothelf, D., Apter, A., & van Praag, H.M. (1997). Measurement of aggression in psychiatric patients. *Psychiatry Research, 71,* 83–95.

Haller, R.M., & Deluty, R.H. (1988). Assaults on staff by psychiatric in-patients. *British Journal of Psychiatry, 152,* 174–179.

Hallsteinsen, A., Kristensen, M., Dahl, A.A., & Eilertsen, D.E. (1998). The Extended Staff Observation Aggression Scale (SOAS-E): Development, presentation and evaluation. *Acta Psychiatrica Scandinavica, 97,* 423–426.

Hare, R.D. (1991). *The Hare Psychopathy Checklist-Revised.* North Tonawanda, NY: Multi-Health Systems.

Harris, G.T. (1989). The relationship between neuroleptic drug dose and the performance of psychiatric patients in a maximum security token economy program. *Journal of Behavior Therapy and Experimental Psychiatry, 20,* 57–67.

Harris, G.T., & Rice, M.E. (1986). Staff injuries sustained during altercations with psychiatric patients. *Journal of Interpersonal Violence, 1,* 193–211.

Harris, G.T., & Rice, M.E. (1992). Reducing violence in institutions: Maintaining behavior change. In R.D. Peters, R.J. McMahon, & V.L. Quinsey (Eds.), *Aggression and violence throughout the life span* (pp. 261–282). Newbury Park, CA: Sage.

Harris, G.T., Rice, M.E., & Preston, D.L. (1989). Staff and patient perceptions of the least restrictive alternatives for the short term control of disturbed behavior. *Journal of Psychiatry and Law, 17,* 239–263.

Harris, G.T., & Varney, G.W. (1986). A ten-year study of assaults and assaulters on a maximum security psychiatric unit. *Journal of Interpersonal Violence, 1,* 173–191.

Harris, S.L., & Ersner-Hershfield, R. (1978). Behavioral suppression of seriously disruptive behavior in psychotic and retarded patients: A review of punishment and its alternatives. *Psychological Bulletin, 85,* 1352–1375.

Harrow, M., Rattenbury, F., & Stoll, F. (1988). Schizophrenic delusions: An analysis of their persistence, of related premorbid ideas, and of three major dimensions. In T.F. Oltmanns & B.A. Maher (Eds.), *Delusional beliefs* (pp. 184–211). New York: Wiley.

Heilbrun, K., Hart, S.D., Hare, R.D., Gustafson, D., Nunez, C., & White, A.J. (1998). Inpatient and postdischarge aggression in mentally disordered offenders. *Journal of Interpersonal Violence, 13,* 514–527.

Hellerstein, D., Frosch, W., & Koenigsberg, H.W. (1987). The clinical significance of command hallucinations. *American Journal of Psychiatry, 144*, 219–221.

Hillbrand, M. (1995). Aggression against self and aggression against others in violent psychiatric patients. *Journal of Consulting and Clinical Psychology, 63*, 668–671.

Hillbrand, M., Spitz, R.T., Foster, H.G., Krystal, J.H., & Young, J.L. (1998). Creatine kinase elevations and aggressive behavior in hospitalized forensic patients. *Psychiatric Quarterly, 69*, 69–82.

Hughes, D.H. (1998). Pharmacologic management of the chronically aggressive psychiatric patient. *Psychiatric Annals, 28*, 367–370.

Infantino, J.A., & Musingo, S.Y. (1985). Assaults and injuries among staff with and without training in aggression control techniques. *Hospital and Community Psychiatry, 36*, 1312–1314.

James, D.V., Fineberg, N.A., Shah, A.K., & Priest, R.G. (1990). An increase in violence on an acute psychiatric ward. *British Journal of Psychiatry, 156*, 846–852.

Junginger, J. (1996). Psychosis and violence: The case for a content analysis of psychotic experience. *Schizophrenia Bulletin, 22*, 91–103.

Kay, S.R., Wolkenfeld, F., & Murrill, L.M. (1988a). Profiles of aggression among psychiatric patients. I: Nature and prevalence. *Journal of Nervous and Mental Disease, 176*, 539–546.

Kay, S.R., Wolkenfeld, F., & Murrill, L.M. (1988b). Profiles of aggression among psychiatric patients. II: Covariates and predictors. *Journal of Nervous and Mental Disease, 176*, 547–557.

Krakowski, M.I., Convit, A., Jaeger, J., Lin, S., & Volavka, J. (1989a). Inpatient violence: Trait and state. *Journal of Psychiatric Research, 23*, 57–64.

Krakowski, M.I., Convit, A., Jaeger, J., Lin, S., & Volavka, J. (1989b). Neurological impairment in violent schizophrenic inpatients. *American Journal of Psychiatry, 146*, 849–853.

Krakowski, M.I., Czobor, P., Carpenter, M.D., Libiger, J., Kunz, M., Papezova, H., Parker, B.B., Schamder, L., & Abad, T. (1997). Community violence and inpatient assaults: Neurobiological deficits. *Journal of Neuropsychiatry and Clinical Neurosciences, 9*, 549–555.

Krakowski, M., Jaeger, J., & Volavka, J. (1988). Violence and psychopathology: A longitudinal study. *Comprehensive Psychiatry, 29*, 174–181.

Kroner, D.G., & Mills, J.F. (1997, February). *The VRAG: Predicting institutional misconduct in violent offenders.* Paper presented at the 50th Annual Meeting of the Ontario Psychological Association, Toronto.

Lanza, M.L. (1992). Nurses as patient assault victims: An update, synthesis, and recommendations. *Archives of Psychiatric Nursing, 6*, 163–171.

Lion, J.R., & Reid, W.H. (Eds.). (1983). *Assaults within psychiatric facilities.* New York: Grune & Stratton.

Maguire, K., Cheung, P., Crowley, K., Norman, T., Schweitzer, I., & Burrows, G. (1997). Aggressive behaviour and platelet ^{3}H-paroxetine binding in schizophrenia. *Schizophrenia Research, 23*, 61–67.

McGuire, M.T., & Troisi, A. (1998). *Darwinian psychiatry.* New York: Oxford University Press.

McNiel, D.E., & Binder, R.L. (1994). Screening for risk of inpatient violence: Validation of an actuarial tool. *Law and Human Behavior, 18*, 579–586.

Menditto, A.A., Beck, N.C., Stuve, P., Fisher, J.A., Stacy, M., Logue, M.B., & Baldwin, L.J. (1996). Effectiveness of clozapine and a social learning program for severely disabled psychiatric patients. *Psychiatric Services, 47*, 46–51.

Noble, P. (1997). Violence in psychiatric in-patients: Review and clinical implications. *International Review of Psychiatry, 9*, 207–216.

Overall, J.E., & Gorham, D.R. (1962). The Brief Psychiatric Rating Scale. *Psychological Reports, 19,* 799–812.

Parkes, J. (1996). Control and restraint training: A study of its effectiveness in a medium secure psychiatric unit. *Journal of Forensic Psychiatry, 7,* 525–534.

Paul, G.L., & Lentz, R.J. (1977). *Psychosocial treatment of chronic mental patients: Milieu versus social-learning programs.* Cambridge, MA: Harvard University Press.

Quinsey, V.L. (1977). Studies in the reduction of assaults in a maximum security psychiatric institution. *Canada's Mental Health, 25,* 21–23.

Quinsey, V.L. (1981). The long term management of the mentally disordered offender. In S.J. Hucker, C.D. Webster, & M. Ben-Aron (Eds.), *Mental disorder and criminal responsibility* (pp. 137–155). Toronto: Butterworths.

Quinsey, V.L., Coleman, G., Jones, B., & Altrows, I. (1997). Proximal antecedents of eloping and reoffending among mentally disordered offenders. *Journal of Interpersonal Violence, 12,* 794–813.

Quinsey, V.L., Harris, G.T., Rice, M.E., & Cormier, C. (1998). *Violent offenders Appraising and managing risk.* Washington: American Psychological Association.

Quinsey, V.L., Marion, G., Upfold, D., & Popple, K.T. (1986). Issues in teaching physical methods of resisting rape. *Sexual Coercion and Assault, 1,* 125–130.

Quinsey, V.L., & Sarbit, B. (1975). Behavioral changes associated with the introduction of a token economy in a maximum security psychiatric institution. *Canadian Journal of Criminology and Corrections, 17,* 177–182.

Quinsey, V.L., Skilling, T., & Rougier-Chapman, C. (1997). *Inter-ministerial population review initiative: Final report.* Submitted to the Ministry of Community and Social Services, Ontario.

Quinsey, V.L., & Varney, G.W. (1977). Characteristics of assaults and assaulters in a maximum security psychiatric unit. *Crime and Justice, 5,* 212–220.

Raja, M., Azzoni, A., & Lubich, L. (1997). Aggressive and violent behavior in a population of psychiatric inpatients. *Social Psychiatry and Psychiatric Epidemiology, 32,* 428–434.

Rasmussen, K., & Levander, S. (1996a). Crime and violence among psychiatric patients in a maximum security psychiatric hospital. *Criminal Justice and Behaviour, 23,* 455–471.

Rasmussen, K., & Levander, S. (1996b). Individual rather than situation characteristics predict violence in a maximum security hospital. *Journal of Interpersonal Violence, 11,* 376–390.

Reid, W.H., Bollinger, M.F., & Edwards, J.G. (1989). Serious assaults by inpatients. *Psychosomatics, 30,* 54–56.

Renwick, S.J., Black, L., Ramm, M., & Novaco, R. (1997). Anger treatment with forensic hospital patients. *Legal and Criminal Psychology, 2,* 103–116.

Rice, M.E., Harris, G.T., Varney, G.W., & Quinsey, V.L. (1989). *Violence in institutions: Understanding, prevention, and control.* Toronto: Hans Huber.

Rice, M.E., Helzel, M.F., Varney, G.W., & Quinsey, V.L. (1985). Crisis prevention and intervention training for psychiatric hospital staff. *American Journal of Community Psychology, 13,* 289–304.

Rice, M.E., Quinsey, V.L., & Houghton, R. (1990). Predicting treatment outcome and recidivism among patients in a maximum security token economy. *Behavioral Sciences and the Law, 8,* 313–326.

Ross, D.J., Hart, S.C., & Webster, C.D. (1998). *Aggression in psychiatric patients: Using the HCR-20 to assess risk for violence in hospital and the community.* Port Coquitlam, BC: Riverview Hospital.

Silver, J.M., & Yudofsky, S.C. (1987). Documentation of aggression in the assessment of the violent patient. *Psychiatric Annals, 17,* 375–384.

Steinert, T., Hermer, K., & Faust, V. (1996). Comparison of aggressive and non-aggressive schizophrenic inpatients matched for age and sex. *European Journal of Psychiatry, 10,* 100–107.

Stermac, L.E. (1987). Anger control treatment for forensic patients. *Journal of Interpersonal Violence, 1,* 446–457.

Stoff, D.M., & Cairns, R.B. (Eds.). (1996). *Aggression and violence: Genetic, neurobiological, and biosocial perspectives.* Mahwah, NJ: Erlbaum.

Tam, E., Engelsmann, F., & Fugure, R. (1996). Patterns of violent incidents by patients in a general hospital psychiatric facility. *Psychiatric Services, 47,* 86–88.

Tardiff, K. (1989). *Concise guide to assessment and management of violent patients.* Washington: American Psychiatric Press.

Thackrey, M. (1987). *Therapeutics for aggression: Psychological/physical crisis intervention.* New York: Human Sciences Press.

Villeneuve, D., & Quinsey, V.L. (1995). Predictors of general and violent recidivism among mentally disordered prison inmates. *Criminal Justice and Behavior, 22,* 397–410.

Volavka, J., Crowner, M.L., Brizer, D., Convit, A., Van Praag, H., & Suckow, R.F. (1990). Tryptophan treatment of aggressive psychiatric inpatients. *Biological Psychiatry, 28,* 728–732.

Yudofsky, S.C., Silver, J.M., Jackson, W., Endicott, J., & Williams, D. (1986). The Overt Aggression Scale for the objective rating of verbal and physical aggression. *American Journal of Psychiatry, 143,* 35–39.

Yudofsky, S.C., Silver, J.M., & Schneider, S.E. (1987). Pharmacologic treatment of aggression. *Psychiatric Annals, 17,* 397–407.

V.L. Quinsey is associated with Queen's University, Kingston, Ontario, Canada.

Author's Note

This chapter was written when the author was supported by a Senior Research Fellowship from the Ontario Ministry of Health.

I wish to thank Jill Atkinson, Brian Jones, and Marnie Rice for commenting on an earlier version of this chapter.

Comments or queries may be directed to Vernon L. Quinsey, Department of Psychology, Queen's University, Kingston, ON K7L 3N6 Canada. Telephone: 613 533-6538. Fax: 613 533-2499. E-mail: <quinsey@psyc.queensu.ca>.

HIGH-RISK FACTORS FOR VIOLENCE

Emerging Evidence and Its Relevance to Effective Treatment and Prevention of Violence on Psychiatric Wards

STÅL BJØRKLY

Introduction

The literature on systematic attempts to reduce violence in psychiatric facilities is not voluminous and, with a few notable exceptions (Corrigan, Yudofsky, & Silver, 1993; Nijman, Merkelbach, Allertz, & a Campo, 1997; Rice, Harris, Varney, & Quinsey, 1989), appears to be of a general nature and lacking in substantiated recommendations for specialized approaches to the prevention of intra-institutional violence per se. Moreover, there is a paucity of studies that report adequate methodology (e.g., controlled studies with double-blind trials) in measuring the efficacy of treatment interventions. Interventions to reduce institutional violence can be organized into various classes such as: drugs, seclusion, mechanical restraint, staff training in crisis intervention, and specific treatment programmes. In another chapter, Dr. Fransson addresses the role of important factors such as social setting, staff atmosphere, work structure, staff competence, seclusion, and risk factors. This chapter will elaborate on the possible impact of three salient risk factors. Space limitations preclude an extensive discussion of other important issues such as contextual differences (short-term vs. long-term treatment), gender differences, and cultural differences.

This chapter focuses on three basic questions that may be useful in attempting to improve treatment and prevention of aggression in the clinical setting. These are: What is our current knowledge of patient characteristics and patient-staff interactions that may increase the risk of violence *(high-risk factors)*? Are there any particular hallmarks pertaining to risk factors that may indicate increased risk of violence *(hallmarks)*? Can such hallmarks be employed to reduce violence in psychiatric wards *(clinical application)*?

High-Risk Factors

The MacArthur Violence Risk Assessment Study defines four categories of risk factors for violence, two categories that are assumed to be of a static nature ("dispo-

S. Hodgins (ed.), Violence among the Mentally Ill, 237–250.
© 2000 *Kluwer Academic Publishers. Printed in the Netherlands.*

sitional" and "historical" factors) and two categories that may be more readily subject to change ("contextual" and "clinical" factors) (Monahan, 1995). This paper concentrates on the latter two categories, among which three factors in particular, and their association to risk of violence in psychiatric patients, have recently been receiving increasing attention. These are: comorbid substance abuse disorder (clinical factors), violence-prone hallucinations and delusions (clinical factors), and limit-setting (contextual factors).

COMORBID SUBSTANCE ABUSE DISORDER

Substance abuse is a significant factor in acts of violence among members of the public who are not psychotic. Recent research findings suggest that it may also be important in assessing the risk of violence among the severely mentally ill (Scott et al., 1998; Steadman et al., 1998). The results of the MacArthur Violence Risk Assessment Study indicate a strong relationship between substance abuse disorder and violence in patients with major mental disorders after discharge from hospital (Monahan, 1995). Swartz et al. (1998) found that patients with major mental disorder and substance abuse problems were twice as likely to have engaged in violent behaviour compared to those without a substance abuse diagnosis. Although there are rare contradictions to this finding (Owen, Tarantello, Jones, & Tenant, 1998; Volavka et al., 1997), a substantial number of studies have found a strong relationship between comorbid substance abuse and risk of violence (Adler & Lidberg, 1995; Coid, 1996; Cuffel, Shumway, Chouljian, & MacDonald, 1994; Eronen, Hakola, & Tiihonen, 1996; Scott et al.; Smith & Hucker, 1994; Wallace et al., 1998).

Questions
Do these findings have any relevance to inpatient treatment? Is comorbid substance abuse disorder per se a risk factor, or do other, related, factors operate with it to induce violence?

VIOLENCE-PRONE HALLUCINATIONS AND DELUSIONS

It has been suggested that studies on the risk of violence in major mental disorder should be examining individual elements of phenomenology (e.g., Buchanan, 1997). Researchers have found an association between certain types of hallucinations and delusions and increased risk of violence across a variety of contexts. Persecutory delusions have predicted violence in patients in a psychiatric secure care unit (e.g., Krakowski & Czobor, 1994). A combination of persecutory and hypochondriacal delusions has been associated with homicide in psychotic patients (e.g., d'Orban & O'Connor, 1989). Violence-inducing auditory hallucinations have been found to be a significant precipitant of violence in psychotic patients (e.g., Junginger, 1995). In a convincing study with several patient groups and a sample of 400 adults who had never received psychiatric services, Link, Andrews, and Cullen (1992) found that current psychotic symptoms predicted recent violence not only in the patient group, but also in the community group. In a large-scale study of a complete resident sample of special hospital patients, Taylor et al. (1998) found that 75% of those with a psychosis were recorded as being driven to commit criminal offences by their delusions. In the absence of delusions, hallucinations had no such effect.

Questions
Are there any specific hallmarks of delusions and hallucinations (e.g., content, theme, loudness) associated with increased risk of violence? If so, how can this information be efficiently applied in the clinical context?

LIMIT-SETTING

There is a limited but growing number of reported studies on antecedents of violent behaviour in psychiatric facilities (Bjørkly, 1993; Cooper & Mendonca, 1989; Kennedy, Kemp, & Dyer, 1992; Linaker & Busch-Iversen, 1995). A substantial number of these have found a relationship between situational factors, such as limit-setting, and inpatient violence (Bjørkly, 1999; Dietz & Rada, 1982; Durivage, 1989; Lee, Villar, Juthani, & Bluestone, 1989). In a study by Sheridan, Henrion, Robinson, and Baxter (1990), 60% of violent episodes in a psychiatric ward were triggered by limit-setting situations. The authors were surprised by the fact that only 20% of violent behaviours were precipitated by hallucinations and delusions, especially since 70% of the patients had a diagnosis of schizophrenia. Armond (1982) and Bjørkly (1999) found that limit-setting situations were precursors of violent incidents in about 60% of the recorded episodes. These results are supported by those of Depp (1983) and Perregaard and Bartels (1992), who found that 78% of a total of 248 episodes were triggered by limit-setting. Although empirical documentation of a relationship between limit-setting and violence is not overwhelming, so far the stability of an "about 60%" finding appears to be justified.

Questions
Can rates of limit-setting interactions be reduced in psychiatric facilities (without negative consequences for the structured treatment milieu)? Can improved communication on the part of the nurse in setting limits help diminish the risk of violence?

Hallmarks

Although a relatively strong association among the three aforementioned risk factors and violence has been documented, evidence is emerging that our attention should be directed to specific hallmarks pertaining to each risk factor. It has been suggested that sorting out such hallmarks may facilitate clinical application of this information to prevent violence.

COMORBID SUBSTANCE ABUSE DISORDER

The results of a majority of investigations strongly support the existence of an association between diagnosis of comorbid substance abuse disorder and increased risk of violence in psychiatric patients. However, this association does not appear strong enough to be a single predictor of high-risk individuals in clinical practice. A sub-group of patients with severe mental disorder fall into a self-perpetuating cycle of substance abuse, illness exacerbation, violent behaviour, and institutional recidivism (e.g., Torrey, 1994). In certain patients, risk of violence appears to be increased by specific patient characteristics concomitant with substance abuse problems. Findings to date suggest that the risk of violence is increased by a combination of substance abuse problems, medication non-compliance, and low insight into the illness (Smith & Hucker, 1994; Swartz et al., 1998; Torrey). Swartz et al. found that patients with both non-compliance and substance abuse problems were more than twice as likely to commit violent acts, while those individuals with only one of these problems were at no greater risk of violence.

The concept of "threat/control override" (TCO) has been advanced to interpret the possible impact of certain psychotic symptoms as precipitants of violence (Link & Stueve, 1994). A high TCO index indicates that the patient feels threatened (others wish to inflict harm) and that his or her internal controls are compromised compre-hensively (one's mind is dominated by forces beyond one's control and the thoughts of others are put into one's head). Findings of a study with more than 300 patients indicate that the combination of substance abuse disorder and TCO symptoms add significantly to the risk of violence (Swanson, Borum, Swartz, & Monahan, 1996).

In sum, there appears to be growing empirical support for the notion that the following three factors, together with a diagnosis of comorbid substance abuse dis-order, increase the risk of violence: low insight into illness, medication non-compliance, and high levels of TCO.

VIOLENCE-PRONE HALLUCINATIONS AND DELUSIONS

Unlike studies of the associations between violence and broad categories of subject characteristics (e.g., age and mental illness), analyses of the relationship between violence and the content and theme of psychotic symptoms can be specific and de-tailed. A small but steadily growing number of studies have focused on persecutory delusions, command hallucinations, and TCO.

Buchanan (1997) found that three areas of phenomenology influenced the likeli-hood of a persecutory delusion being acted upon: (a) patients who were able to identify evidence supporting their delusion, (b) patients who went looking for evi-dence to confirm or refute their belief, and (c) patients who were frightened by their delusions. An association between these characteristics and increased risk of vio-lence has been reported by a number of studies (Kendler, Glazer, & Morgenstern, 1983; Wesseley et al., 1993). A small-scale study by Kennedy et al. (1992) offers provisional support to the violence-triggering effect of fear and anger in delusional disorder. In a record survey of a complete resident sample of special (high security) hospital patients ($n = 1,740$), Taylor et al. (1998) concluded that delusions precipi-tated violent crimes in a very high proportion of patients. The delusions were almost invariably of a persecutory nature. This finding is consistent with those of earlier works (Junginger, 1996; Krakowski & Czobor, 1994; Link & Stueve, 1994; Swanson et al., 1996; Taylor, 1985). The same relationship has been found between persecu-tory delusions and threats of violence (Estroff, Zimmer, Lachicotte, & Benoit, 1994).

The extent to which hallucinations induce violent acts is less clear. Some results tend to suggest that hallucinations are rarely associated with violent acts (Cheung, Schweitzer, Crowley, & Tuckwell, 1997; McNiel, 1994; Taylor, 1985), whereas other findings indicate that violent command hallucinations have the potential to precipitate violent behaviour (Rogers, Gillis, Turner, & Frise-Smith, 1990; Volavka et al., 1997). In particular, some of Junginger's work questions the claim that command hallucinations pose little if any danger (Junginger, 1990, 1995). McNiel notes that where significant positive associations between hallucinations and violence have been shown, it has usually been in the context of other psychotic symptoms. Other studies confirm the existence of a violence-escalating interaction between delusions and hallucinations (Swanson et al., 1996), and even indicate that in the absence of delusions hallucinations appear to have minimal violence-triggering effect (Taylor et al., 1998). This interaction effect is supported by the preliminary finding of a statistically significant relationship between loudness and intrusiveness of hallucinations and intensity of delusions (Hustig & Hafner, 1990).

In a convincing study based on data from the Epidemiologic Catchment Area, Swanson et al. (1996) found that patients reporting TCO symptoms were about twice as likely to engage in violent behaviour as those with only hallucinations or other psychotic symptoms. In a recent study on the understanding of the mechanisms underlying delusions, Freeman and Garety (1999) concluded that delusional distress is not simply related to content but is associated with whether the patient worries about being unable to control thoughts concerning the delusional belief. In a matched study of violent and non-violent schizophrenia patients, Cheung et al. (1997) found that the violent group were more likely to report that the persecutory delusions made them feel angry. Although more empirical support for the role of TCO in violent behaviour is required, it appears to be a promising approach to the analysis of mechanisms underlying persecutory delusions as precipitants of violent behaviour.

To sum up, three hallmarks pertaining to psychotic symptomatology have been gaining steadily growing empirical support as precursors of violent behaviour: fear-inducing persecutory delusions in patients with a strong conviction of other people wishing one harm; fear-inducing persecutory delusions in patients perceiving that their thoughts and actions are controlled by others; fear-inducing persecutory delusions in combination with violent command hallucinations.

LIMIT-SETTING

Clinical studies on the exact nature of patient-staff interactions that may increase the risk of violence in psychiatric wards are scarce (Friis & Helldin, 1994) but steadily growing in number (e.g., Nijman et al., 1997). With few exceptions (e.g., Crowner, Peric, Stepcid, & Ventura, 1995), these studies are retrospective in nature and are not based on direct observation or participant observation of limit-setting situations. However, some findings appear to be stable across studies. A strong relationship between staff-patient communication problems and increased risk of violence is documented by several studies (Owen et al., 1998; Whittington & Wykes, 1996). Shah, Fineberg, and James (1991) argue that authoritarian attitudes on the part of staff and lack of staff-patient communication may elicit violence. Earlier studies reached similar conclusions (e.g., Katz & Kirkland, 1990; Rice et al., 1989). Dubin, Wilson, and Mercer's (1988) survey disclosed that while no psychiatrists using positive talking strategies were injured, one third of those using an aggressive response were injured. Other studies have come to similar conclusions concerning staff acting in a provocative manner (Madden, Lion, & Penna, 1976) or exhibiting high levels of irritability (Edwards & Reid, 1983). In separate studies, Blair (1991) and Flannery, Hanson, Penk, and Flannery (1996) found that inflexible attitudes among staff and inconsistency in setting limits may induce violence. Another study concluded that experienced staff, compared to inexperienced, were significantly more competent in helping patients to control their anxiety, more ready to ask for help, and less reluctant to admit that they were anxious in certain limit-setting interactions (Perregaard & Bartels, 1992). The authors hypothesize that these factors explain the disproportionately low number of violent encounters involving more experienced nurses as opposed to less experienced ones.

Viewed within the limitations set by the small number of empirical studies, there emerge three hallmarks of the exact nature of interpersonal communication that may induce violence in limit-setting situations: authoritarian, inflexible attitudes and poor communication on the part of staff; lack of consistency in setting limits; insufficient recognition of, and failure to address, increased levels of anxiety in patients.

Clinical Application

The basic question in this section is: Can evidence concerning specific hallmarks pertaining to high-risk factors be employed to reduce violence in psychiatric facilities?

COMORBID SUBSTANCE ABUSE DISORDER

Numerous studies have found a dual diagnosis of severe mental illness and substance abuse to be significantly associated with violent behaviour. In general, however, these studies have examined associations only, and therefore their results cannot be interpreted as proof of a causal link between substance abuse and violence. Putting too much weight on substance misuse as a high-risk factor for violence runs the risk of overpredicting violence in this patient group. It has been suggested that specialized security measures for this patient group may substantially reduce risk of violence in psychiatric facilities (Mulvey, 1994). It has also been advocated that higher priority be given to specific training and interventions for management of patients with dual diagnosis (Johnson, 1997). Based on the present survey of the literature, some specific measures can be recommended:
- Patients with comorbid substance abuse disorder and a previous history of violent behaviour should be considered risk patients.
- Patients with a comorbid substance abuse disorder disclosing low insight into illness, medication non-compliance, and high levels of TCO should be considered high-risk patients.

- Measures should be taken to initiate either manual or computerized flagging of the medical records and ward books of such patients. Eichelman (1991) cites a 1989 study by Sparr and colleagues in which implementation of flagging was followed by a 25% decrease in emergency room assaults.
- Direct measures should be taken to make treatment staff aware of the difficulty of improving insight into illness for this particular group of patients. In particular, confronting patients on lack of insight into illness should be kept to an absolute minimum during phases of intoxication and acute abstinence (e.g., Whittington & Wykes, 1994).
- Staff-patient interactions around medication, especially if involuntary administration of medicine is required, should be considered high-risk situations for violence, and handled accordingly.
- Individual risk monitoring, focusing on the relative risk of violence associated with factors such as intoxication or abstinence, should be established.
- Thorough security procedures should be implemented to prevent patients from becoming further intoxicated while hospitalized (e.g., Rice et al., 1989).

VIOLENCE-PRONE HALLUCINATIONS AND DELUSIONS

There seems to be consensus that the main aspect of mental state related to violence is the presence of persecutory delusions, especially those that imply a particular course of action (e.g., Junginger, 1996). The risk of violence appears to be increased in patients who perceive that their thoughts and actions are controlled by others (e.g., Swanson et al., 1996) and if the persecutory delusions are accompanied by violent command hallucinations (e.g., Volavka et al., 1997). Despite the apparent effectiveness of neuroleptics, it is reported that up to 50% of psychotic patients on medication will continue to experience delusions and hallucinations (e.g., Borell, d'Elia, & Orhagen, 1995; Curson, Patel, Liddle, & Barnes, 1988; Roth, Fonagy, Parry, Target, & Woods, 1996) and up to 30–40% of schizophrenic patients on medication will relapse (e.g., Curson et al.; Tarrier, 1992). A growing number of controlled trials have confirmed the effectiveness of cognitive-behavioural techniques (CBTs) aimed at the modification of delusions and hallucinations (Drury, Birchwood, Cochrane, & Macmillan, 1996a, 1996b; Garety, Kuipers, Fowler, Chamberlain, & Dunn, 1994; Kuipers et al., 1998; Tarrier et al., 1993). Systematic attempts to modify individuals' delusions have included verbal questioning, belief modification, stimulus control techniques, and experimental reality testing. Preliminary findings indicate that the presence of "distress factors" such as low self-esteem (e.g., Freeman et al., 1998), high levels of anxiety (e.g., Freeman & Garety, 1999), and anger (e.g., Cheung et al., 1997; Howells, 1989) have an aggravating effect on persecutory delusions. In a well-controlled 18-month follow-up trial, Kuipers et al. found that patients in the CBT treatment group showed a significant and continuing reduction in delusional distress and frequency of hallucinations, whereas the control group did not change from baseline. An extensive (50-study) meta-analysis on the effect of CBTs in the treatment of anger showed a mean weighted effect size of .70 (Beck & Fernandez, 1998). It is suggested that reduction of "distress factors," if substantiated by further research, should be given high priority as a treatment target for the prevention of violent behaviour as well. So far, studies on the efficacy of CBT in treating hallucinations and delusions have involved small samples and the treatments have not been subject to large-scale evaluation. However, there appears to be a consistent trend suggesting that treatment approaches that have focused on cognitions and beliefs associated with the symptom have produced benefits generalizable outside the treatment session, to other symptoms, and over time (e.g., Haddock et al., 1998; Kuipers et al.). Thus, there is emerging empirical evidence for suggesting measures that may contribute to more efficient treatment of patients suffering from "violent" hallucinations and delusions. These measures are:

- Identification of situations and interactions that precipitate "violent" hallucinations and delusions in the individual patient (precipitants).
- Identification of each patient's early warning signs of "violent" delusional thinking and hallucinations (warning signs).
- Implementation of routine staff interventions individually adapted to the patient's precipitants and warning signs (i.e., clinical application of CBTs).
- Application of CBTs to modify delusions and hallucinations in the context of individual therapy.
- Specific treatment interventions to reduce "distress factors"; these seem to be warranted, since low self-esteem, high levels of anxiety, and anger appear to have an aggravating effect on persecutory delusions.

LIMIT-SETTING

It is quite well documented that limit-setting situations are frequent precipitants of violence in psychiatric wards. Efforts to reduce the number of limit-setting interactions may be one consequence of such findings. However, limit-setting is an integral part of a structured treatment approach, which has been demonstrated to be superior to an unstructured approach in the treatment of potentially violent psychiatric patients (e.g., Aquilina, 1991; Flannery et al., 1996; Friis & Helldin, 1994; Katz & Kirkland, 1990). It is argued here that efforts to improve nurses' ability to identify escalating situations, together with measures to improve the quality of staff communication in limit-setting interactions, may reduce both the rate of violence and the number of limit-setting episodes. Accumulated empirical evidence points to the need for further steps to reduce salient aspects of staff communication that are of a violence-inducing nature, and, correspondingly, to increase interpersonal communications that are of a violence-reducing nature. Empirical evidence for the efficacy of staff training programmes is steadily growing. An early comparative study found a ten-fold difference in the assault rate on untrained and trained inpatient staff (Infantino & Musingo, 1985). Another study observed a similar reduction in the assault rate after the staff had been formally trained (Gertz, 1980). Using a therapeutic management protocol, Kalogjera, Bedi, Watson, and Meyer (1989) obtained a 64% reduction in seclusions and restraints on three wards. Their protocol gives detailed suggestions on how staff members should react to patients' disruptive behaviour at an early stage. As far as I know, a recent study by Nijman et al. (1997) is one of the first controlled studies of staff training programmes. It failed to find a strong effect of training on rates of aggression, mainly because there was a marked reduction in frequencies of aggressive behaviour in both experimental (about 60%) and control (about 40%) wards. Nijman et al. concluded that standardized reporting by staff of aggressive episodes may in itself reduce rates of aggression. Similar findings have been reported in other studies (e.g., Nilson, Palmstierna, & Wistedt, 1988). There is an apparent need for further research to improve the content and clinical implementation of standardized staff training programmes. Such programmes should focus on warning signs and situational antecedents of violence, as well as on communication styles aimed at conflict resolution and calming down in limit-setting interactions.

Since violence rarely erupts without warning, staff guidelines for optimal timing of, and criteria for, setting limits are an important factor in an optimal staff intervention procedure. Monitoring of early warning signs in the individual patient may allow for early interventions while the anxiety level is still low in both patient and staff (Tardiff, 1989). There appears to be good empirical evidence that recidivist patients generally show warning signs prior to violent acts in psychiatric wards (Linaker & Busch-Iversen, 1995; Powell, Caan, & Crowe, 1994). While there are numerous studies on demographic variables and violence, there is a deplorable paucity of studies on warning signs.

Although studies on situational and interactional antecedents of violent behaviour are slowly growing in number (e.g., Aquilina, 1991; Nijman et al., 1997; Powell. et al., 1994), very few procedures and forms for measuring violence among psychiatric patients give prominence to situational factors (Bjørkly, 1996). Effective treatment and prevention of violence on psychiatric wards may profit from more comprehensive and accurate monitoring of situational precipitants (Bjørkly, 1999; Noble, 1997; Powell et al.). The following interventions may result in improved patient management in limit-setting situations:

- Accurate monitoring and well-planned interventions pertaining to recurrent warning signs of violent behaviour.
- Accurate monitoring and well-planned interventions pertaining to recurrent situational antecedents of violent acts.
- Non-authoritarian and anxiety-reducing staff interventions.

Concluding Remarks and Some Future Research Issues

This chapter has dealt with recent empirical evidence of a relationship between violence and three variables: diagnosis of comorbid substance abuse disorder, "violent" hallucinations and delusions, and limit-setting. However, a growing number of studies indicate that these variables may be epiphenomena—not themselves directly related to patient violence but indicators of underlying or concomitant variables that are more directly predictive. If these preliminary findings are substantiated by further empirical evidence, a series of new questions emerges.

GENERAL QUESTIONS

Do the three risk factors function simultaneously, or do they emerge sequentially ordered and thus have a dominating impact one at a time? Do these risk factors share a single throughgoing factor that actually accounts for the violence-triggering impact that each factor seems to possess?

COMORBID SUBSTANCE ABUSE DISORDER

Is there a typical violence profile for this patient group, or is substance abuse a general vulnerability factor that lowers patients' tolerance threshold? Are there any recurrent precipitants of violence typical of patients with comorbid substance abuse disorder?

VIOLENCE-PRONE HALLUCINATIONS AND DELUSIONS

Even in recurrently violent patients with auditory command hallucinations, persecutory delusions, and perceived loss of control, these phenomena do not inevitably lead to violence. Are there other concomitant triggers required to produce violence?

LIMIT-SETTING

Limit-setting interactions are striking and are therefore easy for nurses to observe and record. Does this lead to overreporting of limit-setting as a precipitant of violence at the cost of other, more relevant, precursors? Closely related to this question is another: Is limit-setting actually just a final releaser that, in order to induce violence, depends on the accumulated impact of other precipitants?

Despite many unanswered questions and the evident need for more clinical studies, there are adequate grounds to conclude that even at this stage a more systematic clinical application of existing knowledge of high-risk factors may reduce violence on psychiatric wards.

References

Adler, H., & Lidberg, L. (1995). Characteristics of repeat killers in Sweden. *Criminal Behaviour and Mental Health, 5,* 9–13.

Aquilina, C. (1991). Violence by psychiatric in-patients. *Medicine, Science and the Law, 31,* 306–312.

Armond, A.D. (1982). Violence in the semi-secure ward of a psychiatric hospital. *Medicine, Science and the Law, 22,* 203–209.

Beck, R., & Fernandez, E. (1998). Cognitive-behavioral therapy in the treatment of anger: A meta-analysis. *Cognitive Therapy and Research, 22,* 63–74.

Bjørkly, S. (1993). Scale for the Prediction of Aggression and Dangerousness in Psychotic Patients: An introduction. *Psychological Reports, 73,* 1363–1377.

Bjørkly, S. (1996). Report Form for Aggressive Episodes: Preliminary report. *Perceptual and Motor Skills, 83,* 1139–1152.

Bjørkly, S. (1999). A ten-year prospective study of aggression in a special secure unit for dangerous patients. *Scandinavian Journal of Psychology, 40,* 57–65.

Blair, T. (1991). Assaultive behaviour: Does provocation begin in the front office? *Journal of Psychosocial Nursing, 29,* 21–26.

Borell, P., d'Elia, G., & Orhagen, T. (1995). Vad vet patienter med schizofreni om sin sjukdom? (What do schizophrenic patients know about their illness?). *Scandinavian Journal of Behaviour Therapy, 24,* 13–23.

Buchanan, A. (1997). The investigation of acting on delusions as a tool for risk assessment in the mentally disordered. *British Journal of Psychiatry, 70*(suppl 32), 12–16.

Cheung, P., Schweitzer, I., Crowley, K., & Tuckwell, V. (1997). Violence in schizophrenia: Role of hallucinations and delusions. *Schizophrenia Research, 26,* 181–190.

Coid, J.W. (1996). Dangerous patients with mental illness: Increased risks warrant new policies, adequate resources, and appropriate legislation. *British Medical Journal, 312,* 965–966.

Cooper, A., & Mendonca, J. (1989). A prospective study of patient assaults on nursing staff in a psychogeriatric unit. *Canadian Journal of Psychiatry, 34,* 399–404.

Corrigan, P.W., Yudofsky, S.C., & Silver, J.M. (1993). Pharmacological and behavioral treatment for aggressive psychiatric inpatients. *Hospital and Community Psychiatry, 44,* 125–132.

Crowner, M., Peric, G., Stepcic, F., & Ventura, F. (1995). Psychiatric patients' explanation for assaults. *Psychiatric Services, 46,* 614–615.

Cuffel, B.J., Shumway, M., Chouljian, T.L., & MacDonnald, T. (1994). A longitudinal study of substance use and community violence in schizophrenia. *Journal of Nervous and Mental Disease, 182,* 704–708.

Curson, D.A., Patel, M., Liddle, P.F., & Barnes, T.R.E. (1988). Psychiatric morbidity of a long stay hospital population with chronic schizophrenia and implications for future community care. *British Medical Journal, 297,* 819–22.

Depp, F.C. (1983). Assaults in a public mental hospital. In J.R. Lion & W.H. Reid (Eds.), *Assaults within psychiatric facilities.* New York: Grune & Stratton.

Dietz, P.E., & Rada, R.T. (1982). Interpersonal violence in forensic facilities. In J.R. Lion & W.H. Reid (Eds.), *Assaults within psychiatric facilities.* New York: Grune & Stratton.

D'Orban, P.T., & O'Connor, A. (1989). Women who kill their parents. *British Journal of Psychiatry, 154,* 27–33.

Drury, V., Birchwood, M., Cochrane, R., & Macmillan, F. (1996a). Cognitive therapy and recovery from acute psychosis. I: Impact on symptoms. *British Journal of Psychiatry, 169,* 593–601.

Drury, V., Birchwood, M., Cochrane, R., & Macmillan, F. (1996b). Cognitive therapy and recovery from acute psychosis. I: Impact on recovery time. *British Journal of Psychiatry, 169,* 602–607.

Dubin, W.R., Wilson, S.J., & Mercer, C. (1988). Assault against psychiatrists in outpatient settings. *Journal of Clinical Psychiatry, 49,* 338–345.

Durivage, A. (1989). Assaultive behavior before it happens... *Canadian Journal of Psychiatry, 34,* 393–397.

Edwards, J.G., & Reid, W.H. (1983). Violence in psychiatric facilities in Europe and in the United States. In J.R. Lion and W.H. Reid (Eds.), *Assaults within psychiatric facilities.* New York: Grune & Stratton.

Eichelman, B. (1991). Violence toward clinicians. In R. Baenninger (Ed.), *Targets of violence and aggression.* New York: Elsevier.

Eronen, M., Hakola, P., & Tiihonen, J. (1996). Factors associated with homicide recidivism in a 13-year sample of homicide offenders in Finland. *Psychiatric Services, 47,* 403–406.

Estroff, S., Zimmer, C., Lachicotte, W., & Benoit, J. (1994). The influence of social networks and social support on violence by persons with serious mental illness. *Hospital and Community Psychiatry, 45,* 669–679.

Flannery, R.B., Hanson, M.A., Penk, W.E., & Flannery, G.J. (1996). Violence and the lax milieu? Preliminary data. *Psychiatric Quarterly, 67,* 47–50.

Freeman, D., & Garety, P.A. (1999). Worry, worry processes and dimensions of delusions: An exploratory investigation of a role for anxiety processes in the maintenance of delusional distress. *Behavioural and Cognitive Psychotherapy, 27,* 47–62.

Freeman, D., Garety, P.A., Fowler, D., Kuipers, E., Dunn, G., Bebbington, P., & Hadley, C. (1998). The London–East Anglia randomised controlled trial of cognitive-behaviour therapy for psychosis. IV: Self-esteem and persecutory delusions. *British Journal of Clinical Psychology, 37,* 415–430.

Friis, S., & Helldin, L. (1994). The contribution made by the clinical setting to violence among psychiatric patients. *Criminal Behaviour and Mental Health, 4,* 341–352.

Garety, P.A., Kuipers, E., Fowler, D., Chamberlain, F., & Dunn, G. (1994). Cognitive behavioural therapy for drug-resistant psychosis. *British Journal of Psychiatry, 67,* 259–271.

Gertz, B. (1980). Training for prevention of assaultive behavior in a psychiatric setting. *Hospital and Community Psychiatry, 31,* 628–630.

Haddock, G., Tarrier, N., Spaulding, W., Yusupoff, L., Kinney, C., & McCarthy, E. (1998). Individual cognitive-behavior therapy in the treatment of hallucinations and delusions: A review. *Clinical Psychology Review, 18,* 821-838.

Howells, K. (1989). Anger-management methods in relation to the prevention of violent behaviour. In J. Archer & K. Browne (Eds.), *Human aggression: Naturalistic approaches.* London: Routledge.

Hustig, H.H., & Hafner, R.J. (1990). Persistent auditory hallucinations and their relationship to delusions and mood. *Journal of Nervous and Mental Disease, 178,* 264–267.

Infantino, J.A.J., & Musingo, S. (1985). Assaults and injuries among staff with and without training in aggression control techniques. *Hospital and Community Psychiatry, 36,* 1312–1314.

Johnson, S. (1997). Dual diagnosis of severe mental illness and substance misuse: A case for specialist services? *British Journal of Psychiatry, 171,* 205–208.

Junginger, J. (1990). Predicting compliance with command hallucinations. *American Journal of Psychiatry, 147,* 245–247.

Junginger, J. (1995). Command hallucinations and the prediction of dangerousness. *Psychiatric Services, 46,* 911–914.

Junginger, J. (1996). Psychosis and violence: The case for a content analysis of psychotic experience. *Schizophrenia Bulletin, 22,* 91–103.

Kalogjera, I.J., Bedi, A., Watson, W.N., & Meyer, A.D. (1989). Impact of therapeutic management on use of seclusion and restraint with disruptive adolescent inpatients. *Hospital and Community Psychiatry, 40,* 280–285.

Katz, P., & Kirkland, F.R. (1990). Violence and social structure on mental hospital wards. *Psychiatry, 53,* 262–277.

Kendler, K., Glazer, W., & Morgenstern, H. (1983). Dimensions of delusional experience. *American Journal of Psychiatry, 140,* 466–469.

Kennedy, H.G., Kemp, L.J., & Dyer, D.E. (1992). Fear and anger in delusional (paranoid) disorder: The association with violence. *British Journal of Psychiatry, 160,* 488–492.

Krakowski, M., & Czobor, P. (1994). Clinical symptoms, neurological impairment, and prediction of violence in psychiatric inpatients. *Hospital and Community Psychiatry, 45,* 700–705.

Kuipers, E., Fowler, D., Garety, P., Chisholm, D., Freeman, D., Dunn, G., Bebbington, P., & Hadley, C. (1998). London–East Anglia randomised controlled trial of cognitive-behavioural therapy for psychosis. III: Follow-up and economic evaluation at 18 months. *British Journal of Psychiatry, 173,* 61–68.

Lee, H.K., Villar, O., Juthani, N., & Bluestone, H. (1989). Characteristics and behavior of patients involved in psychiatric ward incidents. *Hospital and Community Psychiatry, 40,* 1295–1297.

Linaker, O.M., & Busch-Iversen, H. (1995). Predictors of imminent violence in psychiatric inpatients. *Acta Psychiatrica Scandinavica, 92,* 250–254.

Link, B., Andrews, H., & Cullen, F. (1992). The violent and illegal behaviour of mental patients reconsidered. *American Sociological Review, 57,* 275–292.

Link, B., & Stueve, C. (1994). Psychotic symptoms and the violent/illegal behavior of mental patients compared to community controls. In J. Monahan & H. Steadman (Eds.), *Violence and mental disorder* (pp. 137–159). Chicago: University of Chicago Press.

Madden, D.J., Lion, J.R., & Penna, M.W. (1976). Assaults on psychiatrists by patients. *American Journal of Psychiatry, 133,* 422–425.

McNiel, D.E. (1994). Hallucinations and violence. In J. Monahan & H.J. Steadman (Eds), *Violence and mental disorder: Developments in risk assessment.* Chicago: University of Chicago Press.

Monahan, J. (1995). Violence among mentally ill found to be concentrated among those with comorbid substance abuse disorder. *Psychiatric News, 30*(23), 8–9.

Mulvey, E.P. (1994). Assessing the evidence of a link between mental illness and violence. *Hospital and Community Psychiatry, 45,* 663–668.

Nijman, H.L.I., Merkelbach, H.L.G.J., Allertz, W.F.F., & a Campo, J.M.L.G. (1997). Prevention of aggressive incidents on a closed psychiatric ward. *Psychiatric Services, 48,* 694–698.

Nilson, K., Palmstierna, T., & Wistedt, B. (1988). Aggressive behavior in hospitalized psychogeriatric patients. *Acta Psychiatrica Scandinavica, 78,* 172–175.

Noble, P. (1997). Violence in psychiatric in-patients: Review and clinical implications. *International Review of Psychiatry, 9,* 207–216.

Owen, C., Tarantello, C., Jones, M., & Tenant, C. (1998). Violence and aggression in psychiatric units. *Psychiatric Services, 49,* 1452–1457.

Perregaard, R.N., & Bartels, U. (1992). Violence against staff in mental hospitals. Abstract. *First European symposium on aggression in clinical psychiatric practise.* Psychiatric Institution, Karolinska Institute, Danderyd Hospital, Stockholm: 22–23.

Powell, G., Caan, W., & Crowe, M. (1994). What events precede violent incidents in psychiatric hospitals? *British Journal of Psychiatry, 165,* 107–112.

Rice, M.E., Harris, G.T., Varney, G.W., & Quinsey, V.L. (1989). *Violence in institutions: Understanding, prevention and control.* Toronto: Hogrefe & Huber.

Rogers, R., Gillis, J.R., Turner, R.E., & Frise-Smith, T. (1990). The clinical presentation of command hallucinations in a forensic population. *American Journal of Psychiatry, 147,* 1304–1307.

Roth, A., Fonagy, P., Parry, G., Target, M., & Woods, R. (1996). *What works for whom? A critical review of psychotherapy research.* New York: Guilford.

Scott, H., Johnson, S., Menezes, P., Thornicroft, G., Marshall, J., Bindman, J., Bebbington, P., & Kuipers, E. (1998). Substance misuse and risk of aggression and offending among the severely mentally ill. *British Journal of Psychiatry, 172,* 345–350.

Shah, A.K., Fineberg, N.A., & James, D.V. (1991). Violence among psychiatric inpatients. *Acta Psychiatrica Scandinavica, 84,* 305–309.

Sheridan, M., Henrion, R., Robinson, L., & Baxter, V. (1990). Precipitants of violence in a psychiatric inpatient setting. *Hospital and Community Psychiatry, 41,* 776–780.

Smith, J., & Hucker, S. (1994). Schizophrenia and substance abuse. *British Journal of Psychiatry, 165,* 13–21.

Steadman, H.J., Mulvey, E.P., Monahan, J., Robbins, P.C., Appelbaum, P.S., Grisso, T., Roth, L.H., & Silver, E. (1998). Violence by people discharged from acute psychiatric inpatient facilities and by others in the same neighbourhood. *Archives of General Psychiatry, 55,* 393–401.

Swanson, J.W., Borum, R., Swartz, M.S., & Monahan, J. (1996). Psychotic symptoms and disorders and the risk of violent behaviour in the community. *Criminal Behaviour and Mental Health, 6,* 309–329.

Swartz, M.S., Swanson, J.W., Hiday, V.A., Borum, R., Wagner, R., & Burns, B.J. (1998). Violence and severe mental illness: The effects of substance abuse and nonadherence to medication. *American Journal of Psychiatry, 155,* 226–231.

Tardiff , K. (1989). *Assessment and management of violent patients.* Washington: American Psychiatric Press.

Tarrier, N. (1992). Management and modification of residual positive psychotic symptoms. In M. Birchwood & N. Tarrier (Eds.), *Innovations in the psychological management of schizophrenia* (pp. 148–167). London: Wiley.

Tarrier, N., Beckett, R., Harwood, S., Baker, A., Yusupoff, L., & Ugarterburu, I. (1993). A trial of two cognitive-behavioral methods of treating drug-resistant residual psychotic symptoms in schizophrenic patients. I: Outcome. *British Journal of Psychiatry, 162,* 524–532.

Taylor, P.J. (1985). Motives for offending among violent and psychotic men. *British Journal of Psychiatry, 147,* 491–498.

Taylor, P.J., Leese, M., Williams, D., Butwell, M., Daly, R., & Larkin, E. (1998). Mental disorder and violence: A special (high security) hospital study. *British Journal of Psychiatry, 172,* 218–226.

Torrey, E.F. (1994). Violent behavior by individuals with serious mental illness. *Hospital and Community Psychiatry, 45,* 653–662.

Volavka, J., Laska, E., Baker, S., Meisner, M., Czobor, P., & Krivelevich, I. (1997). History of violent behaviour and schizophrenia in different cultures: Analyses based on the WHO study on determinants of outcome of severe mental disorders. *British Journal of Psychiatry, 171,* 9–14.

Wallace, C., Mullen, P., Burgess, P., Palmer, S., Ruschena, D., & Browne, C. (1998). Serious criminal offending and mental disorder: Case linkage study. *British Journal of Psychiatry, 172,* 477–484.

Wesseley, S., Buchanan, A., Reed, A., Cutting, J., Everitt, B., Garety, P., & Taylor, P. (1993). Acting on delusions. I: Prevalence. *British Journal of Psychiatry, 163,* 69–76.

Whittington, R., & Wykes, T. (1996). "Going in strong": Confrontive coping by staff. *Journal of Forensic Psychiatry, 5,* 609–614.

Stål Bjørkly is Associate Professor, Faculty of Health Sciences, Molde College, Molde, Norway.

Author's Note

Comments or queries may be directed to Stål Bjørkly, Department of Health Care, Molde College, PO Box 308, N-6401 Molde, Norway. Telephone: 47 71 21 40 12. Fax: 47 71 21 40 50. E-mail: <stal.bjorkly@himolde.no>.

VIOLENCE AGAINST OTHERS BY PSYCHIATRIC HOSPITAL INPATIENTS WITH PSYCHOSIS

Prevention Strategies and Challenges to Their Evaluation

PAMELA J. TAYLOR
HANS SCHANDA

The Nature of the Problem

Hospitals are microcosms of society and, as such, have many of society's strengths and weaknesses. Among the weaknesses is the possibility of violence among individuals or groups or against property. Against this background are conflicting expectations or assumptions: first, that hospitals, as places of healing or asylum, should necessarily be safer than the outside world; and second, that hospitals, as places where damaged and stressed people are grouped and, frequently, undergo unpleasant and restricting procedures, must carry greater potential for violent incidents. Violence in hospitals is no more exclusively the preserve of people with a psychiatric disorder than violence elsewhere in the community. However, as there appears to be a small but significant association between some mental disorders and violence, and as one important reason for admission to a psychiatric hospital is the threat of or actual violence, psychiatric hospitals and units might be expected to be disproportionately affected.

A late-1980s British national survey of violence against staff confirmed that in the health service in England and Wales mental handicap and psychiatric workers were particularly at risk (Health Services Advisory Committee, 1987). A year later, the Department of Health and Social Security (1988) reported that at least one in 10 psychiatric patients had assaulted a staff member. Noble (1997) reports an increase in published articles on patient violence and a net increase in inpatient assaults (all victims) over the period 1970 to 1994 in one inner London psychiatric hospital, although the assaults were beginning to fall and plateau by the mid-1980s. Across the Atlantic, in a large state hospital in Maryland during the 1980s, Snyder (1994) found an increase in number and proportion of injuries to staff relative to the hospital patient population—from 5.5 per 100 patients in 1980 to 50.5 in 1989. Also in the United States, a study of five public-sector psychiatric hospitals suggested that injuries as a result of patient violence to nursing staff alone exceeded injury rates from all causes to workers in traditionally high-risk industries such as mining and con-

S. Hodgins (ed.), Violence among the Mentally Ill, 251–275.
© 2000 *Kluwer Academic Publishers. Printed in the Netherlands.*

struction (Love & Hunter, 1996). Edwards, Jones, Reid, and Chu (1988) offer an estimate of comparative rates of inpatient violence between North America and the UK. Their published figures from one UK psychiatric unit yield a rate of 0.39 assaults per bed per year, taking staff and patients together as victims; their cited unpublished data from 14 North American hospitals show a rate of 1.36 assaults per bed year in psychiatric units and 0.28 in non-psychiatric units. Whatever the additional disorder or the institutional influences, inpatient violence rates may be in part reflective of wider community base rates.

Inpatient violence thus appears to pose valid concerns for mental health clinicians. These include the potential for physical and mental pain and disability, as well as adverse effects on staff morale, recruitment, and retention. It is also acknowledged that there are considerable costs involved when violence occurs. These include time lost from work and replacement costs, direct compensation for injury, and, in relation to more serious injuries, perhaps substantial inquiry and/or litigation costs (Hillbrand, Foster, & Spitz, 1996). It is thus arguable that prevention strategies should take account of not only the prevention of violence per se, but also, where it does occur, the minimization of immediate harm, post hoc emotional distress, time lost from work, and escalation of costs. In the UK there is a widespread perception of an unresolved problem. Prior to issuing its first clinical practice guidelines, the Royal College of Psychiatrists (Royal College of Psychiatrists Research Unit [Royal College], 1998) conducted a postal survey of 1,700 people who used, provided, or purchased mental health services in the UK and Ireland. The respondents rated management of imminent violence in clinical practice as their top priority for guidance.

Violence among patients is probably less common than violence to nursing staff but more common than violence to other clinical staff or visitors (James, Fineberg, Shah, & Priest, 1990; Noble & Rodger, 1989). Perhaps consequently, some studies focus exclusively on violence to staff (e.g., Haller & Deluty, 1988). Occasionally people who are designated inpatients may temporarily leave the hospital, with or without the knowledge of staff, and commit violence, sometimes very serious violence, outside the bounds of the hospital. Molnar and Pinchoff (1993) document the risk of harm to self and others among general psychiatric patients absconding from a US urban state hospital. Molnar, Keitner, and Swindall (1985) pose the potential problem in terms of increased risk of medico-legal liability for the hospital staff. Richmond, Dandridge, and Jones (1991) tested an observational checklist as a prevention strategy. In an Austrian high-security hospital, 13% of people with mental illness had committed crimes as inpatients of general psychiatric hospitals, some of them after absconding. Failure to hold inpatients in open hospitals, or at lower levels of security, may constitute a reason for transfer to higher security. Quinsey, Coleman, Jones, and Altrows (1997; see also Quinsey, this volume) quantified absconsion with re-offending by offender patients from specialist forensic hospital units in Ontario, Canada. Just over half of a series of 60 offender patients identified over a 10-year period had re-offended while away from the hospital but still technically inpatients, with the hospital potentially responsible for their acts. Moore (submitted) found that in England over a shorter period (1989–94) there were very few absconsions from high-security hospitals. At one such hospital, low-security accommodation accounted for 10 of the 12 departures from within the hospital perimeter. Other departures (32) were from rehabilitation trips or other necessary trips outside the hospital or during trial leave. With the exception of two patients who were at liberty for 48 hours, all had returned or been retaken within 24 hours. Just one patient committed an offence—an assault against another man in a bar.

Returning to the inpatient setting, there is a lack of clarity about the nature of acts that should be included for study. Some studies focus exclusively on acts of violence resulting in physical injury, others include damage to property, while still others add threats or incorporate general indicators of aggression inclusive of shouting and swearing. There is a general view that inpatient violence is hopelessly under-reported, especially when reliance is placed on incident forms (e.g., Cheung, Schweitzer, Crowley, & Tuckwell, 1997; Lion, Snyder, & Merrill, 1981), but also that there is a differential sensitivity hierarchically, with more complete recording associated with more serious incidents. This raises the question as to whether under-recording is an appropriate explanation for the discrepancy between official records and researcher-observed data. It is arguable that a certain amount of intermittent anger and its expression is normal human behaviour. It is an unusual person who has never shouted, cursed, or banged a door, and yet each of these behaviours might attract a rating on commonly used research instruments—for example, the Overt Aggression Scale (Yudovsky, Silver, Jackson, Endicott, & Williams, 1986). Perhaps the staff judgements that allow for such elements of aggression to be construed as sometimes within the normal range, or at any rate not worthy of an incident form, provide a better estimate of violence—or of behaviours that harm others—than do the research rating scales. At other times it may be important to include aggression that would appear trivial only to the casual observer. Staff may be acutely frightened by it or, if it persists, chronically shaken emotionally, frustrated, and unhappy. Thus the ward atmosphere will be affected regardless of whether physical injury has actually occurred or its degree of severity (Baxter, Hafner, & Holme, 1992; Caldwell, 1992; Cheung et al.; Cooper & Mendonca, 1991). If the threat is great enough, what might have happened becomes as challenging as what actually did happen.

Other major methodological differences among studies—for example, in sampling—render comparisons or meta-analyses unsatisfactory. This makes any generalizable estimate of prevalence elusive, and yet such an estimate would be useful in prevention studies, in effect offering a possible standard against which to evaluate first the baseline in a unit about to test interventions and then any deviations from the unit norms in response to preventive strategies. The suggested trend towards an overall increase in inpatient violence, while interesting for within-study correlations, is not necessarily indicative of a true general increase. These correlations are most useful for their potential to indicate provocative factors—as targets for preventive strategies. James at al. (1990), for example, found an increase in violent incidents over a 15-month period and determined that this best correlated with staffing changes, less qualified and less regular staff being available during the index period. Snyder (1994) linked the increase he observed within a reducing inpatient population to the concentration and circulation of more difficult patients: Healthier patients, who might have offered stability to the social structure of the hospital, were no longer a part of it; overcrowding was more frequent as wards were closed and some specialist treatment settings discontinued—with resultant integration of their patients into the mainstream; there was a higher turnover of those patients who were at their most distressed and disruptive.

The focus of this discussion is the prevention of violence in a psychiatric inpatient unit, where the heterogeneity of patients, staff, settings, and type of violence may be considerable. Nevertheless, the same questions apply: What are the known risk factors, and therefore the potential points for intervention? Are these the same as those for acts of violence committed elsewhere by people with a mental disorder? To what extent does the inpatient environment introduce unique stressors and unique advantages in the management of the threat of violence?

Sources of Information and Boundaries of Interest

The boundaries given for this paper were: *the nature of the target behaviour*—violent acts to others; *the nature of the mental disorder*—the functional psychoses; *the environment*—the hospital inpatient setting; and *the task*—prevention of those violent acts. No limits were placed on the process of review, but a classic systematic review was beyond our resources.

PROCESS OF REVIEW

Computerized literature databases have been criticized for their low sensitivity and low specificity compared with manual searching (e.g., Adams, Power, Frederick, & Lefebvre, 1994), with no evidence of improvement after the first wave of such criticism (Watson & Richardson, 1999). This review, in eschewing database searches, may suffer from bias in choice of sources for review and in limits to period of review, but excludes any selection bias within those sources by encompassing manual search. The major US National Research Council more general review *Understanding and Preventing Violence* (Reiss & Roth, 1993/94) was scanned, as were selected journals as described below; some of our own pertinent research is introduced.

The periodicals selected were among those on the list of the 10 highest-impact psychiatric journals (Howard & Wilkinson, 1998), with three additions. The period reviewed was January 1995 to December 1998. The periodicals selected from among the former group were *Archives of General Psychiatry* (ranked 1), *American Journal of Psychiatry* (2), *Journal of Clinical Psychiatry* (4), and *British Journal of Psychiatry* (6). Specialist psychopharmacological journals and disorder-specific journals were excluded, except, given the focus on psychosis, *Schizophrenia Bulletin,* which yielded nothing. *Archives* yielded no relevant papers at all for the period, *American Journal of Psychiatry* just four papers in the 2 later years, *British Journal of Psychiatry* less, and *Journal of Clinical Psychiatry* just one. The three additions were *Psychological Medicine* (regarded by some as the British equivalent of *Archives*), the North American *Psychiatric Services,* and the British *Psychiatric Bulletin.* The first need not have detained us; the other two were by far the most productive sources. Having identified appropriate articles, we also followed up relevant citations.

THE FOCUS ON VIOLENT ACTS

The review covers only acts of violence against others. It does not include self-harm, which is commonly viewed as being at the opposite end of a violence dimension, although some acts of self-harm may be primarily motivated by aggression towards others, and, perhaps particularly among people with a schizophrenic illness, boundaries between self and others may be sufficiently disturbed that the direction of harm is not clear in the patient's mind. Limiting review to physical acts of violence has face validity; it seems plausible that physical injury is likely to be the most distressing aspect of aggression, but as far as we can tell no one has done the research to confirm this. Certainly, as indicated above, staff do become demoralized by persistent verbal abuse alone from patients, and in clinical practice one encounters patients who present as more distressed by alleged threats and hostility from other patients or from staff than by physical injury. Although we have raised the question that under-recording of verbal aggression may reflect appropriate clinical judgement, how often is the distinction between verbal and physical violence somewhat arbitrary? Verbal aggression tends to occur more commonly among patients who also show physical violence, but verbal aggression without such progression may occur in up to one third of patients (Noble & Rodger, 1989). Could a focus on preventing verbal aggression prevent progression to physical violence? Does permissiveness towards verbal violence diffuse the drive towards physical contact injuries? Could both strategies apply, but differentially to different patient groups? We could find no evidence-based answers.

THE FOCUS ON THE FUNCTIONAL PSYCHOSES

People have been admitted to psychiatric hospitals with a wide range of problems, but taking psychosis as the centre of consideration may become increasingly appropriate. There appear to be trends, at least in inner-city general psychiatric hospital units, to admit preferentially people who have a psychotic illness. It seems likely that people with such illnesses may be over-represented in the violent groups within such settings (e.g., Noble & Rodger, 1989). Even so, a bare majority of residents in this study had a psychosis, and a minority of these became violent in the inpatient setting. In a multi-centre US study, set up to examine post-discharge violence but capturing consecutive inpatient admissions, again a bare majority had a psychotic illness (Steadman et al., 1998). By contrast, in English high-security hospitals, where one of the principal reasons for admission is violence or other dangerous behaviour to others, about two thirds of men, but only half of women, have a psychotic illness (Taylor et al., 1998). A bare majority of violent acts are committed by people with a psychotic illness, but the proportion is greater among those with a personality disorder. It is not necessarily the case that, setting aside the issue of varying the specific treatment according to the nature of the disorder, prevention strategies would be similarly effective across all patient groups. There is a hint of this in the study of Palmstierna, Huitfeldt, and Wistedt (1991), who found that higher resident patient numbers correlated with violent episodes for people with schizophrenia but not other diagnoses.

THE FOCUS ON THE INPATIENT UNIT

Almost all published research on violence in the context of treatment for mental disorder has been conducted within inpatient settings. Increasingly, however, clinical interactions occur among patients and between staff and patients in a community setting. It might be important to focus separately on this setting, given the argument that violence which occurs specifically during clinical interactions, in a clinical relationship, or in "made communities" such as hostels may arise for reasons that are different from those predisposing to wider community violence but different again from those behind inpatient violence, and thus call for different preventive strategies. There are hints of different routes to violence in the psychiatric hospital compared with the wider community.

In their overview of predictive and prospective studies of violent behaviour, Chaiken, Chaiken, and Rhodes (1994) examined research with young offenders, adult offenders, and offenders with mental disorder. Almost invariably the focus was community violence. Only one follow-up study (Steadman & Morrissey, 1982) differentiated subsequent in-hospital (100 of 256 cases) and in-community (28 of 154 cases) violence among men indicted for a felony and found unfit to stand trial. Prior arrests for violence and age at first hospitalization were the criteria associated with community violence but not inpatient violence, while inpatient assaultive men were distinguished by age, race, alcohol problems, and juvenile-crime record.

In the 1980s in New York, Tardiff conducted a series of cross-sectional studies of violence among patients in different circumstances. Not all had a psychotic illness; there is no hint of whether there was any overlap between the samples. The violent subgroup within the inpatient sample contained relatively more women than men and the non-paranoid forms of schizophrenia predominated, with indicators of organic brain dysfunction (Tardiff, 1983). By contrast, there was a strong association between paranoid schizophrenia and violence in the pre-admission sample (Tardiff & Sweillam, 1980). It could be that confinement in the tightly constructed social milieu of an institution is particularly oppressive for those with non-paranoid illnesses. It could also be that those with the more paranoid illnesses were more responsive to specific treatments such as medication, once admitted to hospital, than those with comorbid organic brain syndromes.

Tardiff's more recent work (Tardiff, Marzuk, Leon, & Portera, 1997) explicitly took a longitudinal view of 1,068 consecutive admissions to a university psychiatric hospital over 18 months. There was a strong relationship between pre- and post-hospitalization violence in the sample, with patients who had been violent in the month prior to admission being more than nine times more likely than their previously non-violent peers to be violent to others after discharge. Violence during hospitalization did not differentiate the community violence groups. None of the patients who were physically violent during their stay in hospital were violent after discharge. Although the follow-up reported was brief (2 weeks), it was of the same order as the inpatient stay.

Patients in English high-security hospitals are almost invariably admitted after serious violence, usually leading to a criminal conviction (Taylor et al., 1998). Maden, Curle, Meux, Burrow, and Gunn (1993) found that, excluding the first admission year, two thirds of such patients avoided violence in the hospital. Other longitudinal data also suggest differences between characteristics associated with pre- and post-admission violence (Heads, Leese, Taylor, & Phillips, submitted). Detailed information was available for a subsample of 102 patients with schizophrenia, representing all the female patients of one of the hospitals in the first half of 1993, all the Afro/Anglo-Caribbean men, and a random same-size sample of white, indigenous men. Prior to admission, the violence was three times more likely to have been psychotically, usually delusionally, driven by those in contact with their victim, and the level of violence in these offences was significantly higher than for other groups. At the extreme, significantly more of those living with a partner or family member had committed homicide at least partly in response to delusions. The in-hospital social networks of patients were assessed using the Social Network Schedule (Dunn, O'Driscoll, Dayson, Wills, & Leff, 1990). Seventeen, one quarter of the responding patients, reported no significant social contacts at all within the hospital, and six of these had no outside visitors. Social networks for the others were generally small (mean number of significant contacts, 5; friends or confidants, 3), and nearly one third of these patients reported one or more of their contacts as "upsetting." Nevertheless, there was an inverse relationship between number of social contacts and inpatient violence. Although there was some association between delusions with hallucinations and this violence, there were much stronger associations with severity of negative symptoms and of symptoms of disorganization, such as thought disorder.

These pieces of research thus raise the question as to whether prevention of violence within a hospital setting must be construed as a task different from prevention of violence by people with a mental disorder when they are living in the community.

THE FOCUS ON PREVENTION

In health services, three prevention tasks are now generally recognized (Caplan & Siebert, 1964):

- primary prevention, directed at reducing the incidence of new cases
- secondary prevention, directed at reducing the duration of the disorder or the severity and length of a given episode
- tertiary prevention, designed to reduce the longer-term disability associated with the disorder.

In practice, considering that violence is, almost by definition, an intermittent problem, distinctions between management and prevention might be regarded as somewhat artificial.

Prevention of violence per se is rarely researched, and indeed is difficult to achieve. Even in the relatively controlled and limited environment of the inpatient setting there is a multiplicity of potentially relevant variables. In an ideal scientific model it would be important to select one or two to test, while holding the rest constant. In practice this is virtually impossible. It is essential, if the impact of any hypothetically preventive measure is to be assessed adequately, that there be a sound reference baseline, but is enough understood about natural fluctuations in base rates of violence in hospitals to determine this? Clinicians who feel themselves or their patients to be under significant threat of violence are likely to be particularly reluctant to accept classical models of randomization of patients for research, and have to be persuaded if such work is to take place. There may even be legal implications for them, and for service managers, engaging in research, not least because people who lack real capacity to consent to research are especially likely to fall into groups needed for such research. In the face of so few strictly preventive studies, it is inevitable that some reliance must still be placed on descriptive studies of inpatient violence and studies of the management of violence once it has occurred, but we have tried to focus on preventive aspects.

A useful starting point for generating hypotheses about institutional violence and its prevention is Hinde's (1993) separation of contextual social levels. He suggests that each level has properties that are not relevant to the level below, but that each level affects and is affected by those adjacent to it and by the values, beliefs, and norms of the over-arching sociocultural structures and the physical environment. His levels are:

- individual behaviour
- short-term interactions between individuals
- relationships involving a series of interactions over time between individuals who know each other such that each interaction is affected by previous ones and, often, by the expectation of future ones
- groups
- societies involving a number of distinct or overlapping groups.

In all settings for those with psychosis, preventive measures are likely to depend in part on modifying aspects of the individual's presentation or circumstances; in most short-stay units the characteristics of others around the patient and the quality of their day-to-day interactions will offer a further focus for attention; in longer-stay units these matters will apply, but in addition it will be necessary to take account of evolving relationships, both as they develop in their own right and as they perhaps mirror some aspects of earlier relationship development, inclusive of transference formation. In contrast to many patients with other psychiatric diagnoses and to many prisoners, patients with psychosis rarely cooperate in groups; however, level four is likely to apply to staff. There is some evidence from an observational study—without research intervention—on six wards of one mental hospital, that there is less violence on wards with good leadership, structured staff roles, and predictable routines (Katz & Kirkland, 1990). Around all the personal and social interactional issues, factors in the physical environment will also play a part, inclusive of political, legal, and fiscal considerations as well as the configuration of buildings and availability of weapons or substances of abuse.

Prevention Strategies

SETTING REALISTIC GOALS

No realistic prevention strategy is likely to be completely effective, and it may help staff and patients alike to acknowledge that fact. This is partly a result of the necessity to maintain a balance between safety and quality of life, the latter in part on humanitarian grounds but also potentially in the interests of longer-term safety. As violence to others, by definition, requires the presence of more than one person, complete, indefinite isolation of an assaultive individual, without access to harmful materials, would prevent such harm. It would have an unacceptable cost in terms of civil rights, would almost certainly increase the risk of self-harm, and would pose difficulties in the practical provision of care. Then too, the extent to which violence to others can be reduced, in either frequency or degree, may prove as much a measure of whether any given service is performing its allocated task as a measure of the effectiveness of appropriate strategies. Another simple way of preventing in-hospital violence might be to avoid admitting certain very sick and challenging patients. A high rate of patient-inflicted injuries in an inpatient unit might be evidence of staffing deficiencies, but a low rate might be indicative of failure to maintain an appropriate threshold for admission to the unit. Today's saving on risk of assaultiveness towards hospital staff might be tomorrow's inquiry or litigation after a homicide in the community.

THE PHYSICAL ENVIRONMENT

It is widely suggested that building design contributes substantially to the reduction of risk of assault. Among the features cited as critical are a sense of substantial personal space (Dietz & Rada, 1982), but also good sightlines for staff, attractive presentation and proper maintenance of buildings, opportunities for privacy and peace, and an absence of potential weapons in the building structure or furniture. Most objects can, however, be converted into weapons by people with a mind to do so. There have been suggestions that overcrowding and small ward/unit size in terms of patient numbers resident within one physical space at any one time contribute to violent episodes, but Palmstierna and Wistedt (1995) pose a challenge to the simplistic wisdom that reduction of overcrowding per se is preventive. Palmstierna et al. (1991) observed a psychiatric ward for acutely ill patients over 25 weeks in the mid-1980s. For those patients with schizophrenia who perpetrated at least one serious act of violence, on the days they did so there were significantly more patients on the ward. For non-schizophrenic patients who committed violence, on the days they did so there was no significant difference in the number of patients on the ward. A later study on a psychiatric intensive-care unit found that before and after the number of beds was halved to 10, without other obvious changes in patient type or regimen, there was a fourfold, albeit non-significant, increase in number of incidents. The severity of the attacks was, however, reduced (Palmstierna & Wistedt). The accompanying increase in privacy for patients may have been counterproductive for inter-patient violence. The larger communal spaces and single-room occupancy almost inevitably meant that, on the same staffing levels, observation could not be continuous, and this may have been a factor.

The nature of the daily routine may be construed as provocative, with an absence of rewarding tasks or the occurrence of certain activities, like gathering for meals, targeted as critical. Hunter and Love (1996) describe a management approach (TQM—total quality management) to reducing the frequency of aggressive incidents around mealtimes in a large Californian hospital for offender patients, most of whom had schizophrenia. The strategy included specific evaluation of the nature of the problem *in that setting,* and a response informed by this evaluation. Special incident reports were analysed over 6 months to identify peak times for violent assaults, 15 years to explore weapon use, and 6 months to clarify details of related patient activity. Patients were interviewed in order to take account of their observations. Policies and procedures were reviewed and modified accordingly, and a programme of change was implemented. This focused on mealtimes, as peak times for assault: changing eating utensils, which were commonly being used as weapons; playing music recommended by music therapists as calming; increasing the amount of space available; improving the social skills of those serving the meals; and offering selective opportunities for patients to progress through the dining areas, according to their ability to take responsibility for their behaviour. It almost goes without saying that removal of metal cutlery meant that patients could no longer attack with it, but neither did they attack with the new plastic variety. Of more interest is the fact that the year after implementation of the new policies, compared with the year before, showed a 40% reduction in the number of violent incidents and a saving of nursing time. In order to meet the criticism that, in the absence of randomization of new and old management styles, the change might be construed as part of a natural fluctuation in violence rates, a trend analysis was performed on violent incidents over the preceding 5 years, the result of which was no trend to change in either direction. Limitations in design nevertheless remain. It is not clear whether other, potentially relevant, changes were taking place simultaneously—and in the absence of randomization could not be controlled in analysis. Further, because so many changes were occurring simultaneously it is impossible to know whether all were necessary, or whether any one or two of the changes were the critical ones. For example, the mere fact that patients were consulted about their environment and its management, with some manifest attention to their wishes, could itself have brought about the improvements. However, the face validity of this approach to managing violence is among the highest of any of the studies reviewed, and Hunter and Love do succeed in providing, from evidence of context, a convincing case that the approach has some value.

Attractiveness of environment is a highly subjective concept. Buildings tend to be designed by people with one set of aesthetic values for people who may have quite another but have never been consulted about them. At the least it makes intuitive sense that buildings to be used for clinical purposes should be designed in consultation with the staff who will have to manage the living and working spaces, but very little research has been done on physical environmental qualities.

Patients have complained that the poor physical facilities offered in some hospitals are provocative (e.g., Watson, 1996), and we believe them. Although Watson refers to "institution-induced anger" as only "prolonging hospitalisation," for some patients the reason for this will be that anger is translated into assault. Perhaps it is because environmental conditions as triggers to violence seem so obvious that in the mental health field so little work has been done. Watson, as a long-term user of such facilities, refers to overcrowding, grotesque and unhealthy physical environment, substandard quality and quantity of staff, total inactivity for most patients, lack of or painfully delayed effective therapy, and the grim reality of verbal and physical abuse. She says: "It does not take an investigative commission to assess the damage to already battered and fragile psyches."

We would not advocate use of scarce research monies to seek to establish Watson's point "scientifically"; accommodation such as she describes is unacceptable whether or not it excites violence. There are, however, some relevant quantitative data from educational fields. Rutter, Maughan, Mortimore, and Ouston (1979) studied 12 English schools and confirmed that differences in delinquency rates could not be entirely accounted for either by prevailing socioeconomic factors in the catchment areas or by individual variation among the pupils; therefore, factors in the schools themselves would appear to be relevant. Age and condition of buildings, number of students, amount of space per student, staff-student ratio, and academic emphasis were all excluded as significant variables. The attitudes and approaches of teachers were not. A high amount of punishment and a low amount of praise were the best correlates of antisocial behaviour within schools. Such attributes are not unobserved in hospital staff and may be worthy of special attention in prevention of in-hospital violence.

In the 1990s, perhaps as a side effect of the pre-eminence of community care, disorders in the use of alcohol and other drugs have been shown to occur at least four to five times more frequently among people with schizophrenia than among others (Regier et al., 1990). In turn, alcohol and other drugs are increasingly associated with raising the risk of violence among people with a mental disorder in the community (e.g., Swanson, Holzer, Ganju, & Jono, 1990; Wallace et al., 1998). Yet there has been remarkably little consideration of substance misuse as an environmental factor pre-disposing to violence among psychiatric inpatients. This is not because substance misuse does not occur while people are resident in hospital. The frequency with which it does, however, and the frequency, in turn, with which it is associated with inpatient violent episodes, is not documented. Management of imminent violence is a task closely related to its prevention. The clinical practice guidelines by the Royal College of Psychiatrists (Royal College, 1998) for the UK and Ireland are remarkable for making no mention of alcohol or illicit drugs in the section on environmental management (or anywhere else), notwithstanding an acknowledgement that the basis for most guidelines offered lies in policy and consensus documents collected from around the country rather than in research evidence. This might be taken to suggest that mental health services generally may be in a state of at least official or public denial about the challenge posed by alcohol and illicit substances.

In the UK both alcohol and drug use by residents in open psychiatric units is regarded as a problem in practice, not least because such patients are generally accorded freedom of movement and may go outside the hospital and drink, even if exhorted not to. In closed units the principal problem lies with illicit drugs, which are much more difficult to identify in search procedures, while the bulk of alcohol is generally obvious. Patients may attempt to make their own brews, but again these are relatively easily detected. A further problem is the potential for abuse of some drugs widely used in psychiatric therapy. Antiparkinsonian agents, for example, commonly used to counter the side effects of the conventional anti-psychotic drugs, are favoured by some patients for producing a "high." Occasionally in the unusual marketplace of an isolated or closed institution, almost any drug may be employed as a trading commodity. Such use may be more difficult to detect than that of illegal drugs, which depends on the patient not having been prescribed the drug for identification of misuse in, say, random urine screens.

Strategies likely to be preventive of both inpatient use and violence include clearly stated bans on use in leaflets and notices for patients and their visitors, counselling on likely adverse effects, routine searches of the environment and/or patients, general vigilance by staff, random testing of patients' urine for evidence of drugs or their metabolites, exclusion of users (rarely clinically sound), and sanctions for being found to have used such substances. There appears to be no evidence that any of these strategies have been tested as measures for limiting substance misuse in hospitals, preventing violence, or both, yet doing so would seem relatively straight-forward.

PATIENT-CENTRED FACTORS

Among patients with psychosis, there is considerable evidence that features of psychotic illness are commonly relevant to violent episodes, both within and outside hospital. It is less clear whether the symptoms most provocative of violence are the same regardless of setting. There is evidence that in the most seriously violent of psychotic patients delusions are probably the most important in driving violence in the context of opportunities for them to develop, generally in the course of longer-term social interactions, however limited or pathological those may be (Buchanan et al., 1993; Heads et al., submitted; Taylor, 1998; Taylor et al., 1998). Although such evolving drive may remain a risk in longer-stay institutions, it is otherwise likely to be more important among partly treated or untreated cases in the community. The role of hallucinations in generating violence in the inpatient setting is much less clear, possibly clouded by preventive management strategies (Hellerstein, Frosch, & Koenigsberg, 1987). In the latter study there was no difference between hallucinating and non-hallucinating patients in terms of self- or other-directed violence, but the hallucinating patients were more likely to have received special treatment by staff, including episodes of seclusion and/or 1:1 nursing. Junginger (1995) found that 93 of 370 patients under short-term hospitalization reported having experienced command hallucinations at some time over the 2 years prior to interview; however, only 25 experienced the hallucinations while an inpatient. Again, a possible inpatient/outpatient difference emerged: Although patients in the two groups were almost equally likely to report acting on a command hallucination, the inpatients were significantly less likely to report acting dangerously. This could indicate partial effectiveness of treatment in preventing such behaviour. Patients will not uncommonly report a shift in the emotional impact of their hallucinations or delusions before there is any clearance of those symptoms, but the reports to Junginger suggested environmental impact. Commands experienced in the hospital tended to be specific to the hospital environment, and less dangerous commands were reported.

One or two studies (e.g., Janofsky, Spears, & Neubauer, 1988), inclusive of our work with high-security inpatients (Heads et al., submitted), have suggested that symptoms affecting day-to-day communications, inclusive of disorders of the form of thought and negative symptoms, may become particularly risky when people are brought together at close quarters, as when they are resident in hospital. Still others have cited impulsivity, or perhaps relative disinhibition, as releasing factors, which may or may not operate in conjunction with more typical psychotic features, particularly where frequency of violence is the major problem (Christison, Kirch, & Wyatt, 1991).

It may be arguable that, in terms of violence prevention, the details of which symptoms are more or less associated with breakdown into violence become unimportant if those symptoms are responsive to medication. It is sufficient to acknowledge that symptomatic relief is necessary and urgent on these grounds as well as all others, inclusive of humanitarian grounds and cost. Evaluation of specific treatment of psychosis in the form of medication lends itself particularly if not uniquely well to classic prevention studies. Here at least, randomization of specific treatment mode, and objective measures of both treatment compliance and presumed mediators of violence, could be more readily attempted. Even with regard to the related issue of management of violence, where aggression at least, and often the repetition of violent acts, had been well established, the systematic review of such work by the Royal College of Psychiatrists team (Royal College, 1998) identified only one trial that satisfied all the design criteria specified—namely, randomization, clinician blind, patient blind, more than 20 subjects in each group, follow-up achieved for at least 80% of each study group. This was a study, in essence, of chemical restraint (Thomas, Schwartz, & Petrelli, 1992). Further, other studies still manifest a good deal of confusion in outcome measures. Terms like *difficult, disturbed, aggressive,* and *hostile* are used almost as if interchangeable. They are not, and the evidence that any of them correlate well with actual physical violence is inconsistent. Researchers face a problem, because actual physical violence, even when people are acutely ill and even when relatively trivial episodes are counted, is still an occurrence with too low a base rate for satisfactory measurement in small intervention studies, but surrogate measures cannot be adopted on mere face validity. That said, it may be valid and important to accept other benefits of specific interventions. Volavka et al. (1990) completed a small (20 assaultive patients) double-blind trial of tryptophan as an adjunct to conventional antipsychotic medication. While there was no reduction in the number of violent incidents, there was a significant reduction in the use of injected neuroleptics and sedatives.

There is some suggestion that it may be possible to contain "disruptive behaviour" among patients with psychosis even when the symptoms of the illness are not apparently improved (Kane & Marder, 1993; McEvoy, Hogarty, & Steingard, 1991; Peralta, Cuesta, Caro, & Martinez-Larrea, 1994). Here the measures were, however, of presence or absence of symptoms. It is likely also to be important to measure the impact of symptoms—for example, the extent to which a given psychotic symptom made the patient frightened or depressed (Taylor et al., 1994). It is premature to suggest that neuroleptic medication, and perhaps particularly high-dose neuroleptics, have a direct anti-aggressive effect among patients with a psychosis until this more subtle route of illness mediation has been tested.

While substance misuse among people with psychosis may arise for the same sort of social reasons that it does in anyone else, the disproportionate risk of misuse suggests that the illness itself may be relevant. Patients may use drugs to account for their otherwise inexplicable symptoms, to seek oblivion from the financial and social poverty trap in which so many of those with the more disabling illnesses find themselves, and, perhaps best recorded, as an attempt to relieve those symptoms that the conventional antipsychotics do not relieve—in particular, dysphoria or associated depression—or even that they induce—for example, slowing or anhedonia. One small, open study of a broad-spectrum antipsychotic medication (Buckley, Thompson, Way, & Meltzer, 1994) shows promise in this regard. Among psychotic patients treated with clozapine, those who abused substances did at least as well as those who did not, with little tendency to return to substances of abuse while continuing to take clozapine.

There will be some patients whose psychosis is resistant even to clozapine, and to the new generation of atypical antipsychotics with multi-receptor-site action. Management strategies to reduce the impact of the symptoms with other medications (Barnes, McVedy, & Nelson, 1996; Christison et al., 1991), and/or more psychological approaches such as cognitive or dialectical behaviour therapies, may then be called upon for use with preventive strategies. Three studies have shown that lithium can be a useful adjunct to neuroleptics for patients with symptoms resistant to treatment with neuroleptics alone (Carman, Bigelow, & Wyatt, 1981; Growe, Crayton, Klass, Evans, & Stizich, 1979; Small, Kellams, Milstein, & Moore, 1975). Two small, uncontrolled studies offer a suggestion that lithium may be especially helpful where "aggression" is a feature (Altshuler, Abdullah, & Rainer, 1977; Sheard, 1984). Carbamazepine may offer a similar added advantage in treatment-resistant cases, again perhaps particularly favouring aggressive patients (Okuma et al., 1989), but this is the only one of three double-blind controlled trials to show such an advantage. Tiihonen and Swartz (this volume) carry forward the discussion of the place of medication.

Findings are as yet tentative with respect to psychological approaches, with the main thrust on modification of symptoms (Garety, Kuipers, Fowler, Chamberlain, & Dunn, 1994; Kuipers, 1996; Persaud & Marks, 1995). This may be a particularly promising area for future research. Quinsey (this volume) presents data on the problems of implementing, maintaining, and assessing a token economy scheme in the Canadian maximum-security psychiatric facility within Oak Ridge Hospital.

Clinical impression strongly suggests that the most important indicator of whether a patient who has been seriously violent to another person is ready to leave hospital is whether that patient has developed a capacity to negotiate with professional staff and, where relevant, lay carers or family on issues relating to his or her continuing care and treatment. Beauford, McNiel, and Binder (1997) describe use of a six-point therapeutic alliance scale (Clarkin, Hurt, & Crilly, 1987) to rate the admitting clinician's view of this, from records, in a consecutive series of 328 patients admitted to a university hospital. Patients who went on to display violence within the hospital were significantly more likely to have been rated as poor for therapeutic alliance at admission, even when controlling for demographic and other clinical correlates. The study does not clarify where the deficits arose, and the scale, dependent on clinician reporting of patient attitudes over time, seems open to layers of subjectivity. Frank and Gunderson (1990) emphasise the persistence and therapeutic optimism required in forming a therapeutic alliance with patients with schizophrenia, showing significant gains over 6 months even in unpromising cases. It takes two to form a therapeutic alliance, and it is by no means always the case that the inability to do so rests with the patient, or at least solely with the patient. This work opens up an important channel for evaluation of a preventive strategy which includes assessment of this alliance, *and* assessment-informed work to improve it.

STAFF-CENTRED FACTORS

A number of studies have suggested that younger age, nature of professional disciplinary group (nurses), less experience or skill, poor motivation, lack of choice in working environment, low staff numbers, and instability as a team all have some correlation with the occurrence of inpatient violence. As it is often the case that the most junior and least experienced staff of any discipline are the ones in most contact with the patients, it is hardly surprising that these may be the groups numerically most at risk of being victims. However, when time at risk is taken into account some of the differences may disappear. For example, Carmel and Hunter (1991) confirmed that, on this basis, the *rate* of attack of psychiatrists was similar to that of nurses. Most of the other characteristics have been derived intuitively, although James et al. (1990) inferred the role of temporary staff from evidence that there had been a 240% increase in violent incidents in one acute psychiatric inpatient ward over a 15-month period, while patient characteristics and admission rates and bed occupancy had remained constant. There had been a 50% reduction in permanent staff with a concomitant increase in agency nurses. This may be a reflection less of skills than of the importance of teamwork on the part of staff and familiarity with the patients in treatment at any one period.

A model used more than once for the evaluation of the effectiveness of staff training is relative counts of violent incidents in units where staff have and have not been trained in the management of violence. Rice, Harris, Varney, and Quinsey (1989) present a very detailed description of a staff training course for controlling violent incidents, the development of which had been informed by extensive review within and without the maximum-security unit in Ontario's Oak Ridge Hospital. The difficulties in evaluating such a programme are apparent. They are illustrative of the point that human systems are not readily subject to the laboratory conditions beloved of quasi-scientific purists demanding only randomized controlled trials, and conversely that even if such conditions can be obtained they may bear little resemblance to real life, and thus have potentially limited application in practice. An immediate advantage in violence reduction and hospital staff working days lost has been documented on wards with such trained staff, but not sustained (see also Quinsey, this volume).

Carmel and Hunter (1990) simply describe the difference between incidents on nine wards in a state forensic hospital in California where 60% or more of the staff had undergone training in the management of violence, compared with 18 wards where the proportion of such specifically trained staff was lower. There was no difference in frequency of violent incidents per bed, but the rate of injury to staff was significantly different, suggesting no overall prevention gained by, say, the confidence and skills engendered by training, but some prevention of harm.

Phillips and Rudestam (1995) conducted a tiny study but one in which staff volunteers had been randomly assigned to one of three groups—eight men received didactic training in just over 4 hours, eight men received didactic and physical skills training for the same period, and eight men received no training but were evaluated, before and after, using the same instruments, which included measures of fear and hostility as well as role play and a count of actual ward-based assaults for up to 2 weeks after the training period. There was a significant reduction in fear and expressed hostility only in the doubly trained group, but a hierarchy of involvement in actual assaults. The doubly trained group had a collective record of 23% fewer assaults than those who received only didactic training, who in turn had 20% fewer assaults than those without training.

Smoot and Gonzales (1995) describe a comparison between two inpatient state hospital units for patients with recidivist tendencies to "aggression." In one unit a training programme was introduced to increase staff empathy for patient needs, while in the other no change was introduced. The experimental unit showed a decrease in staff turnover, less sick leave, fewer incidents of restraint and seclusion, and a reduction of $63,000 in expenditure.

There is little doubt that various staff activities may be perceived by patients as aversive. Not least of the problems that staff face is that a judgement of imminent violence may lead to an approach by a staff member that is perceived as threatening and that constitutes the final trigger for an assault. Whittington and Wykes (1994) examined the precursors to 100 violent assaults by interviewing the staff concerned within 72 hours of the incident. Over half had been preceded by some action to prevent harm or absconding, request for an activity, or negative verbal statements. Many patients perceive as punitive certain procedures designed to safeguard them, such as seclusion or restraint. There is a risk that they may be used that way, but we did not find any studies that explored seclusion rates in relation to rates of violent incidents or that clarified the direction of any relationship. It is possible that units which have an over-reliance on seclusion are provocative of patient violence; it is also possible that units which have to contain any violence without the availability of such segregation of the person who has been violent may, like those where staff feel ill-equipped for other reasons, have a worse record for the number or quality of incidents. One-to-one nursing care, received favourably among one small group of suicidal inpatients, most of whom were suffering from depression (Pitula & Cardell, 1996), appears also to have received one mention for patients with a propensity for violence. Vartiainen, Vuorio, Halonen, and Hakola (1995) report that 36% of residents in high-security hospitals had found seclusion or restraint helpful. Anecdotally, patients in one English high-security hospital, the majority of whom have schizophrenia, commonly complain that 1:1 nursing is oppressive. It also creates tensions for them, because the extra nursing usually has to be done without additional resources, so some of their peers give them a hard time for absorbing too much staff attention. Seclusion (being locked alone in a purpose-designed room) is rarely used in this setting, but patients in particular distress not uncommonly ask to spend time in the room, or to sleep in it without the door being locked, and may be allowed to do so. It may be that response to these various provisions is determined more by staff presentation than the actual interventions or facilities.

Lancee, Gallop, and McCaye Toner (1995) studied styles of limit-setting among nurses. A consecutive series of consenting patients, 1 week after admission to hospital, were exposed to 24 role-playing situations with nurse actors over two sessions. The styles tested were: belittlement, platitudes, generic responses, solutions without options, explanation of rules without possible courses of action, solutions with options, expressions of concern without options, and expressions of concern with options. The approach was artificial, so may not be generalizable to real practice; however, the results have face validity for such potential. For all diagnostic groups, belittlement generated significantly more anger than the other styles, and affective involvement *with options* significantly less. For the nearly one third of patients with schizophrenia, the intermediate states could not be differentiated.

While much interaction with potentially violent patients may take place in an acute inpatient setting, most with functional psychotic illnesses will require long-term professional care and treatment. Where serious violence has occurred, this may even be mandatory. There is an extensive literature on the relationship between the course of schizophrenia and qualities in the family environment (Kavanagh, 1992). People appear more prone to relapse in families with high expressed emotion (EE), often particularly negative emotions and highly correlated with criticism of the person with schizophrenia, than those in a low-EE setting (Bebbington & Kuipers, 1994). People in long-term residency in hospital, or in long-term managed care in the community, may come to relate in similar ways to professional carers—and the former, perhaps, to other patients. Moore, Ball, and Kuipers (1992) explored EE in staff working with the long-term adult mentally ill. Among 35 staff in key worker relationships with 61 patients, almost all with chronic schizophrenia, 15 of the staff showed high EE. This was more dependent on the attributes of the patient than of the staff member, suggesting that it was not a primary or enduring trait in the worker. Even in this small sample, aggressive behaviour by the patient was one of the significant correlates of criticism and high staff EE. In an independent, smaller series, Oliver and Kuipers (1996) report similar findings. Stark, Lewandowski, and Buchkremer (1992) add a finding of sex difference in staff responses to patient characteristics, and observed that patients with a poorer outcome at 2 years could be distinguished by the quality of therapist-patient relationship at the end of the primary therapeutic interaction. Recognition of the development of high EE in a relationship could offer points of intervention in staff training, ongoing support, and supervision, with prevention of subsequent violent responses by the patient among the potential benefits.

There is little in the literature on a related and potentially important issue—the relative preventive value of specific staff interventions after a serious incident. Instigation of the process of prosecution of the offending patient may be a tool used with increasing frequency (Volavka et al., 1995). Eleven percent of Volavka's series went to jail or prison—thus preventing their inpatient repetition of violence in the short term, but notions of preventative value in any more general sense have been explored in theory only (Till, 1998). An incident inquiry, by the clinical team concerned or independent of it, is de rigueur, although the value of the lessons to be learnt from such incident reports or inquiries is unresearched and unclear. Single cases rarely make a good basis for altering practice in general. That is partly why research according to strict criteria and with substantial sample sizes is needed and valued. There is, however, a real dilemma here. Probably the most consistent finding in studies of the frequency of violence in inpatient settings is that a small number of patients account for a large number of the incidents. To give examples at possible extremes of service, Owen, Tarantello, Jones, and Tennant (1998) studied all 855 patients admitted during 105 weeks of data collection in four acute psychiatric units for adults and one psychogeriatric unit in Sydney, Australia. There were 1,289 incidents, perpetrated by 174 individuals, but just 20 of these people accounted for 67% of them. At Broadmoor high-security hospital, there were 575 men and 147 women resident at some time between April 1, 1994, and March 31, 1999. There were 16,000 incidents recorded during that period, when all categories are taken into account, inclusive of verbal aggression and self-harm. Two hundred and ninety-four men (51%) and 102 women (69%) had at least one act of actual physical violence recorded, but 63 men (11%) accounted for 1,638 (72%) of violent assaults against others, and six men for nearly one quarter of the total. One woman appeared over 800 times in incident reports for the period, with 600 of those incidents being personal assaults on staff and fellow patients. It stretches credibility that the same strategies that might be effective in the prevention of violence among the larger group with one or two episodes of violence are likely to work for the outliers at either extreme. Such strategies may be wholly unnecessary and unduly restrictive or expensive for the non-violent, but inadequate for the very persistently assaultive. Intervention research does not generally separate these groups.

MANAGING THE SOCIAL NETWORK

Various indicators show that factors in a patient's social network, even as an inpatient, may predispose to violence and therefore offer points for intervention. Studies of potential modifiers of social skills or capacity for communication are conspicuous by their absence in this context, although in clinical practice this has proved no bar to offering options such as social skills groups. Perhaps too little attention has been paid to more fundamental aspects of communication among the inpatients most vulnerable to becoming violent—those for whom disorders of the form of language (as a surrogate for disorder of thought) are regarded as almost pathognomic. The absence of a social network within a hospital setting, far from indicating a group of patients at lower risk of violence, indicates perhaps a group with the greatest communication problems and the greatest chance of moving to violent action without warning (Heads et al., submitted).

Patients with a social network outside the hospital present a different order of problem. It is those relationships which appear to be particularly violence-prone in the community (Estroff, Swanson, Lachicotte, Swartz, & Bolduc, 1998) that may be best protected by hospital admission, but perhaps only for its duration, and the capacity of a subgroup of relatively intact patients with psychosis to repeat pathological attachments should not be underestimated. It is likely that these appear particularly in longer-stay units for offender patients, where there is also time for such relationships to develop. The nature of the phraseology here, peppered with "probablies" and "it is likely thats," confirms how slight the database is. Another area for exploration is that of treatment of traumatic stress and family management. In an English national review of health and social services for mentally disordered offenders and others requiring similar services (Department of Health, Home Office, 1992), one of the guiding principles was that patients should be cared for as near as possible to their own homes or families if they have them. This was not an evidence-based principle. A substantial minority even of patients in high security with schizophrenia had suffered neglect or emotional or physical abuse at the hands of their families throughout childhood (Heads, Taylor, & Leese, 1997). In the US, Cascardi, Mueser, DeGiralomo, and Murrin (1996) report a high rate of attack on patients by partners (63%) or other family members (46%) in the year prior to admission to ordinary psychiatric facilities. There are no systematic data relating inpatient violence to family visits to the hospital, but certainly in individual cases in English high-security hospitals preventive management strategies have to include additional support, whether chemical, psychological, or both, before and after such visits if damage to the fabric of the hospital, to other patients, or to staff is to be avoided. Conversely, much of the most serious violence that these patients have inflicted, inclusive of homicide, has taken place within the family, or at the widest in the local community. Patients recovering from their psychosis find it exceptionally hard to accommodate what they have done, and the traumatized survivors at home may have no less severe symptoms of post-traumatic stress disorder and its often accompanying rage. These combinations too can affect inpatient safety. That experience of significant trauma and directly resultant disorder, commonly unrecognized and untreated, is not, however, unique to offender patients (Mueser et al., 1998).

Conclusions

Far too much guidance in the field of preventing inpatient violence depends on principle, consensus statements, and "self-evident" advice. "High impact" psychiatry journals publish nothing on prevention in this area, and little that is directly relevant. There are real barriers to effective research, including staff anxieties, perhaps legitimate, about maintaining safety while the research is carried out. Real consent on the part of patients is likely to be genuinely problematic in this group, with a likelihood that patients without capacity are particularly likely to cluster in the groups of interest. Nevertheless, research with such groups is necessary given the evidence suggesting that key factors associated with inpatient violence may differ from those associated with violence in the wider community.

The low base rate of violence provides another challenge, but "hostility" and "anger" do not necessarily represent equivalents. Then too, the violence to be prevented is almost certainly heterogeneous in type and in predisposing factors, even within a hospital setting. The individuals who are unusual within the population account for the highest frequency, but each such case may be too atypical for generalization. Strategies which may be more helpful for larger numbers of less frequently or exceptionally violent patients may have to be devised and tested separately.

A feature of disorder or disease is that it tends to narrow the repertoire of responses. Even among people with a mental illness, however, routes to violent behaviours are generally complex, and solutions accordingly so too. Evaluation of necessarily multifaceted interventions for complex problems is beyond the scope of most researchers, partly because techniques are likely to call for special skills, but also because large sample sizes will be needed for the power analyses involved, and thus only multi-centre trials hold a prospect of answers. While randomized controlled trials of some elements of practice may be an attainable goal, full management packages and such central concepts as "negotiating safety" (Stanko, 1990, 1993), with the implied necessity for retention of flexibility in relationships and arrangements, do not lend themselves readily to such trials, which, if achieved, may still mislead in the field. Double blindness is applicable only where it is feasible—generally in relation to medication.

In spite of all these challenges to research, and the limitations of the research published so far, there do seem to be indicators of intervention points. Plausible, testable strategies for prevention through environmental modification include consultation with staff and patients about their setting, hospital-specific review of patterns of incidents and their circumstances to inform strategy, attention to staff attitudes, and prevention of use of non-prescribed psychoactive substances. Staff attitudes and skills appear to be the most important of the institutional environment factors in the prevention of violence. That said, prevention strategies are usually complex, and the few evaluations that are available do not distinguish between the effect of a package and the effect of its component parts. Persistence in accumulating small steps in knowledge and efforts at multi-centre collaboration are surely the principal ways forward.

References

Adams, C.E., Power, A., Frederick, K., & Lefebvre, C. (1994). An investigation of the adequacy of Medline searches for randomised control trials (RCT) of the effects of mental health care. *Psychological Medicine, 24,* 741–748.

Altshuler, K.Z., Abdullah, S., & Rainer, J.D. (1977). Lithium and aggressive behaviour in patients with early total deafness. *Diseases of the Nervous System, 38,* 521–524.

Barnes, T.R.E., McVedy, C.J.B., & Nelson, H.E. (1996). Management and treatment of schizophrenia unresponsive to clozapine. *British Journal of Psychiatry, 169*(Suppl 31), 31–40.

Baxter, E., Hafner, R.J., & Holme, G. (1992). Assaults by patients: The experience and attitudes of hospital nurses. *Australian and New Zealand Psychiatry, 26,* 567–573.

Beauford, J.E., McNiel, D., & Binder, R.L. (1997). Utility of the initial therapeutic alliance in evaluating psychiatric patients' risk of violence. *American Journal of Psychiatry, 154,* 1272–1276.

Bebbington, P., & Kuipers, L. (1994). The predictive utility of expressed emotion in schizophrenia: An aggregate analysis. *Psychological Medicine, 24,* 707–718.

Buchanan, A., Reed, A., Wessely, S., Garety, P., Taylor, P.J., Grubin, D., & Dunn, G. (1993). Acting on delusions. 2: The phenomenological correlates of acting on delusions. *British Journal of Psychiatry, 163,* 77–82.

Buckley, P., Thompson, P., Way, L., & Meltzer, H.Y. (1994). Substance abuse among patients with treatment resistant schizophrenia: Characteristics and implications for clozapine therapy. *American Journal of Psychiatry, 151,* 385–389.

Caldwell, M. (1992). Incidence of PTSD among staff victims of patient violence. *Hospital and Community Psychiatry, 26,* 838–839.

Caplan, N.S., & Siebert, L.A. (1964). Distribution of juvenile delinquent intelligence test scores over a thirty-four-year period. *Journal of Clinical Psychology, 20,* 242–247.

Carman, J.S., Bigelow, L.B., & Wyatt, R.J. (1981). Lithium combined with neuroleptics in chronic schizophrenic and schizoaffective patients. *Journal of Clinical Psychiatry, 42,* 124–128.

Carmel, H., & Hunter, M. (1990). Compliance with training strategy in managing assaultive behavior and injuries from in-patient violence. *Hospital and Community Psychiatry, 41,* 558–560.

Carmel, H., & Hunter, M. (1991). Psychiatrists injured by patient attack. *Bulletin of the American Academy of Psychiatry and Law, 19,* 309–316.

Cascardi, M., Mueser, K.T., DeGiralomo, J., & Murrin, M. (1996). Physical aggression against psychiatric inpatients by family members and partners. *Psychiatric Services, 47,* 531–533.

Chaiken, J., Chaiken, M., & Rhodes, W. (1994). Predicting violent behavior and classifying violent offenders. In A.J. Reiss & J.A. Roth (Eds.), *Understanding and preventing violence. Vol. 4: Consequences and control* (pp. 217–295). Washington: National Academy Press.

Cheung, P., Schweitzer, I., Crowley, K., & Tuckwell, V. (1997). Violence in schizophrenia: Role of hallucinations and delusions. *Schizophrenia Research, 26,* 181–190.

Christison, G.D., Kirch, D.G., & Wyatt, R.J. (1991). When symptoms persist: Choosing among alternative somatic treatments for schizophrenia. *Schizophrenia Bulletin, 17,* 217–245.

Clarkin, J.F., Hurt, S.W., & Crilly, J.L. (1987). Therapeutic alliance and hospital treatment outcome. *Hospital and Community Psychiatry, 38,* 871–875.

Cooper, A.J., & Mendonca, J.A. (1991). A prospective study of patient assaults in Canada. *Acta Psychiatrica Scandinavica, 84,* 163–166.

Department of Health, Home Office. (1992). *Review of health and social services for mentally disordered offenders and others requiring similar services. Final summary report.* Cm. 2088. London: HMSO.

Department of Health and Social Security. (1988). *Violence to staff. Report of the DHSS Advisory Committee on Violence to Staff.* London: Author.

Dietz, P.E., & Rada, R.T. (1982). Battery incidents and batterers in a maximum security hospital. *Archives of General Psychiatry 39,* 31–34.

Dunn, M., O'Driscoll, C., Dayson, D., Wills, W., & Leff, J. (1990). The TAPS Project. 4: An observational study of the social life of long-stay patients. *British Journal of Psychiatry, 157,* 842–848.

Edwards, J.G., Jones, D., Reid, W.H., & Chu, C. (1988). Physical assaults in a psychiatric unit of a general hospital. *American Journal of Psychiatry, 145,* 1568–1571.

Estroff, S.E., Swanson, J.W., Lachicotte, W.S., Swartz, M., & Bolduc, M. (1998). Risk reconsidered: Targets of violence in the social networks of people with serious psychiatric disorders. *Social Psychiatry and Psychiatric Epidemiology, 33*(Suppl 1), S95–S101.

Frank, A.F., & Gunderson, J.G. (1990). The role of the therapeutic alliance in the treatment of schizophrenia: Relationship to course and outcome. *Archives of General Psychiatry, 47,* 228–236.

Garety, P.A., Kuipers, L., Fowler, D., Chamberlain, F., & Dunn, G. (1994). Cognitive behavioural therapy for drug resistant psychosis. *British Journal of Medical Psychology, 67,* 259–271.

Growe, G.A., Crayton, J.W., Klass, D.B., Evans, H., & Stizich, M. (1979). Lithium in chronic schizophrenia. *American Journal of Psychiatry, 136,* 454–455.

Haller, R.M. & Deluty, R.H. (1988). Assaults on staff by psychiatric in-patients: A critical review. *British Journal of Psychiatry, 152,* 174–179.

Heads, T., Leese, M., Taylor, P.J., & Phillips, S. (submitted). Schizophrenia and serious violence: An exploration of interaction between social context, symptoms and violence. Available from authors: T. Heads, Ealing, Hammersmith & Fulham Mental Health Trust, Southall, Middlesex UB1 3EU UK.

Heads, T.C., Taylor, P.J., & Leese, M. (1997). Childhood experiences of patients with schizophrenia and a history of offending/violent behaviour. *Criminal Behaviour and Mental Health, 7,* 117–130.

Health Services Advisory Committee. (1987). *Violence to staff in the health services.* Health and Safety Commission. London: HMSO.

Hellerstein, D., Frosch, W., & Koenigsberg, H.W. (1987). The clinical significance of command hallucinations. *American Journal of Psychiatry, 144,* 219–221.

Hillbrand, M., Foster, H.G., & Spitz, R.T. (1996). Characteristics and costs of staff injuries in a forensic hospital. *Psychiatric Services, 47,* 1123–1125.

Hinde, R.A. (1993). Aggression at different levels of social complexity. In P.J. Taylor (Ed.), *Violence in society* (pp. 31–36). London: Royal College of Physicians of London.

Howard, L., & Wilkinson, G. (1998). Impact factors of psychiatric journals. *British Journal of Psychiatry, 172,* 457.

Hunter, M.E., & Love, C.C. (1996). Total quality management and the reduction of inpatient violence and costs in a forensic psychiatric hospital. *Psychiatric Services, 47,* 751–754.

James, D.V., Fineberg, N.A., Shah, A.K., & Priest, R.G. (1990). An increase in violence on an acute psychiatric ward: A study of associated factors. *British Journal of Psychiatry, 156,* 846–852.

Janofsky, J.S., Spears, S., & Neubauer, D.N. (1988). Psychiatrists' accuracy in predicting violent behaviour on an inpatient unit. *Hospital and Community Psychiatry, 39,* 1090–1094.

Junginger, J. (1995). Command hallucinations and the prediction of dangerousness. *Psychiatric Services, 46,* 911–914.

Kane, J.M., & Marder, S.R. (1993). Psychopharmacologic treatment of schizophrenia. *Schizophrenia Bulletin, 19,* 287–302.

Katz, P., & Kirkland, F.R. (1990). Violence in social structure on mental hospital wards. *Psychiatry, 53,* 262–277.

Kavanagh, D.J. (1992). Recent developments in expressed emotion and schizophrenia. *British Journal of Psychiatry, 160,* 601–620.

Kuipers, E. (1996). The management of difficult to treat patients with schizophrenia, using non-drug therapies. *British Journal of Psychiatry, 169*(Suppl 31), 41–51.

Lancee, W.J., Gallop, R., & McCaye Toner, B. (1995). The relationship between nurses' limit-setting styles and anger in psychiatric in-patients. *Psychiatric Services, 6,* 609–613.

Lion, J.R., Snyder, W., & Merrill, G.L. (1981). Under-reporting of assaults on staff in a state hospital. *Hospital and Community Psychiatry, 33,* 497–498.

Love, C.C., & Hunter, M.E. (1996). Violence in public sector psychiatric hospitals: Benchmark in nursing staff injury rates. *Journal of Psycho-social Nursing, 34,* 30–34.

Maden, A., Curle, C., Meux, C., Burrow, S., & Gunn, J. (1993). The treatment and security needs of patients in special hospitals. *Criminal Behaviour and Mental Health, 3,* 290–306.

McEvoy, J.P., Hogarty, G.E., & Steingard, S. (1991). Optimal dose of neuroleptic in acute schizophrenia. *Archives of General Psychiatry, 48,* 739–745.

Molnar, G., Keitner, L., & Swindall, L. (1985). Medicolegal problems of elopement from psychiatric units. *Journal of Forensic Sciences, 30,* 44–49.

Molnar, G., & Pinchoff, D.M. (1993). Factors in patient elopements from an urban state hospital and strategies for prevention. *Hospital and Community Psychiatry, 44,* 791–792.

Moore, E. (submitted). A descriptive analysis of incidents of absconding and escape from English high-security hospitals 1989–1994. Available from author: Broadmoor Hospital, Crowthorne, Berkshire RG45 7EG UK.

Moore, E., Ball, R.A., & Kuipers, L. (1992). Expressed emotion in staff working with the long-term adult mentally ill. *British Journal of Psychiatry, 161,* 802–808.

Mueser, K.T., Goodman, L.B., Trumbetta, S.L., Rosenberg, S.D., Osher, F.C., Vidaves, R., Auciello, P., & Foy, D.W. (1998). Trauma and posttraumatic stress disorder in severe mental illness. *Journal of Consulting and Clinical Psychology, 66,* 493–499.

Noble, P. (1997). Violence in psychiatric in-patients: Review and clinical implications. *International Review of Psychiatry, 9,* 207–216.

Noble, P., & Rodger, S. (1989). Violence by psychiatric in-patients. *British Journal of Psychiatry, 155,* 384–390.

Okuma, T., Yamashita, I., Takahashi, R., Itoh, A., Kurihara, M., Otsuki, S., Watanabe, S., Hazamura, H., & Inanaga, K. (1989). The double-blind study of adjunctive carbamazepine versus placebo on excited states of schizophrenia and schizoaffective disorders. *Acta Psychiatrica Scandinavica, 80,* 250–259.

Oliver, N., & Kuipers, E. (1996). Stress and its relationship to expressed emotion in community mental health workers. *International Journal of Social Psychiatry, 2,* 150–159.

Owen, C., Tarantello, C., Jones, M., & Tennant, C. (1998). Violence and aggression in psychiatric units. *Psychiatric Services, 49,* 1452–1457.

Palmstierna, T., Huitfeldt, B., & Wistedt, B. (1991). The relationship of crowding and aggressive behavior on a psychiatric intensive care unit. *Hospital and Community Psychiatry, 42,* 1237–1240.

Palmstierna, T., & Wistedt, B. (1995). Changes in the pattern of aggressive behaviour among inpatients with changed ward organisation. *Acta Psychiatrica Scandinavica, 91,* 32–35.

Peralta, V., Cuesta, M.J., Caro, F., & Martinez-Larrea, A. (1994). Neuroleptic dose and schizophrenic symptoms: A survey of prescribing practices. *Acta Psychiatrica Scandinavica, 90,* 354–357.

Persaud, R., & Marks, S.I. (1995). The pilot study of exposure control of chronic auditory hallucinations in schizophrenia. *British Journal of Psychiatry, 167,* 45–50.

Phillips, D., & Rudestam, K.E. (1995). Effect of non-violence self-defense training on male psychiatric staff members' aggression and fear. *Psychiatric Services, 46,* 164–168.

Pitula, C.R., & Cardell, R. (1996). Suicidal inpatients' experience of constant observation. *Psychiatric Services, 47,* 649–651.

Quinsey, V.L., Coleman, G., Jones, B., & Altrows, I. (1997). Proximal antecedents of eloping and reoffending among mentally disordered offenders. *Journal of Interpersonal Violence, 12,* 794–813.

Regier, D.A., Farmer, M.E., Rae, D.S., Locke, B.Z., Keith, S.J., Judd, L.L., & Goodwin, F.K. (1990). Comorbidity of mental disorders with alcohol and other drug abuse. *Journal of the American Medical Association, 264,* 2511–2518.

Reiss, A.J., & Roth, J.A. (Eds.). (1993/94). *Understanding and preventing violence. Vols. 1–4.* Washington: National Academy Press.

Rice, M.E., Harris, G.T., Varney, G.W., & Quinsey, V.L. (1989). *Violence in institutions: Understanding, prevention and control.* Toronto: Hogrefe & Huber.

Richmond, I., Dandridge, L., & Jones, K. (1991). Changing nurse practice to prevent elope-ment. *Journal of Nursing Care Quality, 6*, 73–81.

Royal College of Psychiatrists Research Unit. (1998). *Management of imminent violence: Clinical practice guidelines to support mental health services.* Occasional paper OP41. London: Royal College of Psychiatrists.

Rutter, M., Maughan, B., Mortimore, P., & Ouston, J. (1979). *Fifteen thousand hours.* London: Open Books.

Sheard, M.H. (1984). Clinical pharmacology of aggressive behavior. *Clinical Neuropharma-cology, 7*, 173–183.

Small, J.G., Kellams, J.J., Milstein, V., & Moore, J. (1975). A placebo-controlled study of lithium combined with neuroleptics in chronic schizophrenic patients. *American Journal of Psychiatry, 132*, 1315–1317.

Smoot, S.L., & Gonzales, J.L. (1995). Cost-effective communication skills training for state hospital employees. *Psychiatric Services, 46*, 819–822.

Snyder, W. (1994). Hospital downsizing and increased frequency of assault on staff. *Hospital and Community Psychiatry, 45*, 378–380.

Stanko, E. (1990). *Everyday violence.* London: Pandora.

Stanko, E.A. (1993). Everyday violence and experience of crime. In P.J. Taylor (Ed.), *Vio-lence in society* (pp. 169–180). London: Royal College of Physicians.

Stark, F.M., Lewandowski, L., & Buchkremer, G. (1992). Therapist-patient relationship as a predictor of the course of schizophrenic illness. *European Psychiatry, 7*, 161–169.

Steadman, H.J., & Morrissey, J. (1982). Predicting violent behaviour: A note on cross valida-tion study. *Social Forces, 61*, 475–483.

Steadman, H.J., Mulvey, E.P., Monahan J., Robbins, P.C., Appelbaum, P.S., Grisson, T., Roth, L.H., & Silver, E. (1998). Violence by people discharged from acute psychiatric in-patient facilities and by others in the same neighborhoods. *Archives of General Psychiatry, 55*, 393–401.

Swanson, J.W., Holzer, C.E., Ganju, V.K., & Jono, R.T. (1990). Violence and psychiatric disorder in the community: Evidence from the Epidemiologic Catchment Area surveys. *Hospital and Community Psychiatry, 41*, 761–770.

Tardiff, K. (1983). A survey of assault by chronic patients in a state hospital system. In J.R. Lion & W.H. Reid (Eds.), *Assaults within psychiatric facilities* (pp. 3–19). New York: Grune & Stratton.

Tardiff, K., Marzuk, P.M., Leon, A.C., & Portera, L. (1997). A prospective study of violence by psychiatric patients after hospital discharge. *Psychiatric Services, 48*, 678–681.

Tardiff, K., & Sweillam, A. (1980). Assault, suicide and mental illness. *Archives of General Psychiatry, 37*, 164–169.

Taylor, P.J. (1998). When symptoms of psychosis drive serious violence. *Social Psychiatry and Psychiatric Epidemiology, 33*, S47–S54.

Taylor, P.J., Garety, P., Buchanan, A., Reed, A., Wessely, S., Ray, K., Dunn, G., & Grubin, D. (1994). Delusions and violence. In J. Monahan & H. Steadman (Eds.), *Violence and mental disorder: Developments in risk assessment* (pp. 161–182). Chicago: University of Chicago Press.

Taylor, P.J., Leese, M., Williams, D., Butwell, M., Daly, R., & Larkin, E. (1998). Mental disorder and violence: A special (high security) hospital study. *British Journal of Psy-chiatry, 172*, 218–226.

Thomas, H.J., Schwartz, E., & Petrelli, R. (1992). Droperidol versus haloperidol for clinical restraint of agitated and combative patients. *Annals of Emergency Medicine, 21*, 407–413.

Till, U. (1998). The prosecution of psychiatric inpatients for assault: Benefits and ethics. *Psy-chiatric Care, 5*, 219–224.

Vartianinen, H., Vuorio, O., Halonen, P., & Hakola, P. (1995). The patients' opinions about curative factors in involuntary treatment. *Acta Psychiatrica Scandinavica, 91,* 163–166.

Volavka, J., Crowner, M., Brizer, D., Convit, A., Van Praag, H., & Suckow, F. (1990). Tryptophan treatment of aggressive psychiatric inpatients. *Biological Psychiatry, 28,* 728–732.

Volavka, J., Mohammad, Y., Vitrai, J., Connolly, M., Stefanovic, M., & Ford, M. (1995). Characteristics of state hospital patients arrested for offenses committed during hospitalization. *Psychiatric Services, 46,* 796–800.

Wallace, C., Mullen , P., Burgess, P., Palmer, S., Ruschera, D., & Browne, C. (1998). Serious criminal offending and mental disorder. *British Journal of Psychiatry, 172,* 477–484.

Watson, B.E. (1996). Can institution-induced anger prolong hospitalization for patients who repress anger? *Psychiatric Services, 47,* 363–364.

Watson, R.J.D., & Richardson, P.H. (1999). Accessing the literature on outcome studies in group psychotherapy: The sensitivity and precision of Medline and Psyc INFO bibliographic data base searching. *British Journal of Medical Psychology, 72,* 127–134.

Whittington, R., & Wykes, T. (1994). Violence in psychiatric hospitals: Are certain staff prone to being assaulted? *Journal of Advanced Nursing, 19,* 219–225.

Yudovsky, S.C., Silver, J.M., Jackson, W., Endicott, J., & Williams, D. (1986). The Overt Aggression Scale for the objective rating of verbal and physical aggression. *American Journal of Psychiatry, 143,* 35–39.

Pamela J. Taylor is Professor of Special Hospital Psychiatry, Department of Forensic Psychiatry, Institute of Psychiatry, London, UK, and is associated with Broadmoor Hospital, Crowthorne, Berkshire, UK. Hans Schanda is Professor, Justizanstalt Göllersdorf, Göllersdorf, Austria.

Authors' Note

We are very grateful to Martin Butwell for assistance with special hospital inpatient violence figures, Estelle Moore for assistance with references, and Christine Tonks for ensuring that there really was a manuscript.

Comments or queries may be directed to Pamela J. Taylor, Department of Forensic Psychiatry, Institute of Psychiatry, Denmark Hill, London SE5 8AF UK. Telephone: 44 134 475 4398. Fax: 44 134 475 4385. E-mail: <p.taylor@iop.kcl.ac.uk>.

EFFECTIVE TREATMENT STRATEGIES FOR PREVENTING VIOLENCE ON PSYCHIATRIC WARDS

GÖRAN FRANSSON

Introduction

This paper is an effort to discuss practical solutions to the problem of violent incidents on psychiatric wards. The main source is personal experience from many years of forensic psychiatry and the idea that almost none of the knowledge found in the scientific literature can be implemented in practice if we do not consider organizations as a whole.

This discussion touches upon technical security, staff, theoretical framework, structure and rules, routines and procedures, risk assessment and risk management, treatment planning, staff-patient interaction, seclusion, restraint, and humour. This simplification is a deliberate attempt to provide a backbone that will be acceptable and useful in as many institutions as possible.

Violence on psychiatric wards seems to be increasing. Psychiatric emergency wards are now one of the most dangerous places to work—not in terms of fatalities, but in terms of the number of assaults. However, this really does not have to be so. It is actually possible to treat violent, mentally ill patients easily, comfortably, and with a sense of reasonable security. In attempting to reach an ideal state of staff-patient interaction, one must consider the entire spectrum of influential factors. These factors must work together optimally, from the design of the building to daily interactions on the wards. "Violence is not simply a product of mental illness or of an antisocial personality. It is also a consequence of the social settings and relationships in which people find themselves" (Warren & Beadsmoore, 1997). All aspects of social life, psychopathology, and treatment interaction influence one another, and all determine the frequency and character of violence.

Technical Security

The appearance of forensic psychiatric hospitals the world over varies from structures that resemble 19th-century prisons to comfortable, modern facilities that provide personal integrity for the patient along with the necessary security. Yet these vast differences in setting are rarely discussed when one treatment model is compared with

S. Hodgins (ed.), Violence among the Mentally Ill, 277–288.

another. Many institutions, especially forensic hospitals, rely heavily on technically advanced security systems. Modern techniques should be used whenever appropriate of course, but we should carefully consider how they are used. If we exaggerate our expectation of day-to-day violence with technical surveillance that is too obvious, we may get just the behaviour we are trying to avoid. In reality such surveillance is no more necessary in a maximum security forensic hospital than in a general psychiatric emergency ward. Perimeter safety can be ensured by the ability to "think safety," keeping doors locked and checking visitors carefully to minimize the risk of contraband entering the hospital. If sophisticated mechanical safety devices other than personal alarms are used, they should be confined to protection of the perimeter.

Too often, forensic psychiatric settings feature a prison atmosphere. It is not always possible to build comfortable wards that provide maximum personal integrity, but at least we can eliminate much of the prison environment. There is no proof that the presence of internal video cameras and security staff, or the absence of paintings, flowers, and comfortable furniture, provides more safety than a less sterile environment. We must remember that, for periods of varying length, the ward is actually home to the patients; it may be artificial, but it is a place for privacy and recreation as well as therapy. Repressive surroundings can have a counter-therapeutic effect.

Staff

The staff is the principal tool in managing a non-violent psychiatric ward and should be chosen very carefully. Patient influence on staff can be enormously powerful, and both personal integrity and stability are essential for the job. Staff members must also have the sensitivity to observe and respond to signals from patients and the ability to handle the resulting countertransferences. According to Adler, Kreeger, and Ziegler (1983), staff "must share a common value system with regard to violence." They must firmly believe that there is no room for physical aggressiveness within the hospital system. There should never be a permissive attitude towards violence. A staff member who disagrees with these principles will experience difficulty setting limits, confronting inappropriate conduct, and establishing clear and consistent rules of behaviour. A patient who is confused or who lacks self-control needs the constraining influence of staff refusal to permit physical aggressiveness. If staff fail to provide such influence firmly and consistently, a patient may force the staff to exert the control he or she needs. Whether a ward is violent or peaceful is a function of staff competence.

Warren and Beadsmoore (1997), in their comparison of violent and peaceful wards, found that

> [violent wards were] characterized by an atmosphere of distrust, with limited and often hostile communication between staff and patients. Most meetings and activities appeared at unscheduled times. Staff responsibilities were not clearly defined and patients were not sure whom to approach about their problems and requests. Staff morale was low and staff communication and support were poor. Staff constantly complained about their workload, patients, the hospital, and psychiatrists.... In contrast, peaceful wards had regular meetings and activities that were scheduled and followed closely. Everybody was aware of

what was happening and when. Staff responsibilities were clearly defined and staff functioned in a coordinated fashion. The patients knew who was responsible for what and teamwork predominated.

It is as simple as that. The problem is how to get it to work in practice.

Theoretical Framework

Theories serve the purpose of presenting a common goal for treatment as well as bringing the staff together to work as a team towards this goal. Many institutions with ambitious treatment objectives for the mentally ill have created complex theoretical frameworks, in some cases almost approaching religious dogma. The results have been rivalry within the institution, unclear management strategies, and conflicts among representatives of different opinions. Ideally, staff members should possess the qualities of good parents—solidity and sensitivity—for stability and empathy are the best resources in everyday treatment. Ideology should be limited to acceptance of: the equality of all human beings; the idea that all biological organisms, including human beings, are capable of individual development; and the notion that whatever a person does or has done is within the range of human behavioural possibilities —something we may have done ourselves under particular circumstances serves to enhance our respect for the patient and to facilitate respectful communication. If these ideas are used as a foundation, general and individual treatment strategies can then be built based on science and experience.

Structure and Rules

Rules provide a framework for an efficient and nurturing structure on the ward. The work structure must be very clear, leaving no doubt about its purpose and its ability to protect both staff and patients from violent acts, while reassuring all concerned that every effort is being made to rehabilitate the patients. The ward must be structured simply enough so that everyone understands the reason why something has been done. There should be few rules, as too many rules tend to stifle spontaneity and may result in rigidity on the part of the staff. Each ward should formulate its own rules, since many different conditions must be satisfied, both legally and as a function of local tradition. However, the goal should always be to provide a safe workplace, to clearly identify the responsibilities of each worker, and to allow enough leeway for positive social interaction among ward inhabitants. Also, it must be borne in mind that rules are made for the purposes of security and development, not repression.

The following rules were found to be very useful following a ward crisis. They may serve as an example of how to build structure and define roles.

Long-term treatment of mentally ill violent patients requires careful planning, some firm rules for safety, a pleasant working environment, and results. A staff that feels safe and secure can achieve anything.

1. *Nothing is more important than the safety of the staff.* When necessary, all safety measures, including restraint and seclusion, are readily available.
2. *Violence and threats are never accepted on the ward.* This must be made clear to everybody, both staff and patients.
3. *All decisions concerning safety are made at the weekly staff meeting.* No leaves or paroles, for example, may be granted at any other time.
4. *Staff meetings are scheduled every week.* The patients must be informed about when they can meet with their physician and have their questions answered.
5. *All available staff must attend weekly staff meetings.* Short-term risk assessment requires information from several observers to obtain the full picture.
6. *The head nurse is the ward administrator.*
7. *The chief physician is in charge of medical issues.* He or she never interferes in routine or nursing matters.
8. *The responsible physician can always be reached.*
9. *All important nursing changes come about as a result of the experience of the nursing staff.* It is the responsibility of the management to make proper use of their ideas.

Rule 8 is important in wards for long-term care, where the authority and support of the responsible physician can inspire confidence among staff. This physician can also be expected to know the patient much better than a colleague on duty from another ward; this facilitates swift, correct decision-making in delicate matters. In practice, disturbances are very few when the entire staff know their individual duties and need this extra security only to be able to work with a measure of confidence.

Routines and Procedures

Ward competence is tested the moment a new patient arrives. From then on, the staff has a crucial influence on the risk for violence. Incidents will occur as long as we are dealing with human beings, but prevention begins with proper reception of the new patient, who will most definitely remember those first moments.

Admissions staff must keep it in mind that psychotic patients have very limited resources for adapting to a new environment. The fantasies and expectations of first-time patients concerning psychiatric institutions are probably no different from those of the rest of the population. New patients might be afraid of the staff, and even more afraid of fellow patients, who, they rightly assume, have problems dealing with their aggressions just as they do. They must be assured that nothing will happen to them—an assurance that cannot be made credibly if there is a high rate of violent incidents, as is mostly the case. If they cannot rely on the staff to keep them safe, they will have to consider ways of defending themselves.

The presumed violent patient must be approached in a calm, direct, and friendly manner, while being given no doubt that the staff is in full control of the situation. Such a patient can instil fear in even the most experienced staff members if they know the patient has a violent record, but, rationally, such staff also know that whatever happens they will be able to handle the situation. After a routine search for drugs, weapons, and other contraband, the psychiatrist is called in for the first examination.

It is important that the patient not have to wait long for this first interview. Prompt attention from the responsible psychiatrist is not only a sign of respect for the patient, but also an opportunity to gather information about the patient's status on arrival. Also, schizophrenic patients have a distorted conception of time, and waiting can become almost unbearable in this situation, which might result in unnecessary aggressive outbursts and animosity towards the staff.

In many institutions, the physician is alone when he or she carries out the admission examination. Although this practice indicates respect for confidentiality, it becomes questionable if the cost is an act of aggression on the part of the patient. The first interview is probably the most dangerous one. A study by Ruben, Wolkon, and Yamamoto (1980) of physical attacks on psychiatrists found that almost all attacks occurred during the initial examination. However, aggression is not likely to occur in a relaxed atmosphere with sufficient staff to guarantee everyone's safety. Psychiatric treatment involves teamwork, which requires that staff be fully informed at all times and participate in as much of the professional work as possible.

The interview should be carried out with the patient located near the door so he or she does not feel trapped in a situation that is threatening in itself. The interviewer should not be within reach of the patient, and must be able to take immediate action should the patient attack.

A useful way to conduct the interview is with the interviewer and the patient on opposite sides of a rectangular table. The table should be long enough to seat up to three staff members on each side, depending on the expected degree of aggression. The chairs should be comfortable and the atmosphere relaxed. In such a setting the interviewer is unlikely to show fear or anxiety, as this could reinforce the patient's own fears. Contact between patient and interviewer will be intimate, but there will be no opportunity for attack, since the staff on each side can easily restrain the patient in the event of an assault.

Six bodyguards is of course a bit exaggerated in practice. I have used the maximum number of staff on one occasion only, when I had to confront an elite athlete suffering from schizophrenia who had assaulted me severely a short time earlier. The assault could easily have been avoided if the medical record had been read properly: The patient had been transferred to the ward after threatening to kill his former psychiatrist, and during the course of his illness he had attacked every doctor who tried to medicate him.

The first interview has several purposes: it provides cues for a primary diagnosis; it serves as a means of establishing a good relationship between psychiatrist and patient; and it clearly demonstrates what may be expected from the psychiatrist-patient relationship. The interview should not be long, since even the best interviewer runs the risk of behaving in a confusing manner under the influence of a very disorganized patient. Several brief, clear interviews with the potentially aggressive patient during the first few days are preferable to a single long interview immediately upon admission.

Risk Assessment and Risk Management

During the first interview, steps are taken towards making a risk assessment based primarily on symptoms and attitude. At examination, historical data are already known; where there is a history of violence, the patient is a risk by definition. However, short-term risk assessments based on historical data are not very accurate; additionally, if history is the only consideration, most patients on the ward—at least in forensic psychiatry—are probably high-risk patients.

Historical data are considered the most reliable means of predicting risk. However, among violent individuals, history of violence is often similar from one person to another. More and more authors are now suggesting that clinical factors and risk factors be added to make the predictions more valid. A small study by Strand, Belfrage, Fransson, and Levander (1999) used the HCR-20 (Webster, Douglas, Eaves, & Hart, 1997) to retrospectively assess two matched groups of discharged forensic psychiatric patients, one that had relapsed into violent criminality and one that had not. Contrary to previous research findings, it was shown that risk management factors were more predictive of violence than historical factors. Even though this project was concerned with long-term predictions, the results are sufficient incentive to carefully plan risk management from the very start of treatment. In addition, a prospective study of violence prediction within the correctional system was conducted by Belfrage, Fransson, and Strand (in press). We found that the HCR-20 historical subscale containing items that generally are regarded as the most robust in prediction of violence risk had low predictive validity, whereas clinical items had good predictive validity and risk management items had the overall highest predictive validity.

Implementation of the HCR-20 at the Forensic Psychiatric Hospital in Sundsvall, Sweden (Belfrage, 1998), has provided staff with a simple and stimulating tool for risk identification and management. The variable R items (plans lack feasibility, exposure to destabilizers, lack of personal support, non-compliance with remediation attempts, stress) lend themselves to immediate planning to reduce the risk of violence. Using just a few, valid, items is essential in the clinical setting, where there is little time for extra work. The simplicity of the coding sheet is useful for presenting the assessment to the patient, and it describes ways to reduce risk behaviour, and thus eventually to gain freedom or other benefits. More complex behaviour confrontations will be discussed below. On the whole, the research project has enhanced staff observation to an unexpectedly high degree, with many positive side effects for daily treatment.

Treatment Planning

The risk assessment should serve not only as an identification tool for the violent patient, but also as an inspiration and guide for treatment planning and progressive risk management. The first version of the risk assessment should be finished after 2 weeks, with revisions being made continuously during the course of treatment. The first treatment plan should be made as soon as the patient's problems are clearly defined and the patient has recovered sufficiently to participate in the planning process.

Where possible, treatment programmes should be developed together with the patient. Patients' suggestions should be respected as much as possible, with the goal of defining clear and understandable steps for dealing with their problems. With the violent patient, careful risk management is as important for planning as psychiatric diagnoses and status. Starting with the patient's present situation and allowing a reasonable amount of time, doctor and patient plan and agree on a treatment programme tailored to the patient's particular situation. Just as important as the medical treatment are planned activities such as work or study projects. Drinkwater and Gudjonsson (1989) found that patients spent 60% of their time unoccupied or asleep on the ward and another 8% passively involved (e.g., watching television). Only 8% of their time was spent on social behaviour. During periods without planned activities, violent behaviour was four times higher, and other behaviours prohibited by staff (e.g., breaking ward rules or being verbally abusive) were also higher. Thus in order to provide meaningful activities for their patients, long-term-care facilities must be equipped with resources for study, work, and recreation.

Heilbrun (1997) discusses the advantages of management models over prediction models in risk assessment, and concludes that management models have clear benefits for the clinician in planning treatment. He offers the following possibilities:

Rather than being the object of a prediction, the patient is a
- full participant in a process that
- specifies the target behaviour clearly and
- enlists the patient's participation in working towards a (risk-reduction) goal,
- the achievement of which is within the patient's control;
- in the management model, progress is directly related to reward, lack of progress to absence of reward, thus
- it is easier for the patient to understand, relying as it does more on achievement of goals and less on "clinical judgement."

Staff-Patient Interaction

Staff members must be skilled in interpersonal communication. When personal destructive feelings take over, the result is almost always a provocative situation, even if violent acts occur only in a minority of cases. Relationship security must encompass working through the dynamics that are always at play on the ward. The immediate conscious reaction to a threat of violence is fear. The short-term reaction is loss of composure. The long-term reaction is denial and projection caused by unconscious anger or rage. Thus if staff react poorly at the time of aggression, they will react poorly over time, particularly if their feelings result in vindictive or punitive acts against the patient—who may become aggressive again, thus reactivating the staff member's fear and rage (Maier, 1986). This vicious circle must be broken at an early stage. Staff must learn to identify feelings of fear and rage as a normal response to working with aggressive patients, and they must learn and recognize the concept of countertransference and projective identification.

Provocations are commonly described as occurring mainly when a patient has been denied a request (Bjørkly, 1993). This is an example of an occasion when communications skills are essential. A clear, respectful, non-negotiable response can have a reassuring, even comforting, effect, since all too often the patient has heard vague excuses and explanations and is most likely cautiously asking for a favour. A response can have one meaning for staff and another, very different, meaning for the patient. Never use the words "perhaps" or "maybe" in answer to a patient's request, or you run the risk of raising false expectations that may lead to aggressive outbursts, which will ultimately have a divisive effect on the staff. Use the words "yes" or "no," or, when these are not sufficient, "I don't know." Also, always try to make a distinction between demands and needs. Demands that are satisfied are continuously followed by new and increased demands that must be met with a clear and distinct "no." Then there will be more room for meeting real needs, such as confidence and limits.

An article by Maier (1996), "The role of talk down and talk up," discusses the verbal management of threatening behaviour. The title refers to techniques used in Maier's two categories of threatening behaviour: "threats that are parts of an escalating process in which the patients reflect intense emotion, and threats that are part of a controlling process, which are often made in an unemotional way and are intended to capture the fantasy of the person threatened to gain some control over them for future gain." The first type is called "hot" because of the obvious emotion, the second "cold" because of the lack of emotion (Dubin, 1992, p. 20). Understanding the differences in motivation should make it easier to understand the different management techniques.

Concerning the "hot" threats, Maier (1996) breaks up the process of threatening behaviour, from feeling frustrated to becoming physically aggressive, into five stages, starting with changes in the minor motor muscles, proceeding to physical aggression, and ending in relaxation. The first goal of the clinician entering into this escalating process must be to buy sufficient time for the patient to lose adrenaline. In order to do this, the clinician must know how to talk down the patient, to help him or her regain self-control and thus make the situation safer for them both. To do so, the clinician must first make sure that the patient can hear and respond to his or her voice. Patients under the influence of drugs or alcohol are not good candidates for being talked down, since it is uncertain whether their attention can be held sufficiently.

The first step in the talking-down procedure is setting the stage. Use an assertive voice and accept body buffer zones to give the patient the space he or she needs while maintaining the necessary contact.

The second step is characterized by overdosing: For the time being, every effort is made to overdose the patient with agreement. This technique is open to discussion, since it may constitute something of a double-edged sword. While agreeing with the patient, we must remember not to accept threats or violence. We cannot agree to ideas that must be abandoned as soon as the patient has calmed down. This dilemma can be handled if we can always find acceptable alternatives to unacceptable ideas; otherwise we might give a false impression that will severely impair the relationship with the patient. There is another exception to the rule. When we have a good relationship with a patient and can see that his or her verbal aggression has elements of testing our ability to endure and confront, we can answer the aggression with even stronger means than his or her own.

A schizophrenic patient once told me very aggressively that I had given him too much medicine and had blocked every effort he had made to get discharged from the hospital as well as every project he sought to embark on. I replied, with all the strength in my voice that I could muster: "I have given you everything you have been able to accept. I have lowered your doses of medicine and as a result you became psychotic. I have sent you on leave several times and you have always paid me back by using narcotics. I have listened to your every suggestion about studies, work, and so on, and you have always failed me. So just shut up and blame yourself instead."

Usually the strength of the counterattack will take the edge off the patient's aggressiveness. The most common response is a burst of laughter. It must be stressed, though, that this kind of intervention must be made with the utmost confidence and must be based on a solid relationship with the patient. We must be very careful about becoming emotional with a patient, as we run the risk of losing self-control, but if we have genuine concern for the patient and are good actors we can successfully use emotional arguments.

Concerning the talking-down procedure, Maier (1996) warns us against the tendency to argue with patients, as this will give them reason to continue focusing their anger on the clinician. Instead, try to divide the patient's energy by offering choices about alternative methods of handling the situation. Each time the patient is given a choice, he or she is meant to pause and cognitively consider the options, and each pause decreases the amount of energy behind the anger and leads to self-control.

We can also use the lowest form of agreement, agreeing to disagree, which works more often than not, and then start setting constructive limits and return the ward to a normal state. The idea of taking patients down instead of talking them down may be a real option during the entire process, but should not be implemented until the process of talking down has failed.

Once the patient has regained self-control—either immediately or after a short time when they might have gained a more objective perspective on their behaviour —they must be calmly confronted about what has happened. Then they can identify the stressors that led to their aggression and learn other ways to cope with their anger.

Patients with personality disorders often use cold threats in order to manipulate or gain control of others. They might begin by making personal comments about the physician, then identify the physician's home address or the names of his or her children, and eventually make comments about the physician of such a personal nature that he or she might not be willing to share them with colleagues. If the physician fails to share such behaviour with somebody, the patient can establish a secret relationship with the doctor that can have a binding effect and serve to distort his or her judgement. Thus, sharing the secret is the first step in managing the process. If the threats escalate to insinuations about hurting the doctor's family, the feelings they arouse can act as a powerful impediment to effective management. Then the staff must confront the patient about how the threat was perceived, in order to clarify the mechanisms the patient has used to gain favour and manipulate the staff. Often the staff can teach the patient more effective ways of getting what he or she wants.

Seclusion

In a review, Soloff, Gutheil, and Wexler (1985) found that seclusion practices varied widely, depending on the population served and the philosophical approach of the hospital staff. It was more often used to contain behaviour that might lead to violence than to control violent behaviour itself. The authors conclude that there is overwhelming empirical support for using seclusion and restraint to keep disruptive behaviour from progressing to violence, but that the decision to do so should be based on sound clinical judgement.

In an earlier paper, Soloff (1987) discusses physical control in clinical practice. He states that "defense of the therapeutic milieu and preservation of order are important staff responsibilities. Clinically and legally, the treatment team has a duty to each patient to provide a treatment atmosphere that is both safe and conducive to recovery and rehabilitation." Seclusion is somewhat controversial and may even serve as a symbol of oppressive psychiatry. This is understandable considering the many different ways in which it is administered, but seclusion does not mean solitary confinement. It is a means of segregating a potentially dangerous individual for as long as he or she behaves aggressively. It also provides an option for meeting the patient alone in a situation brought about by his or her destructive behaviour and in which therapeutic confrontations may be very useful. Properly carried out, seclusion is a tool for long-term management of aggression and preservation of the ward structure.

Voluntary seclusion is preferable to compulsory seclusion, but, should it become necessary, seclusion must be forced upon the patient without hesitation. If seclusion is to be undertaken safely, without physical harm to the patient or staff and without psychological damage to the patient, the following procedures are crucial:

- Sufficient staff must be present to let patients know that if they do not walk without resistance they will be gently but easily overwhelmed.
- There must be no discussion about other options once the decision to seclude is made. These can be discussed once the patient is secluded.
- Seclusion must be as brief as possible. Patients usually calm down within hours. In extreme cases, seclusion must be carried out for longer periods. Open-area seclusion (Bjørkly, 1995) should be used wherever possible.
- Seclusion procedures must be reviewed regularly to ensure that they are not being used improperly—for example, as a means of punishment. Patients who have been secluded on multiple occasions, for some reason, must be identified so that patterns of self-destructive tendency can be sought. Poor staff-patient interaction may cause a patient to become violent as a means of gaining attention.

Seclusion procedures are necessary, and, if administered correctly, have a clear treatment value. On the other hand, they are time-consuming, sometimes risky, and sometimes harmful to the patient's confidence in the staff. Thus they should be kept to a minimum.

Restraint

Restraint is not really a treatment strategy but the final recourse when the usual vigilance or interventions have failed. It is the most severe physical intervention and should be used accordingly. It becomes necessary if a patient is so violent that there is an immediate threat of assault or self-mutilation. The administration of restraint entails a high risk of violence or, in an acute situation or when staff are not properly trained, combative wrestling. Like seclusion, restraint can trigger violent behaviour. Low levels of activity and social behaviour on the ward may result in a situation in which any form of physical contact constitutes a reward for the patient (Gudjonsson & Drinkwater, 1986). The frequency of physical restraint may be reduced through the use of contact skills for good staff-patient interaction.

Finally, in a good ward atmosphere and with the right patient, physical restraint may have a surprisingly positive effect on staff and patient alike. The following quotation is from medical records kept by the late Dr. Niko Nägele at the Sundsvall Forensic Psychiatric Hospital.

> On one single occasion the entire staff, both male and female, piled up on top of him in one big happy heap. After 10 minutes they all got up and went about their duties. Since then the patient has never been responsible for any destructive actions.

I guess they just had plain fun at the time, and having fun together must be one of the most effective treatments of violence there is.

Humour

It is extraordinary that the concept of humour is never discussed in the scientific literature on ward violence. Humour can be defined as a sense of proportion—not a very common characteristic among aggressive patients. A humorous approach on the ward can help patients to achieve a sense of proportion, aside from the very beneficial effect of allowing them to have fun. Patients who have lived in emotional isolation for a long time become more sociable when they interact with staff through the right kind of humour. To have fun and laugh also means to be able to lose control in a harmless way, which can be a very rewarding experience for many patients. Anything can be made into a joke. There are no forbidden subjects or situations as long as there is a relationship and as long as the patient feels liked by the staff and sees that the staff, like the patient, can be the subject of a joke. The only exception is the very paranoid patient, who can misinterpret a joke and act destructively. Like all powerful instruments, humour should be used cautiously. However, correctly applied, it is invaluable.

References

Adler, W.N., Kreeger, C., & Ziegler, P. (1983). Patient violence in a private psychiatric hospital. In J.R. Lion & W.H. Reid (Eds.), *Assaults within psychiatric facilities* (pp. 81–89). New York: Grune & Stratton.

Belfrage, H. (1998). Implementing the HCR-20 scheme for risk assessment in a forensic psychiatric hospital: Integrating research and clinical practice. *Journal of Forensic Psychiatry, 9,* 328–338.

Belfrage, H., Fransson, G., & Strand, S. (in press). Prediction of violence within the correctional system using the HCR-20 risk assessment scheme. *Journal of Forensic Psychiatry.*

Bjørkly, S. (1993). Scale for the prediction of aggression and dangerousness in psychotic patients: An introduction. *Psychological Reports, 73,* 1363–1377.

Bjørkly. S. (1995). Open-area seclusion in the long-term treatment of aggressive and disruptive patients: An introduction to a ward procedure. *Psychological Reports, 76*(1), 147–57.

Drinkwater, J., & Gudjonsson, G. (1989). The nature of violence in psychiatric hospitals. In C.R. Hollin & K. Howells (Eds.), *Clinical approaches to violence* (pp. 287–310). Chichester: Wiley.

Dubin, W. (Chair). (1992). *Clinician safety* (Task Force Report #33). Washington: American Psychiatric Press.

Gudjonsson, G.H., & Drinkwater, J. (1986). Intervention techniques for violent behavior. *Issues in Criminological and Legal Psychology, 9,* 38–48.

Heilbrun, K. (1997). Prediction versus management models relevant to risk assessment: The importance of legal decision-making context. *Law and Human Behavior, 21*(4), 347–359.

Maier, G.J. (1986). Relationship security: The dynamics of keeper and kept. *Journal of Forensic Sciences, 31,* 603–608.

Maier, G.J. (1996). Managing threatening behavior: The role of talk down and talk up. *Journal of Psychosocial Nursing, 34,* 25–30.

Ruben, I., Wolkon, G., & Yamamoto, J. (1980). Physical attacks on psychiatric residents by patients. *Journal of Nervous and Mental Diseases, 168,* 243–245.

Soloff, P.H. (1987). Physical controls: The use of seclusion and restraint in modern psychiatric practice. In L.H. Roth (Ed.), *Clinical treatment of the violent person* (pp. 119–137). New York: Guilford.

Soloff, P.H., Gutheil, T.G., & Wexler, D.B. (1985). Seclusion and restraint in 1985: A review and update. *Hospital and Community Psychiatry, 36,* 652–657.

Strand, S., Belfrage, H., Fransson, G., & Levander, S. (1999). Clinical and risk management factors in risk prediction of mentally ill offenders—more important than historical data? *Legal and Criminological Psychology, 4,* 67–76.

Warren, J., & Beadsmoore, A. (1997). Preventing violence on mental health wards. *Nursing Times, 93*(43), 47–48.

Webster, C., Douglas, K., Eaves, D., & Hart, S. (1997). *HCR-20: Assessing the risk of violence, Version 2.* Vancouver: Simon Fraser University and Forensic Psychiatric Services Commission of British Columbia.

Göran Fransson is Chief Psychiatrist, Sundsvall Forensic Psychiatric Hospital, Sundsvall, Sweden.

Author's Note

Comments or queries may be directed to Göran Fransson, Sundsvall Forensic Psychiatric Hospital, Box 880, S-851, 24 Sundsvall, Sweden. Telephone: 46 60 18 1406. Fax: 46 60 18 2240. E-mail: <fransson@sto.erudite.se>.

Section IV

PREVENTING VIOLENCE IN CORRECTIONAL FACILITIES

MAJOR MENTAL DISORDER AND VIOLENCE IN CORRECTIONAL SETTINGS

Size, Specificity, and Implications for Practice

DAVID J. COOKE

The impact of violence on a prison is not hard to discern: Staff and prisoners are physically injured and may become psychologically disturbed, property is destroyed, regimes and programmes are disrupted and thereby impoverished, violent prisoners are not only incarcerated for longer but held in more expensive conditions (Cooke, 1992a; Goetting & Howsen, 1986; Porporino, 1986). Institutional violence may be contagious, leading to epidemics of violence (Lion, Madden, & Christopher, 1976). The more public forms of violence—rooftop demonstrations, riots, and hostage takings—may undermine public confidence in the criminal justice system in general and the prison system in particular (Porporino). Prison violence is a significant problem.

In this chapter I will consider four issues pertaining to major mental disorder and violence in prisons. First, what is the evidence that major mental disorder plays a role in violence in prisons? Is there an effect, and how big is that effect? Second, is it possible to identify specific types, or elements, of major mental disorder that are particularly important for violence? Third, is it possible to move from general descriptions of violence towards an understanding of the forms of violence that are, in some sense, produced by major mental disorder? Fourth, while the preceding issues are relevant to our theoretical understanding of the illness-violence link, it is important to consider the practical implications of any findings. An overarching theme of the Advanced Study Institute (ASI) was the "effective prevention...of violence." In the final section I will consider what the research literature tells us about the management of mentally disordered prisoners who have the potential to be violent.

Does Major Mental Disorder Influence Violence?

The link between major mental disorder and violence is one of the more contentious issues in forensic mental health: While the general public does not doubt the existence of a link, the academic community is less certain. Historically, two positions could be discerned: the "absence of proof' position and the "proof of absence" position. In earlier days, Monahan argued that no firm conclusions could be drawn about

S. Hodgins (ed.), Violence among the Mentally Ill, 291–311.

the relationship because of the inadequacy of the evidence available (Monahan, 1981). By way of contrast, others have argued that the evidence available is sufficient to support the conclusion that there is no link between major mental illness and violence (Teplin, 1985).

Following an influential United Kingdom government inquiry into homicidal violence by the mentally disordered, the Chair, Dr. John Reed, stated, "The great majority of mentally ill people and those with learning disability present no increased danger to others," and argued further, "The best predictors of the future offending among mentally disordered people are the same as those for the rest of the population—previous offending, criminality in the family, poor parenting, etc." (Reed, 1997, p. 4). From this perspective, if there is an effect of mental illness on violence it appears to be a small effect, and factors other than major mental disorder may have greater saliency.

For the sake of simplicity I will review the literature using only one measure of association between major mental disorder and violence—that is, the odds ratio. The odds ratio estimates the odds of violence in the "at risk group" and divides it by the odds of violence in the "not at risk group." Odds ratios vary between 0 and ∞. An odds ratio of 1 indicates no association between a putative risk factor and outcome; epidemiologists consider that odds ratios of 2.5 or greater indicate that the association is of some practical importance (Fleiss, Williams, & Dubro, 1986). The advantages of the odds ratio as a measure of effect size are well summarized by Haddock, Rindskopf, and Shadish (1998):

> The key benefits of the odds ratio are its invariance across sampling methods, the fact that it is not affected by unequal sample sizes, its invariance when either rows or columns or the four-fold table are multiplied by a constant, and its compatibility with logistic regression or loglinear models that already use the odds ratio as the measure of association. Finally, the odds ratio is not affected by differences in the marginal distribution of the four-fold table. No other effect size measure (e.g., raw or standardized difference between proportions successful in each group) has all these benefits. (p. 343)

EVALUATING THE EVIDENCE

In a study of a male penitentiary population in Quebec, Côté and Hodgins (1992) interviewed 460 subjects using a French translation of the Diagnostic Interview Schedule (DIS). Eighty-seven people in their sample had committed one or more homicides; the odds ratio between schizophrenia and homicide was 2.55 ($\chi^2 = 4.85$, $p = 0.028$)—that is, in this study the odds ratio was modest but large enough to be regarded as having some practical and policy implications.

Unfortunately, as with many areas of research, the generalizability of findings is a problem in this field. This can be illustrated by considering a further study. Dell, Robertson, James, and Grounds (1993) carried out a study in England in which the participants were female remand prisoners. Of these, 196 were identified as having psychiatric difficulties on the basis that the prison psychiatrist considered them to have psychiatric difficulties, or because they were referred to an outside agency, or, finally, because they required a psychiatric court report. Psychotic illness was assessed using ICD-9 criteria. Estimation of the odds ratio indicated that the link between psychosis and homicide was small and non-significant—that is, 0.38 (χ^2 = 2.55, p = ns); further, the effect was in the opposite direction to that obtained by Côté and Hodgins (1992). The English female remand prisoners who were charged with homicide were less likely to be psychotic than those not charged with homicide.

These sets of results are not remarkable; however, they highlight the difficulties in this field: The effects appear to be small, and they vary with sample, definition of disorder, and definition of violence—thus, the generalizability of any effect is poor. It is in situations such as this that meta-analytic techniques can be of great benefit. Meta-analysis is a set of statistical methods for systematically reviewing a large number of research studies: The methods serve to control for the biases inherent in traditional qualitative reviews, and they allow quantification of effects (e.g., Cohen, 1988; Glass, McGraw, & Smith, 1981). The techniques simplify complexity—complexity abounds in the literature on mental disorder and violence. For example, studies differ on characteristics such as: the offender group targeted, sampling procedures, comparison groups, types of disorder considered, assessment procedures used, severity of violent behaviour targeted, institutional context, quality of design, and, finally, national and juridical background. Despite these difficulties, meta-analytic techniques make it possible to more precisely quantify the effect of major mental disorder and violence.

Douglas and Hart have produced a very important meta-analytic review on the link between major mental disorder and violence; in this review they estimate 269 effect sizes from 105 studies that they identified in the literature (Douglas & Hart, in press). Using the procedures of meta-analysis, they were able to evaluate the overall effect and examine the impact of diagnostic and methodological procedures on the estimates of effect size. The overall association between psychosis and violence that was estimated from the 269 effect sizes indicated that the median odds ratio was 2.73; thus the risk of violence was increased somewhere between two and a half and three times if psychosis was present. The setting in which the study took place was an important factor. Douglas and Hart distinguished amongst civil psychiatric, forensic psychiatric, community, and correctional settings. The largest number of studies were in civil psychiatric settings and the median odds ratio was 2.5; community settings were next highest with a median odds ratio of 2.94; forensic psychiatric settings were the next highest with a median odds ratio of 3.65; and finally the 15 studies with 23 effect sizes in correctional settings had a median effect size of 4.09. Correctional settings produced the largest of the median effect sizes observed; however, it should also be noted that the effect is highly variable, with the inter-quartile range for the odds ratios being between 2.55 and 16.10.

Thus, on the face of it, the association between psychosis and major mental illness is stronger in correctional settings. This stronger effect, however, may not be what it first appears. On the one hand there are methodological factors that make the correctional studies likely to provide a more accurate estimate of the association, whereas on the other hand there are effects of comorbidity with criminogenic factors that may serve to inflate the measured association. The institution-based studies tended to be methodologically more sound: They were more likely to have prospective designs than the community studies, they were more likely to be based on clinical interviews rather than merely on chart reviews, they were more likely to rely not merely on official records—for example, offences against prison discipline or criminal records—but to utilize self-report measures as well. As would be expected, the use of multiple sources for assessing violence increased the estimated effect size (Monahan & Steadman, 1994b). By way of contrast, there are factors that may have served to enhance the apparent association between psychosis and violence. Returning to Reed's comment quoted above, "The best predictors of the future offending among mentally disordered people are the same as those for the rest of the population—previous offending, criminality in the family, poor parenting, etc." (Reed, 1997, p. 4), a difficulty with the findings of an apparently stronger relationship in correctional settings is that it may not be major mental disorder that is influencing the relationship but rather criminogenic risk factors. Many of the higher odds ratios emerged when the prison groups were compared to data that were obtained in the Epidemiologic Catchment Area (ECA) survey (Swanson, 1994); this procedure was used when no non-psychotic or non-violent comparison group was available in the original study. Within a prison setting the level of criminogenic risk factors will be higher than in the general population. The association between psychosis and violence may appear stronger than it is because of the higher rates of comorbid disorders or conditions, including personality disorders—for example, psychopathy, antisocial personality disorder, and borderline personality disorder—substance abuse and dependence, poor anger control, and impulsivity.

It is noteworthy that all of the studies in the Douglas and Hart (in press) meta-analysis looked at the violence of prisoners—the violent history of those who are incarcerated—rather than the violence of individuals while they are in prison. This is not surprising. It is an accurate reflection of the literature: There are very few systematic studies in English of the relationship between major mental disorder and violence committed by prisoners while they are in prison. Again, the results of the available studies are equivocal.

Toch and Adams (1986) examined the violence perpetrated by prisoners while in prison: They considered all male inmates in New York State prisons who were released in the year between July 30, 1982, and September 1, 1983. In order to estimate rates of prison violence, they used reported violations of prison rules as a measure of disruptive behaviour and computed annual rates of disciplinary infractions. Toch and Adams were interested in the impact of mental health on prison violence. They used type of mental health care as their dependent measure; prisoners were categorized as receiving outpatient services, inpatient services, or no mental health services. The authors assumed that the more intensive the care received, the more severe the prisoner's mental health problem.

Unfortunately, the results provided by the authors do not allow the estimation of effect sizes. However, examination of the violent infraction rate demonstrates an association with type of mental health service received (Annual rate of violent infractions, Hospitalized = 0.8, Outpatient = 0.7, No Services = 0.5). Those who were hospitalized or who received outpatient services had a higher rate of violent infractions than those who received no mental health service. Toch and Adams (1986) obtained the most recent psychiatric diagnosis made prior to the prisoner's release;

this was used as an indicator of the type of mental health problem that the prisoner had suffered from. Those with Adjustment Disorder with associated Conduct Disturbance and those with Antisocial Personality Disorder had substantially higher mean infraction rates; those with Schizophrenia were slightly higher than others.

On the face of it, these results imply an association between mental disorder and violence in prisons. Unfortunately, the results of this study are open to other interpretations. The problem lies in the primary measure of psychiatric morbidity—namely, whether the prisoner received mental health services. It may be that the apparent association between mental disorder and violence is that a subgroup of mentally disordered are disruptive and thus regarded as being suitable cases for treatment. The prisoner who sits quietly hallucinating in his cell is less likely to be referred for treatment.

Porporino and Motiuk (1995) endeavoured to tackle this potential problem of selection bias by examining the prison infractions of prisoners derived from a large sample of male federal inmates in Canada. The psychiatric condition of the prisoners was assessed using the DIS. Thirty-six prisoners with major mental disorder—that is, meeting DIS lifetime criteria for a manic episode, schizophrenia, or schizophreniform disorder—were matched with 36 prisoners without such disorders, matching being carried out in terms of age, offence, and length of sentence. Porporino and Motiuk found no association between disorder and violent infractions while in prison, the odds ratio being 1.21 ($\chi^2 = 0.09$, p = ns). Thus, in this carefully controlled, albeit small, study the association between these forms of major disorder and violence was not apparent.

In a study of the rate of psychological disturbance in the Scottish prison system, I used the Schedule for Affective Disorders–Lifetime Version to collect information from a systematic representative sample of 307 prisoners—both male and female (Cooke, 1994, 1995, 1998). I examined the history of offending within prison during the prisoner's current sentence. In order to simplify the data, I subjected them to principal component analysis (Comrey & Lee, 1992). Two dimensions of prison infractions were evident: violent offending, which was specified by staff assaults, prisoner assaults, and hostage taking; and non-violent offending, which appeared to be an escape component, being specified by escape attempts, possession of drugs, and roof-climbing (Cooke, 1994).

Table 1. Odds ratio of psychiatric disorder and violent offending in Scottish prisons (Cooke, 1994)

RDC Criteria Life Prevalence	All males $n = 246$	Serving 2 years or more $n = 119$	Serving 5 years or more $n = 72$
Major disorders	1.9	2.2	2.9
Suicidal/parasuicidal	2.1	2.8	3.5
Psychopathy	2.6	5.4	14.2

For the purposes of illustration, I have calculated the odds ratios of the associations between some diagnostic groupings and the violent offending component. The lifetime prevalence of psychotic disorders was very low; therefore, the major disorders were mostly major depressive episodes. The odds ratios for all the males, males serving 2 years or more, and males serving 5 years or more are presented separately. It would appear from these data that violent infractions are weakly associated with major disorders, the effect being clearer in those serving longer sentences. This effect of sentence length may well be an effect of criminogenic factors being more prevalent in those serving longer sentences, reflecting Reed's (1997) contention that the best predictors of future offending are to be found not in the domain of the mental disorders but in other domains.

The prevalence of suicidal or parasuicidal behaviour was relatively high in this sample. Violence to self showed an association with violent infractions in prison. Psychopathy was assessed with the PCL-R (Hare, 1991); as might be expected, high scores on this instrument were more strongly associated with violence than were the other diagnoses; however, there may be a degree of circularity here, with the nature of violent behaviour affecting rating of certain of the PCL-R items.

In summary, the evidence on the violence of prisoners, particularly that from the meta-analysis of Douglas and Hart (in press), indicates that there is a weak but reliable association between major mental illness and lifetime history of violence. However, when it comes to violence committed by prisoners, while in prisons, I consider that the jury is still out. Perhaps the Scottish verdict of "not proven" is appropriate here. Uniquely in Scotland, in criminal court cases people may be found guilty, not guilty, or the case is not proven. The cynics say that the not proven verdict means that the jury thinks you are guilty but there is not quite enough evidence to prove it. Perhaps this is the case with mental disorder and violence within prison.

I would like to conclude this first section by considering the practical, as distinct from the theoretical, importance of the link between major mental disorder and violence in prisons. It is important to point out that many of the studies that show a link are North American. From a European perspective—or perhaps a British perspective—the link between major mental disorder and violence is of less practical concern in prison populations because the prevalence of these disorders is very low in prisons. Several studies attest to the validity of this position. Gunn, Maden, and Swinton (1991) assessed the prevalence of psychiatric disorder in a sample of 1,769 sentenced prisoners in England and Wales. The prisoners were interviewed by experienced forensic psychiatrists who used a standardized measure of mental state. They found that only 34, or 2%, of their sample were suffering from psychosis; this contrasts with 10% who were adjudged to be suffering from personality disorder and 23% suffering from substance misuse. Davidson and his colleagues carried out a study of disorder in the Scottish remand population (Davidson, Humphreys, Johnstone, & Owens, 1995). Their results echo those of Gunn et al. in that they found that only 2.3% of their sample were suffering from what they termed "major psychiatric disorder." In two studies in Scottish prisons, one published and one unpublished, I have found low prevalence rates for psychotic disorders (Cooke, 1994). In the first study, the prevalence of psychosis as defined using Research Diagnostic Criteria (Endicott & Spitzer, 1978) was 0.4%. In a recent study of violence in 250 adult male prisoners the prevalence rate of psychosis was 0.0%. These low rates, rates not dissimilar to general population prevalence rates, probably reflect the fact that the deinstitutionalization movement has been less aggressively pursued in the UK in general, and in Scotland in particular, when compared with North America. As a consequence of its low base rate, major mental disorder cannot be regarded as an important predictor of violence in British prisons.

Do Specific Aspects of Major Mental Disorder Influence Violence?

In the previous section I considered, by necessity, the global associations between major mental disorder and violence. In this section I will consider how our understanding of the apparently small, but statistically significant, link between major mental disorder and violence can be improved. In essence, I will examine the question of whether there are types or elements of major mental disorder that are important in relation to violence.

It is a well-established principle in epidemiology that the plausibility of a causal association between a putative cause and a putative effect is enhanced if the specificity of the relationships can be enhanced (e.g., Cooke, 1989b; Susser, 1973)—for example, by showing that specific features of major mental illness are linked to specific forms of violence. An example from the literature on smoking and illness may illustrate this point more clearly. In the early 1950s, Doll and Hill (1952) published their classic study of the effects of smoking on causes of death. Initially, they considered all types of smoking and all causes of death and found an odds ratio of 1.3; then they refined the putative-cause side of the equation and found that focusing on cigarette smoking alone raised the effect size to 1.7; finally, they examined the effect of cigarette smoking on one cause of death—lung cancer—rather than all causes, and obtained an effect size of 32. Thus, by removing forms of smoking with limited etiological significance for lung cancer, Doll and Hill increased the plausibility of a causal link between cigarette smoking and lung cancer.

Research concerned with major mental disorder should be more specific. Douglas and Hart (in press) make the point cogently: "We would also recommend that future research abandon the general question 'Is psychosis associated with future risk of violence?' in favor of a more complex and sophisticated question, such as 'What particular symptoms of psychosis, under which situational circumstance in combination with which personal factors, are associated with increased risk of various kinds of violence'." Their comment echoes McNeil (1994), who indicates that a broader approach is required to the number of levels of analyses that are adopted: "More generally, research needs to evaluate whether the most useful level of analysis is the symptom (e.g., hallucinations) or the diagnosis (e.g., schizophrenia)" (p. 197).

The Douglas and Hart (in press) meta-analytic study lends some support to this strategy, indicating that the specificity of the relationship between mental disorder and violence is improved when mental disorder is defined more narrowly. They found a gradation in effect sizes as they moved from the global towards the more specific (i.e., unspecified psychosis, odds ratio = 1.94; schizophrenia, odds ratio = 2.73; affective psychosis, odds ratio = 2.81; psychotic symptoms, odds ratio = 3.45). It would appear that increasing specificity increases the magnitude of the effect.

A dramatic illustration of this point comes from Link and Stueve's (1994) study in which they examined the relationship between violence and one type of symptom—namely, threat/control-override (TCO), symptoms to do with being dominated by forces beyond your control, thought insertion, and the belief that people are trying to do you harm. They also looked at the effects of other psychotic symptoms as a separate scale. Use of a weapon over the previous 5 years was differentially linked with type of symptom: Non-TCO symptoms had a marginal effect, with an odds ratio of 1.88, whereas the respective odds ratio for TCO symptoms was a substantial 19.22. This focus on specific types of symptoms appeared to be a very promising approach; however, attempts to replicate the results have perhaps tempered the enthusiasm with which they were initially received. Swanson, Borum, Swartz, and Monahan (1996) sought to extend the work of Link and Stueve. They examined the impact of TCO symptoms on risk for violence in a extremely large community sample. Violence since 18 years of age was the dependent variable. The association of TCO symptoms was far more modest here than in the previous study (odds ratio = 2.9): This effect was greater than for both Non-TCO symptoms (odds ratio = 1.8) and a diagnosis of major mental disorder (odds ratio = 1.7). By way of comparison, a diagnosis of Alcohol or Drug abuse disorder had a substantially stronger effect (odds ratio = 5.1). Finally, the effect of TCO symptoms did not replicate in the MacArthur field trial study (Steadman et al., in press) nor in a Scottish prison study alluded to below.

Thus, within the violence literature there is evidence based on diagnostic classes and some evidence based on symptoms, but I wish to argue that there is another way—a third way—based on the recent research into the symptom dimensions or syndromes that appear to underpin psychotic disorders. The term *syndrome* can be used in several senses. In this context I am using it to denote a set of symptoms that occur together and that can be distinguished from other sets of co-occurring symptoms: I am not using the term to denote a diagnostic group. Unlike McNiel (1994), I would argue that focusing on an intermediate level somewhere between the symptom level and the diagnostic-group level might be most productive in increasing our understanding of violence.

In his classic paper on the classification of depression, Eysenck (1970) indicates that it is possible to define syndromes in this sense using factor analytic studies of symptoms. Factor analytic techniques refine the constructs in an empirical rather than an ad hoc manner. The extremely heterogeneous set of symptoms that come together to define psychotic illnesses can be refined into syndromes; aspects of the disorder that are not important to the putative link between the disorder and violence can be excluded. The inclusion of irrelevancies in any measure of disorder merely serves to degrade or attenuate any measured relationship (Cook & Campbell, 1979).

There is support for this approach in other research into major mental disorders; unfortunately, it does not appear to have been exploited in violence research. For example, Ratakonda, Gorman, Yale, and Amador (1998) argue: "Despite multiple major and minor modifications to their symptom compositions, diagnostic groupings based on the categorical model remain etiologically uninformative. There is no clear demarcation between different diagnoses...psychopharmacological agents treat specific symptoms or symptom groups rather than specific diagnostic categories"

(p. 79). I would argue that the links between the categorical model and violence are also uninformative.

Other models are available. Over the last few years there has been growing evidence that schizophrenic symptoms, and psychotic symptoms more broadly, can be conceptualized as occurring in three syndromes. Grube, Bilder, and Goldman (1998) carried out a meta-analysis of 10 published factor analytic studies that had examined the dimensional structure—or syndromes—of schizophrenic symptoms. Using an exploratory method—principal component analysis—they extracted three components that confirmed and extended the clinical descriptions of schizophrenia that emerged in the 1980s. They described these components as Positive Symptoms, Negative Symptoms, and Conceptual Disorganization. Positive Symptoms were defined by hallucinations and delusions, Negative Symptoms were defined by affective flattening, alogia, avolition, anhedonia, and attentional impairment, and, finally, Conceptual Disorganization was defined by positive formal thought disorder and bizarre behaviour. Examination of Grube et al.'s final factor solution indicates that there were cross-loadings—that is, some symptoms had small but significant secondary loadings on other factors. This suggests that the simple three-factor orthogonal solution may not be the best possible solution.

In a methodologically more sophisticated paper, Dollfus and Everitt (1998) applied confirmatory factor analytic methods to evaluate the goodness of fit of the three-factor model, but in addition they considered a four-factor model that included "relationship difficulties." Confirmatory factor analysis allows comparison of the goodness of fit of different models. Dollfus and Everitt determined that a four-factor hierarchical model fitted their data significantly better than the three-factor model proposed by Grube et al. (1998). The additional "Relational factor" was specified by inability to feel intimacy and having relationships with friends and peers.

There are two further notable aspects to this model. First, Dollfus and Everitt (1998) found that positive and negative symptoms were not correlated; this means, as Crow (1985) argues, that the negative and positive dimensions vary independently even when they co-occur in the same patient. Second, positive formal thought disorder was linked to the Positive Symptom syndrome as well as the Conceptual Disorganization syndrome.

It is important to note that the recent research indicates that these dimensional structural models of symptoms are not peculiar to schizophrenia; there is evidence that the same models can generalize to psychotic disorders other than schizophrenia. Ratakonda et al. (1998) used data from the DSM-IV field trial samples that contained 221 patients with schizophrenia and 189 patients with related psychotic disorders. They carried out principal component analysis with orthogonal rotation on the data from the two groups separately and concluded, by an "eyeball" test, that the same structures could be observed in the two groups. While a more robust test of factor similarity would be appropriate, there does appear to be evidence that the syndromes generalize across the psychotic disorders.

These factors or syndromes do not appear to be mere statistical fictions. Ratakonda et al. (1998) indicate that the three distinct syndromes have differential associations with specific biological, neuropsychological, course, and treatment response variables. For example, in a longitudinal study Arndt, Andreasen, Flaum,

Miller, and Nopoulos (1995) found that symptoms within each of the three syndromes varied together—exacerbating or remitting together—but overall the three syndromes changed independently of one another.

Basso, Nasrallah, Olson, and Bornstein (1998) demonstrated that the three-dimensional model of psychosis has different neuropsychological correlates. For example, the negative symptoms were associated with a wide range of deficits in intelligence, executive function, memory, and sustained attention. The deficits associated with the disorganization symptoms were more focused on attention span and sensory motor function: They found no associations between neuropsychological functioning and positive symptoms of schizophrenia. In a study of the association of the three dimensions to aspects of rehabilitation, Smith et al. (1997) found that the dimensions were differentially related to the impact of rehabilitative efforts; for example, negative symptoms were associated with ratings of readiness for rehabilitation, whereas disorganization symptoms influenced participation in rehabilitation efforts and positive symptoms had the strongest influence on global functioning.

Consideration of these distinct dimensions, and their interactions, may improve our understanding of the manner in which major mental disorder can produce violence. While many people have argued that the positive symptoms drive the patient towards violence, there are clearly other dimensions that are important. Junginger (1996), for example, argues: "The content and themes of a patient's psychotic symptoms can be thought of as a blueprint for action. Whether a patient acts on this blueprint, however, apparently is determined by a number of other factors" (p. 97).

For example, both the relationship items/symptoms that specify the dimension in the Dollfus and Everitt (1998) analysis may well have relevance for violence; if an individual is unable to feel intimacy, then one of the impediments to being violent is absent.

There is a significant literature on the advantages and disadvantages of a syndromal approach to research as against a symptom approach. I will not review that literature here; however, I believe, for the purposes of explicating the link between major mental disorder and violence, there are several advantages that accrue from taking this syndromal approach (Mojtabai & Reider, 1998; Van Os et al., 1999). These advantages are as follows: the clustering of symptoms has an empirical basis rather than being ad hoc; higher reliability of measurement is likely, because measurement is based on aggregates of related symptoms rather than individual symptoms; and more stable measurement of underlying traits will result, and this will lead to greater generalization across studies. All these advantages should clarify the associations between syndromes and outcome—in this case, violence.

Disaggregating the Forms of Violence

Violence is a complex phenomenon; it can be described and measured along many dimensions (e.g., Monahan & Steadman, 1994a). The violent act may be described merely at the behavioural level: what was involved—kicking, punching, stabbing, shooting. The range of acts carried out and the frequency, or density, of the violent behaviour might be considered. The apparent motivation for the act might be assessed: Was it an instrumental act designed to obtain a specific end, or was it a reactive act, a consequence of a discharge of emotion? The description of violence will vary with the sources of information—official records, self-report, collateral report, or observation. The location of the violent behaviour may be considered—institutional or community. The target may be described—family, strangers, or professionals. These are just some of the dimensions considered, but it should be clear that there can be multidimensional accounts of violent behaviour. It is important, therefore, to describe violence systematically. This is a significant problem in violence research: "Another recurring problem in risk assessment research is the lack of precision produced by not disaggregating criterion violence into meaningful subtypes. The predictors of one form of violence may be quite different from the predictors of another" (Monahan & Steadman, 1994a, p. 10). This quotation highlights the problem of specificity: Elements or syndromes of major mental illness may be important for different types of violence. I would like to illustrate this point with an analysis of data from a Scottish study of 250 male prisoners that a colleague, Christine Michie, and I have been carrying out (Michie & Cooke, 1999). In this violence prediction study we used many of the MacArthur instruments as well as the SCID-I, SCID-II, and PCL-R.

Early in the analysis, it became apparent that even when only the nature and frequency of violent behaviour was considered violence was not a simple, unidimensional, or coherent construct. In order to assess the severity and extent of an individual's history of violent behaviour we used the MacArthur Community Violence Instrument. This is quite a simple procedure used by the interviewer to discover the extent to which an individual has engaged in violence. The participant is asked if someone has been violent to them in a particular manner, then if they have done the same thing to someone else. For example, the first question is, "Has anyone thrown something at you?" Then they are asked, "Have you thrown something at anyone?" The process continues in this manner for nine questions, the last of which is, "Have you done anything else that might be considered violent?" The research interviewers prompt by giving examples: "Have you ever driven at anyone, tortured anyone or pushed someone through a window?"

Initially we treated the scale as unidimensional—going from the apparently least severe to most severe violent behaviours. We became concerned, however, that the scale might be measuring more than one construct or trait, so we decided to test this hypothesis using confirmatory factor analysis (CFA). We conducted the analysis using EQS (Bentler & Wu, 1995) to determine whether a one-factor model fitted the data—that is, whether the scale could be considered unidimensional. The quality of fit was estimated using multiple measures of fit, because each measure has limitations and there are no agreed methods for absolutely determining goodness of fit (Kline, 1998). The one-factor model did not provide an acceptable fit to the data (Michie & Cooke, 1999).

Exploratory factor analysis suggested that there were two types of violent behaviour being measured by this scale. Using a variety of techniques, including Item Response Theory methods, we tested a two-factor hierarchical model of violent behaviour (Michie & Cooke, 1999; Steinberg & Thissen, 1996; Van der Linden & Hambleton, 1996). The first factor is made up of two items and one testlet (see Figure 1). Testlets occur when pairs or clusters of items are much more closely associated than would be expected by their relationships with the underlying latent trait. The testlet in this case contained items concerning threatening with a knife or gun and using a knife or gun. The other two items that defined this factor were having thrown an object and an item pertaining to other serious violence: Examples provided by the participants included hanging people off bridges, strangling victims with a telephone cable, and pouring petrol over someone and then setting them alight. This factor appears to have to do with serious forms of violence and, in particular, the use of weapons; we defined it as Weapon Aggression.

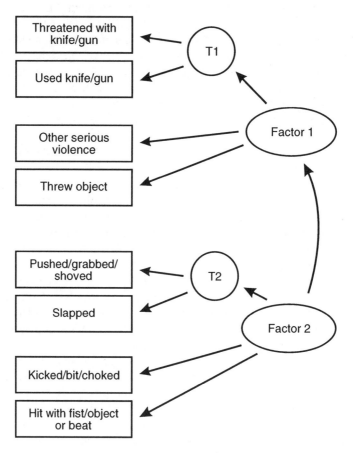

Figure 1. Correlated factor of violence derived from the MacArthur Community Violence Instrument

The second factor entailed the testlet of having pushed, grabbed, or shoved and having slapped—these violent behaviours appear to make up something between one and two items; and the individual items of kicked, bit, and choked, together with the item hit with a fist or object or beat; this appears to be a non-weapon factor, with the violence entailed being less serious. This model provided an excellent fit to the data (Michie & Cooke, 1999). These analyses suggest that even when violence is considered in terms of simple behavioural acts there is complexity; we appeared to be dealing with not one but two types of violence.

I would like to proceed to illustrate the value of disaggregating violence in this way in relation to the dimensions of psychosis I described above. Unfortunately, although our study focused on major mental disorder the prevalence of symptoms in this Scottish prison sample was too low to assist in this issue. I can, however, illustrate the same methodological point using some new results from PCL-R data in this sample.

The PCL-R is the instrument of choice for measuring psychopathic traits (Hare, 1991; Stone, 1995). Using confirmatory analysis of over 3,000 cases and three measures of psychopathy, we have developed a three-factor model of psychopathy (Cooke & Michie, 1999b). Using both statistical criteria derived from item response analyses (Cooke & Michie, 1997, 1999a; Cooke, Michie, Hart, & Hare, 1999) and theoretical consideration, we developed a hierarchical structural model using 13 of the PCL-R items. Examination of factor 1 indicated that it measures interpersonal style being specified by two testlets, the first testlet being defined by the items "glibness and superficial charm" and "grandiose sense of self-worth" and the second testlet being defined by the items "pathological lying" and "conning/manipulative." We have called this Arrogant and Deceitful Interpersonal Style. Factor 2 represents an affective factor being specified by two testlets, the first testlet defined by the items "shallow affect" and "callous/lack of empathy" and the second testlet defined by "lack of remorse of guilt" and "failure to accept responsibility." We have called this Deficient Affective Experience. Factor 3 represents a behavioural factor specified by two testlets, the first defined by three items, "need for stimulation/proneness to boredom," "impulsivity," and "irresponsibility," and the second testlet defined by "parasitic lifestyle" and "lack of realistic, long-term goals." We have called this Impulsive and Irresponsible Behavioural Style. Given that all these first-order factors contribute to a higher order factor, and this factor showed high factor saturation, we consider that this higher order factor can be defined as Psychopathy. This model not only fitted the data well but also was cross-validated across culture, and across methods for measuring psychopathy.

Removing seven of the 20 items has the advantage of removing items that could add circularity to the argument that psychopathy influences violence; the items to do with offending—for example, early behavioural problems, juvenile delinquency, or criminal versatility—were removed from the model.

Examination of Figure 2 indicates that the 13-item PCL-R score had an odds ratio of 7.31 with total aggression—that is, the total score derived from the MacArthur Screening Instrument. When violent behaviour is disaggregated into two facets—Weapon Aggression and Non-Weapon Aggression—the specificity of effect is clear: the odds ratio for Weapon Aggression was 9.7, compared with 3.2 for Non-Weapon Aggression.

When psychopathy is disaggregated into different facets, differences in the strength of relationships emerge. The Deficient Affective Experience facet has the strongest link, whereas the Arrogant and Deceitful Interpersonal Style has the weakest association. The maximum odds ratio is smaller than that for the simple association between the 13-item PCL-R and Weapon Aggression. This can probably be

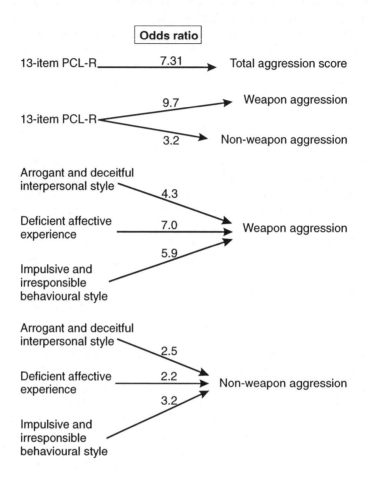

Figure 2. Specificity of effect for three-factor hierarchical model of psychopathy and dimensions of violence derived from the MacArthur Community Violence Instrument

accounted for by two things: First, the whole is probably greater than the sum of the parts; the hierarchical psychopathy factor probably contributes to the relations. Second, the factors are only measured using a few items, so unreliability may be attenuating the relationships. For completeness, if Non-Weapon Aggression is considered, it appears that the only odds ratio above 2.50 is that relating to the Impulsive and Irresponsible Behavioural Style facet.

To conclude this penultimate section, there are potential benefits to be gained by disaggregating both the syndromes of major mental disorder and the syndromes of violence.

What Steps Can We Take to Reduce Violence in Prisons?

An overarching theme of the ASI was the "Effective prevention...of violence." In an ideal world those with major mental illness would be in hospital and not in prison; in the real world this is not always possible. One line of attack is to treat the symptoms, or clusters of symptoms, that drive the offending through the use of medication or through the use of cognitive-behavioural techniques. Unfortunately, in a prison environment symptoms may go undetected; indeed, those suffering from certain symptoms may endeavour to hide the symptoms in what is a hostile environment.

It is important to remind ourselves that violence comes about not merely as a consequence of individual characteristics—symptoms, personality traits, and so forth —but also as a consequence of situational or institutional variables. I was privileged to work in a unit for some of the most violent men in Scottish prisons, the Barlinnie Special Unit. One of the many things that I learned there was the importance of situational determinants of violence (Cooke, 1989a, 1992b, 1997). Men were taken from locked-down conditions and moved to a more liberal regime where they had some say in the running of the regime, where the traditional guard-prisoner relationships were broken down, and where they had greater access to visitors. Their level of violence dropped dramatically. Situational factors were probably responsible—often this is not recognized: "With all our attention to the individual, we tend to underestimate the prison setting as a powerful influence on day-to-day inmate behavior" (Clements, 1982, p. 79).

Unfortunately, compared with the research on individual characteristics, there has been little systematic research carried out on institutional factors; the evidence must, therefore, be derived from practice, experience, and quasi-experimental work (Cooke, 1991, 1992b; Ditchfield, 1991; Porporino, 1986; Rice, Harris, Varney, & Quinsey, 1989).

What are the critical variables? It is a platitude, but platitudes sometimes contain truth, that the quality of staff—their approach, experience, training, and morale—is crucial. This is not a new idea. In 1847 a Scottish prison inspector emphasized the importance of the approach adopted by staff: "In some prisons an unusual degree of good conduct is induced, and the number of punishments kept low, by the personal influence of the officers, and their care in reasoning with prisoners before resorting to punishment" (Inspector of Prisons for Scotland, 1847, p. 5).

Regimes that encourage communication between staff and inmates, that break down the coercive mechanisms of control and replace these with more objective and professional approaches to prisoners' grievances, reduce violence (Cooke, 1989a, 1991). One concrete approach is to implement staff-inmate committees that not only provide both groups—at times—with mutual goals, but also reduce tension by providing the opportunity to ventilate grievances and come to mutual solutions.

Staff require the skills to approach prisoners in a positive way; these skills can be acquired through both experience and training. Evidence from both secure hospitals and prisons indicates that less experienced staff are more likely to be assaulted than experienced staff. For example, Davies and Burgess (1988), in a study in a Birmingham prison, found that staff who were assaulted had, on average, significantly less experience than those who were not assaulted. It appears that the experienced staff were less concerned with losing face and were more subtle and flexible in their approach; they were less likely to promote violence through rigidity; they knew when to support rather than confront; they knew when to stick to the rules and when to waive the rules. Clearly, the role of prison officer/guard should be more than that of a turnkey; they should provide support and supervision. This can best be achieved by giving staff responsibility for ensuring that services for a prisoner's specific needs are accessed through a case-management or a personal-officer scheme. Such schemes provide the prisoner with a social support system and improve staff-inmate communication. Fortunately, it is not necessary to wait until these skills are absorbed through experience. Effective prisoner-management skills can be taught, with subsequent reductions in the rate of assaults. Rice et al. (1989) have provided an excellent handbook for staff trainers.

Staff morale is another critical variable; it is hard to measure yet both the clinical and penal literatures highlight its importance. If staff are demoralized they do not give their full attention to those in their care, and their tensions are transmitted to the inmates. Lion et al. (1976) indicate that poor staff morale and heightened inter-staff conflict are conspicuous precursors of epidemics of violence. Good management is the key to maintaining morale; junior staff should be properly supported by senior staff, and all staff should have the opportunity to discuss their feelings of fear and anger towards those in their charge; teamwork should be emphasized.

While the qualities of the staff are of pre-eminent importance, other institutional characteristics also play a role. The institutional environment can promote or moderate violence. Overcrowding is one of the most studied variables, perhaps merely because it is relatively easy to measure. The research literature is unclear; yet with individuals prone to violence overcrowding should be avoided. In overcrowded conditions the prisoner is unable to control or avoid unwanted interaction and stimulation; staff are unable to monitor interactions; prisoners cannot be protected from a primary pain of confinement—being with other prisoners. The mix of prisoners is also important. Quay (1983) distinguishes between "heavy" and "light" prisoners—between predators and prey—and demonstrates that avoiding "toxic mixes" of these types reduces the rates of inmate-staff and inmate-inmate assaults.

Others have argued that in creating suitable "mixes" it is important to attempt to accommodate the personal preferences of inmates (Rice et al., 1989). Younger inmates generally prefer the opportunity for more social interaction, whereas older inmates prefer greater privacy. Prisoners prone to major mental illness may prefer quieter regimes. As Toch and Adams (1986) note: "Explosivity, rebelliousness, and other disruptiveness may be situationally responsive. In a predatory environment a victim-prone person can be hounded into preemptive aggression or into explosive panic... Safety—both actual and subjective—may be impossible to come by" (p. 16).

The empirical evidence suggests that size does not matter: The rates of violence are similar in large and small prisons (Porporino, 1986). This may be true for the generality of prisoners; however, clinical evidence suggests that so-called difficult prisoners are less likely to be violent if they are living in small groups (Cooke, 1991).

Change is threatening. Porporino (1986) elegantly demonstrates that turnover, or transiency, in prison populations appears to be a critical variable. Attempts should be made to limit transiency. In a rapidly changing population, normal social structures are not maintained; challenges to prisoner hierarchy are more frequent; natural wariness of new and potentially dangerous prisoners is heightened; normal prison trading relationships in drugs, money, tobacco, and gambling are more risky; prison staff behave in a more disciplinary manner. But it should be emphasized that just as prisoner transiency can affect the operation of the regime, so can staff transiency; the use of temporary staff should be eschewed, as it can promote violence.

Meaningful regime activity reduces frustration and provides stimulation. The general frustrations of life in many institutions—limited visiting opportunities, lack of meaningful work, limited access to education, poor food—act as significant situational stimuli to violence. King (1991) examined the rates of assault in an English and in an American maximum security prison. He argued the lower rates of assault in the American prison could be attributed to the quality of the regime: more out-of-cell activities, greater disposable income, more frequent and better-quality visits, and in-cell television. Behaviour may have been improved not merely because the quality of life was improved, but also because inmates had more to lose.

To limit this exposure, management structures must ensure that administrative uncertainty is minimized. There is empirical evidence that low rates of institutional disturbance flow from effective institutional management. Effective management should reduce the uncertainties that pervade the institutional lives of inmates—uncertainty produced by inconsistent application of rules, uncertainty about how to achieve parole, uncertainty about how to obtain access to treatment, education, or training (Gentry & Ostapiuk, 1988; Pelissier, 1991; Schnell & Lee, 1974; Ward, 1987). Rules need to be in place, and it is important that these rules are clear and unambiguous, and are applied fairly.

In conclusion:

1. Major mental disorder appears to have limited impact on the violence of prisoners; we still do not have enough convincing evidence that major mental disorder significantly affects violence while prisoners are in prison.
2. We could improve our understanding of the apparent association between major mental disorder and violence by paying attention to the recent research concerning syndromes of psychotic disorders.
3. Equally, we need to pay more attention to analyzing the forms that violence can take.
4. Finally, as clinicians we need to realize that often we can be as effective—or perhaps even more effective—in reducing violence by influencing the situational determinants of violence as by merely treating individual prisoners.

References

Arndt, S., Andreasen, N.C., Flaum, M., Miller, D., & Nopoulos, P. (1995). A longitudinal study of symptom dimensions in schizophrenia: Predictions and patterns of change. *Archives of General Psychiatry, 52*(May), 352–359.

Basso, M.R., Nasrallah, H.A., Olson, S.C., & Bornstein, R.A. (1998). Neuropsychological correlates of negative, disorganized and psychotic symptoms in schizophrenia. *Schizophrenia Research, 31,* 99–111.

Bentler, P.M., & Wu, E.J.C. (1995). *EQS for Windows.* Encino, CA: Multivarate Software Inc.

Clements, C.B. (1982). The relationship of offender classification to the problems of prison overcrowding. *Crime and Deliquency, 28,* 72–81.

Cohen, J. (1988). *Statistical power analysis for the behavioural sciences (2nd ed.).* New York: Academic Press.

Comrey, A.L., & Lee, H.B. (1992). *A first course in factor analysis (2nd ed.).* Hillsdale, NJ: Erlbaum.

Cook, T.D., & Campbell, D.T. (1979*). Quasi-experimentation, design and analysis issues for field settings.* Chicago: Rand McNally College Publishing.

Cooke, D.J. (1989a). Containing violent prisoners: An analysis of the Barlinnie Special Unit. *British Journal of Criminology, 29*(2), 129–143.

Cooke, D.J. (1989b). Epidemiological and survey methods. In G. Parry & F. Watts (Eds.), *A handbook of skills and methods in mental health research* (pp. 287–315). London: Erlbaum.

Cooke, D.J. (1991). Violence in prisons: The influence of regime factors. *Howard Journal of Criminal Justice, 30,* 95–109.

Cooke, D.J. (1992a). The psychological impact of prison riots on prison staff in Scotland. In S. Boddis (Ed.), *Prison service psychology conference: Conference proceedings* (pp. 133–143). London: HMSO.

Cooke, D.J. (1992b). Violence in prisons: A Scottish perspective. *Forum on Corrections Research, 4,* 23–30.

Cooke, D.J. (1994). Psychological disturbance in the Scottish prison system: Prevalence, precipitants and policy. Edinburgh: SHHD.

Cooke, D.J. (1995). Psychological disturbance in the Scottish prison system: A preliminary account. In G. Davie, S. Lloyd-Bostock, M. McMurran, & C. Wilson (Eds.), *Psychology, law and criminal justice: International developments in research and practice.* Berlin: De Gruyter.

Cooke, D.J. (1997). The Barlinnie Special Unit: The rise and fall of a therapeutic experiment. In E. Cullen, L. Jones, & R. Woodward (Eds.), *Therapeutic communities for offenders* (pp. 101–120). London: Wiley.

Cooke, D.J. (1998). The development of the Prison Behavior Rating Scale. *Criminal Justice and Behavior, 25*(4), 482–506.

Cooke, D.J., & Michie, C. (1997). An item response theory analysis of the Hare Psychopathy Checklist–Revised. *Psychological Assessment, 9*(1), 3–14.

Cooke, D.J., & Michie, C. (1999a). Psychopathy across cultures: North America and Scotland compared. *Journal of Abnormal Psychology, 108*(1), 55–68.

Cooke, D.J., & Michie, C. (1999b). Refining the construct of psychopathy: Towards a hierarchical model. Unpublished manuscript.

Cooke, D.J., Michie, C., Hart, S.D., & Hare, R.D. (1999). The functioning of the Screening Version of the Psychopathy Checklist–Revised: An item response theory analysis. *Psychological Assessment, 11*(1), 3–13.

Côté, G., & Hodgins, S. (1992). The prevalence of major mental disorders among homicide offenders. *International Journal of Law and Psychiatry, 15,* 89–92.

Crow, T.J. (1985). The two-syndrome concept: Origins and current status. *Schizophrenia Bulletin, 11,* 471–485.

Davidson, M., Humphreys, M., Johnstone, E., & Owens, D.G.C. (1995). Prevalence of psychiatric morbidity among remand prisoners in Scotland. *British Journal of Psychiatry, 167*(4), 545–548.

Davies, W., & Burgess, P.W. (1988). Prison officers' experience as a predictor of risk of attack: An analysis within the British prison system. *Medicine, Science and the Law, 28,* 135–138.

Dell, S., Robertson, G., James, K., & Grounds, A. (1993). Remands and psychiatric assessments in Holloway prison. 1: The psychotic population. *British Journal of Psychiatry, 163*(634), 640–646.

Ditchfield, J. (1991). *Control in prison: A review of the literature.* London: HMSO.

Doll, R., & Hill, A.B. (1952). A study of the aetiology of carcinoma of the lung. *British Medical Journal, 2,* 1271–1286.

Dollfus, S., & Everitt, B.S. (1998). Symptom structure in schizophrenia: Two, three or four-factor model. *Psychopathology, 31,* 120–130.

Douglas, K.S., & Hart, S.D. (in press). Psychosis as a risk factor for violence: A quantitative review of the research. *Psychological Bulletin.*

Endicott, J., & Spitzer, R.L. (1978). A diagnostic interview: The schedule for affective disorders and schizophrenia. *Archives of General Psychiatry, 35,* 837–844.

Eysenck, H.J. (1970). The classification of depressive illness. *British Journal of Psychiatry, 117,* 241–250.

Fleiss, J., Williams, J.B.W., & Dubro, A.F. (1986). The logistic regression analysis of psychiatric data. *Journal of Psychiatric Research, 20,* 145–209.

Gentry, M., & Ostapiuk, E.G. (1988). The management of violence in a youth treatment centre. In Anonymous, *Clinical approaches to aggression and violence: Issues in criminological and legal psychology No. 12.* Leicester: British Psychological Society.

Glass, G.V., McGraw, B., & Smith, M.L. (1981). *Meta-analysis in social research.* Beverly Hills, CA: Sage.

Goetting, A., & Howsen, R.M. (1986). Correlates of prisoner misconduct. *Journal of Quantative Criminology, 2,* 49–67.

Grube, B.S., Bilder, R.M., & Goldman, R.S. (1998). Meta-analysis of symptom factors in schizophrenia. *Schizophrenia Research, 31,* 113–120.

Gunn, J., Maden, A., & Swinton, M. (1991). Treatment needs of prisoners with psychiatric disorders. *British Medical Journal, 303,* 338–341.

Haddock, C.K., Rindskopf, D., & Shadish, W.R. (1998). Using odds ratios as effect sizes for meta-analysis of dichotomous data: A primer on methods and issues. *Psychological Methods, 3*(3), 339–353.

Hare, R.D. (1991). *Manual for the Revised Psychopathy Checklist.* Toronto: Multi-Health Systems.

Inspector of Prisons for Scotland. (1847). *1844 annual report.* Edinburgh: HMSO.

Junginger, J. (1996). Psychosis and violence: The case for content analysis of psychotic experiences. *Schizophrenia Bulletin, 22*(1), 91–103.

King, R.D. (1991). Maximum-security custody in Britain and the USA: A study of Gartree and Oak Park Heights. *British Journal of Criminology, 31,* 126–152.

Kline, R.B. (1998). Principles and practice of structural equation modeling. New York: Guilford.

Link, B.G., & Stueve, A. (1994). Psychotic symptoms and the violent/illegal behavior of mental patients compared to community controls. In J. Monahan & H.J. Steadman (Eds.), *Violence and mental disorder: Developments in risk assessment* (pp. 137–159). Chicago: University of Chicago Press.

Lion, J.R., Madden, D., & Christopher, R.L. (1976). A violence clinic: Three years' experience. *American Journal of Psychiatry, 133,* 432–435.

McNiel, D.E. (1994). Hallucinations and violence. In J. Monahan & H.J. Steadman (Eds.), *Violence and mental disorder: Developments in risk assessment* (pp. 183–202). Chicago: University of Chicago Press.

Michie, C., & Cooke, D.J. (1999). *The structure of violent behavior: A hierarchical model of the MacArthur Community Violence Screening Instrument.* Unpublished manuscript.

Mojtabai, R., & Reider, R.O. (1998). Limitations of the symptom-orientated approach to psychiatric research. *British Journal of Psychiatry, 173*(9), 198–202.

Monahan, J. (1981). *Predicting violent behavior: An assessment of clinical techniques.* Beverly Hills, CA: Sage.

Monahan, J., & Steadman, H. (1994a). Towards a rejuvenation of risk assessment research. In J. Monahan & H.J. Steadman (Eds.), *Violence and mental disorder: Developments in risk assessment* (pp. 1–17). Chicago: University of Chicago Press.

Monahan, J., & Steadman, H.J. (1994b). *Violence and mental disorder: Developments in risk assessment (1st ed.).* Chicago: University of Chicago Press.

Pelissier, B. (1991). The effects of a rapid increase in a prison population: A pre- and post-test study. *Criminal Justice and Behaviour, 18,* 427–447.

Porporino, F.J. (1986). Managing violent individuals in correctional settings. *Journal of Interpersonal Violence, 1,* 213–237.

Porporino, F.J., & Motiuk, L.L. (1995). The prison careers of mentally disordered offenders. *International Journal of Law and Psychiatry, 18*(1), 29–44.

Quay, H.O. (1983). *Standards for adult correctional institutions.* Washington: Federal Bureau of Prisons.

Ratakonda, S., Gorman, J.M., Yale, S.A., & Amador, X.F. (1998). Characterization of psychotic conditions: Use of the domains of psychopathology model. *Archives of General Psychiatry, 55*(Jan), 75–81.

Reed, J. (1997). Risk assessment and clinical risk management: The lessons from recent inquiries. *British Journal of Psychiatry, 170*(32), 4–7.

Rice, M.E., Harris, G.T., Varney, G.W., & Quinsey, V.L. (1989). *Violence in institutions: Understanding, prevention and control.* Toronto: Hans Huber.

Schnell, J.F., & Lee, J.F. (1974). A quasi-experimental restrospective evaluation of a prison policy change. *Journal of Applied Behavioural Analysis, 7,* 483–496.

Smith, T.E., Rio, J., Hull, J.W., Hedayat-Harris, A., Goodman, M., & Anthony, D.T. (1997). Differential effects of symptoms on rehabilitation and adjustment in people in schizophrenia. *Psychiatric Rehabilitation Journal, 21*(2), 141–143.

Steadman, H., Silver, E., Monahan, J., Appelbaum, P., Robbins, P.C., Mulvey, E.P., Grisso, T., Roth, L.H., & Banks, S. (in press). A classification tree approach to the development of actuarial violence risk assessment tools. *Law and Human Behavior.*

Steinberg, L., & Thissen, D. (1996). Uses of Item Response Theory and the testlet concept in the measurement of psychopathology. *Psychological Measurement, 1*(1), 81–97.

Stone, G.L. (1995). Review of the Hare Psychopathy Checklist–Revised. In J.C. Conoley & J.C. Impara (Eds.), *Twelfth mental measurement yearbook* (pp. 454–455). Lincoln: Buros Institute.

Susser, M. (1973). *Causal thinking in the health sciences.* New York: Oxford University Press.

Swanson, J.L. (1994). Mental disorder, substance abuse, and community violence: An epidemiological approach. In J. Monahan & H.J. Steadman (Eds.), *Violence and mental disorder: Developments in risk assessment* (pp. 101–136). Chicago: University of Chicago Press.

Swanson, J.W., Borum, R., Swartz, M.S., & Monahan, J. (1996). Psychotic symptoms and disorders and the risk of violent behaviour in the community. *Criminal Behaviour and Mental Health, 6*(4), 317–338.

Teplin, L.A. (1985). The criminality of the mentally ill: A dangerous misconception. *American Journal of Psychiatry, 142,* 593–599.

Toch, H., & Adams, K. (1986). Pathology and disruptiveness among prison inmates. *Journal of Research in Crime and Delinquency, 23,* 7–21.

Van der Linden, W.J., & Hambleton, R.K. (1996*). Handbook of modern item response theory.* New York: Springer.

Van Os, J., Gilvarry, C., Bale, R., Van Horn, E., Tattan, T., White, I., & Murray, R. (1999). A comparison of the utility of dimensional and categorical representations of psychosis. *Psychological Medicine, 29*(2), 595–606.

Ward, D.A. (1987). Control strategies for problem prisoners in American penal systems. In A.E. Bottoms & R. Light (Eds.), *Problems of long-term imprisonment.* Aldershot: Gower.

David J. Cooke is associated with Glasgow Caledonian University and the Douglas Inch Centre, Glasgow, Scotland, UK.

Author's Note

I would like to express my gratitude to Mark Davidson, Kevin Douglas, Stephen Hart, John Marshall, and John Monahan for their comments on an earlier draught. I would like to thank Christine Michie for her assistance with the statistical analyses.

The violence data were collected with support from the Chief Scientist's Office of the Scottish Office (Grant Number KPR/OPR/18/5). We would like to thank Lorraine Philip and Elaine Carr for collecting the data, and the Scottish Prison Service, in particular the Governor, Roger Houchin, and staff of H.M. Prison, Barlinnie, for facilitating data collection.

Comments or queries may be directed to David J. Cooke, Department of Clinical Psychology, Douglas Inch Centre, 2 Woodside Terrace, Glasgow G3 7UY Scotland, UK. Telephone: 44 141 211 8000/8006. Fax: 44 141 211 8005. E-mail: <djcooke @rgardens.u-net.com>.

EFFECTIVE TREATMENT FOR DISTURBED VIOLENT PRISONERS?

HANS TOCH

Observers in the media conceive of prisons as hotbeds of predation and violence, redolent with rapes, riots, and carnage. Such portraits can be overdrawn. For example, Ouimet (1999) points out that in the United States between 1984 and 1989 the prison homicide rate for corrections officers was 2.91 per 100,000, while the homicide rate for the US population was 8 per 100,000. Miners, truck drivers, and construction workers were more likely than prison staff to die on the job (p. 28).

Inmate misbehaviour, or violent misbehaviour in prisons, is not endemic, but follows an attenuated J curve with an extended tail.[1] The stem of this curve represents the majority of prisoners, whose custodial involvements are consistently negligible. The tail—which is steeper than usual in a J curve—comprises hard-core aggressors and redundant violators of assorted rules and regulations.[2]

When a prison system has mental health services its clients will reliably have more adjustment problems than the other prisoners. Inmates who are emotionally disturbed will be under-represented in the stem of the "J" and over-represented in its foot and tail (Toch & Adams, 1989). Moreover, at the extreme tip of the tail—where the legendary trouble-makers of the system are located—the disturbed prisoners will tend to predominate. In the US state of Washington, for example, 40 chronic violators were nominated by prison staff as being "behaviourally disturbed." Most of the members of this select group (62%) showed "evidence of serious mental illness" (Lovell & Jemelka, 1998). Twenty years earlier, a group of 356 New England prisoners had been identified as special management problems; 53% (195 of the inmates) were diagnosed as seriously disturbed. Hartstone, Steadman, Robbins, and Monahan (1984), who cite these data, conclude that "clearly, a major source of conflict in volatile prison settings are mentally disordered inmates. These inmates present problems with which prison officials usually are not prepared or trained to cope" (p. 281).

In this paper I shall consider the question of what prisons can do about the disturbed prisoners who are situated in the tail of the misbehaviour distribution. I shall refer to these subjects of my concern as "disturbed disruptive prisoners" (Toch, 1982). In doing so, I mean to imply that when disturbed prisoners become involved in violence they are not effectively dealt with if their clinical problems and their violent behaviour are addressed separately.

S. Hodgins (ed.), Violence among the Mentally Ill, 313–337.

The routine use of the prison disciplinary machinery to punish prisoners who are transparently disturbed is especially unseemly. Among the experts most acutely aware of this fact are the prison staff who are doing the punishing of the prisoners (Toch & Adams, 1987). One result has been a tendency for custodial staff in prisons to solicit mental health consultation, to the discomfiture of some of the mental health staff whose assistance is invoked.

One reason for discomfiture is that disturbed disruptive prisoners are frequently difficult and recalcitrant patients who oscillate between destructive and self-destructive behaviour; another reason is that we know little about disturbed disruptive syndromes and have difficulty producing long-term changes in the prison behaviour of offenders using conventional treatment approaches. Chronic disruptive prisoners who receive mental health services tend to return to being disruptive at some point after they have received them.

It is nevertheless tempting to postulate the amenability to mental health intervention of disruptive prisoners. For example, two officials of the US Bureau of Prisons have proposed a three-fold classification of violent inmates, with one category reserved for those prisoners who are presumed to require "clinically oriented treatment to address their emotional or behavioral problems" (Innes & Verdeyen, 1997, p. 2). The authors envisage a two-step process for these disturbed violent prisoners. They write that "the symptoms of the disorder must be managed before inmates in this group can benefit from special correctional programs" (p. 6).

The same authors prescribe a contrasting one-step process for another group of violent prisoners, whom they define as "psychopathic." About this group of inmates, they contend:

> The available evidence suggests that no program or treatment now available can be effective in influencing the behavior of this type of person.... In our view, the most appropriate and effective correctional response for such inmates is to assess carefully the level of custody needed to protect staff and other inmates from them. (Innes & Verdeyen, 1997, p. 4)

One fly in this prescriptive ointment is that conjoint diagnoses of psychosis and psychopathy—either in tandem or concurrently—are widely prevalent. The assumption of untreatability of personality disorders also encourages the use of the psychopathy (or antisocial personality) designation for disturbed prisoners who are obnoxious, ungrateful, or uninviting. One manifestation of such bias is the fact that patients who are committed from prison to hospital diagnosed as schizophrenic frequently are discharged from the hospital to the prison suffering from—on paper, at least—psychopathy or an antisocial personality disturbance (Toch & Adams, 1989). This transmutation is facilitated by the fact that applicable diagnostic criteria and psychometric psychopathy measures systematically highlight offensive behaviour that is deemed serious or persistent, which raises the probability of disturbed disruptive prisoners earning the appellation (Toch, 1998), no matter what else may be wrong with them.

Unreliability of diagnoses is one of many reasons why those who deal with disturbed violent offenders often tell us that they find the diagnoses of such offenders unhelpful as guides to assessment and treatment. Decades ago, Kozol, Boucher, and

Garofalo (1972) pointed out that "the terms used in standard psychiatric diagnosis are almost totally irrelevant in the determination of dangerousness" and that "the descriptions of the aggressor in action is often the most valuable single source of information" (pp. 383–384). More recently, Rice and Harris (1993) wrote that:

> All important clinical and administrative issues pertain to symptoms and other problems experienced by disturbed inmates and not to diagnosis per se.... In several studies of psychiatric patients...we examined subjects' clinical presentation with cluster analysis. In every case, clinically useful (with respect to treatment and supervision needs) subgroups depended not upon psychiatric diagnosis but instead upon current interpersonal problems, skill deficits, criminal history, and current symptomatology.... We conclude that treatment decisions cannot and should not be based solely or directly upon diagnosis. (p. 93)

There are also many disturbed prisoners who never come to the attention of clinicians or who have escaped their taxonomic endeavours. Though misbehaving inmates may be more likely than others to be referred for diagnosis (Hartstone et al., 1984), the level of violence and of eccentricity in diagnosed and undiagnosed disturbed disruptive prisoners is frequently indistinguishable. Prisoners in adjoining cells who issue the same shrill and incoherent threats may have wildly discrepant mental health records, and behavioural histories of diagnosed and undiagnosed inmates may describe patterns of irrational assaults and self-mutilations that appear similarly cryptic and unmotivated.

From the point of view of lay custodial staff, behaviour that on the face of it is tinged with eccentricity makes the prisoner presumptively disturbed. Given this sensible tautology, inmates who engage in delusionally motivated assaults, obsessive self-mutilations, or seemingly out-of-control tantrums are referred to mental health staff, with the expectation that they will be classified as mentally ill and accepted as clients. This expectation is frequently disconfirmed to the disappointment of the officers. Of course, corrections officers know that professional judgements need not mirror common sense. They also understand that prisoners who stand diagnosed as mentally ill can at times engage in violence that has nothing to do with their pathology, though the latter may help get the prisoners into situations that they feel must be violently resolved.

Disciplining Disturbed Prisoners

Violence in prisons is invariably responded to with punishment. Prison staff punish individuals who violate prison rules, and more severely punish those who commit more serious violations.

The emphasis in disciplinary dispositions is on the harm that the prisoner has done, and equivalent harm calls for comparable penalties. However, this does not mean that one need be completely oblivious to questions relating to motivation, intent, and state of mind. Prison hearing officers are likely to feel especially ill at ease if the prisoner who has committed an eccentric offence seems not to be in possession of his or her faculties at the time of the hearing. But where discretion is exercised in mitigation of punishment of such persons, the reasons for the decisions are often left deliberately unclear. We may not be told, for example, whether a lenient disposition reflects some doubt about level of culpability (such as whether a despondent prisoner who sets his bed on fire while occupying it is guilty of premeditated arson) or concerns about whether the prisoner can tolerate extended confinement.

In the US and many other countries there is no insanity defence in penal institutions, and no requirement that prisoners who are charged with offences be deemed competent to participate in their own defence.[3] Nor does the law demand that prison staff consider whether the disposition facing the prisoner could affect the prisoner adversely, which is often presumptively the case (Kupers, 1999).

There are many qualifications and exceptions, however. Some courts have become concerned with the adequacy of correctional mental health services, and in that connection have taken an interest in florid psychotics who reside untreated in punitive segregation cells. In New York State, for example, mental health personnel are required to monitor the condition of disturbed offenders who are confined, and to treat them when they have problems. The courts have also provided for off-the-record consultation of mental health staff where such testimony is deemed relevant by hearing officers.

Where mental health staff become thus involved, their role may pose ethical conflicts or become a source of controversy. A recent incident—which is ongoing as I write—illustrates the dilemmas that can arise:

> A resident of a prison mental health unit announces that she is embarking on an unauthorized expedition. She attempts to walk through the officer who obstructs her exit, and strikes the officer in the head. The civilian supervisor who presides over her hearing describes the inmate as "drooling." He takes testimony from mental health staff, as he is required to do given the fact that the prisoner appears disturbed and is a mental health client. Following this testimony, the hearing officer announces that he is dismissing the charges based upon the advice of the mental health staff and his own observations.
>
> In the aftermath of this incident, corrections officers manifest predictable displeasure, arguing that assaults on staff must carry tangible consequences. A union official protests what he describes as a blatant incursion of mental health professionals into custody matters. The mental health staff indicate, in reply, that they see themselves as providing information only, rather than as dispensing advice and/or counsel.

The prisoner involved in the incident is a long-term resident of the unit who has an extensive history of pathologically tinged assaults, for which she has served segregation terms. These experiences, however, have not tempered the chronicity of her violent involvements.

On past occasions the prison (whose warden is a redoubtable correctional innovator) has made it a point to involve assault victims in arriving at disciplinary dispositions. Staff victims of inmate assaults have therefore been consulted during the hearing phase, and, if modifications of segregation terms are considered, at subsequent junctures. "Accidental" encounters of assaulted staff members and the disturbed prisoners who assaulted them are arranged. These encounters provide occasions for reconciliation and learning. Interventions of this kind are restorative and beneficial to all parties concerned. They typify an approach in which crises can serve as learning opportunities for individuals and institutions.

Dismissing charges is unfortunately not an across-the-board option in prisons, where penalties are seen as having deterrent value. Prisoners who decompensate in a segregation cell may be committed to a forensic hospital, but most often must serve the remainder of their sentence after discharge. In theory it is, of course, possible for the clock not to stop during the hospital stay, since hospitalization is not a vacation undertaken at the request of the inmate nor an intermission from confinement. But logic does not dictate correctional policy.

SUPERMAX, SUPERSTRESS SETTINGS

A recent development that poses special problems for disturbed prisoners is the advent of the "maxi-maxi" or "supermax" institution. This type of prison is not in fact new: It is a technologically advanced version of an austere prison fortress such as Alcatraz (opened in 1934) in which "the worst of the worst" prisoners could be sequestered (Hershberger, 1998). The fortress, end-of-the-road prison provides for social and physical isolation, for "hard-edged solitude" (Clines, 1994). The experience purveyed to the inmate is one of sensory deprivation, eventlessness, and monotony.

The mental health implications of supermaximum confinement have become obvious as maxi-maxi prisons have proliferated. The issue reached the US courts in a landmark case, *Madrid v. Gomez,* decided in 1995. This case focused on a famous California prison, Pelican Bay, dedicated in 1989 and described as "state of the art" and "a model for the rest of the nation." The judge who decided the case instead wrote that the prison "may press the outer borders of what most humans can psychologically tolerate."[4] With regard to disturbed inmates, the judge contended that confinement at Pelican Bay was "the mental equivalent of putting an asthmatic in a place with little air to breathe" ("Judge," 1995).

The judge in *Madrid v. Gomez* pointed out that punitive segregation settings invariably contain disproportionate numbers of mentally ill prisoners. He wrote that "since inmates suffering from mental illness are more likely to engage in disruptive conduct, significant numbers of mentally ill inmates in the California prison system are ultimately transferred to the Pelican Bay SHU." He found that the conditions in the setting "cause mentally ill inmates to seriously deteriorate; other inmates who are otherwise able to psychologically cope with normal prison routines may also begin decompensating in the SHU" (cit. Cohen, 1995, p. 90).

The judge in this case recognized that stressful confinement settings can have differential impacts. He conceded that "for an occasional inmate, the SHU environment may actually prove beneficial," but concluded that the concern must be with prisoners for whom "the conditions...will likely lead to serious mental illness or a massive exacerbation of existing mental illness" (cit. Cohen, 1995, p. 91).

This solicitude about the exacerbation of symptoms under stress need not be limited to the effects of the most extreme supermaximum settings. Variations on the paradigm can cause counterpart problems. New York State, for example, has ostensibly mitigated supermax confinement by housing two prisoners to a cell. In commenting on this practice, Gonnerman (1999) asks, "What could be worse than spending 23 hours a day in a cell? Try spending 23 hours a day in a cell with somebody else." She notes that "Pelican Bay State Prison in California is in the midst of eliminating this practice because 10 prisoners have killed their cell mates in the last few years" (p. 38).

The most conservative response to the problem of the iatrogenic effects of isolation has been to intensify mental health services to prisoners who are confined in maxi-maxi settings. A more innovative solution to the problem is combined screening at intake (to keep vulnerable inmates out of the setting) and periodic screening of all prisoners serving time in SHUs ("Ohio," 1998).

A mixed custody-mental health model that has been considered at several historical junctures is that of modified disciplinary segregation settings for disturbed prisoners. In such settings, prisoners' interpersonal difficulties can plausibly be addressed as they serve segregation time and prepare themselves for re-integration into the prison population. An American version of this strategy was the design for Adjustment Centers in California in the 1960s (Fox, 1958); a Canadian version was the concept of Special Handling Units in the 1970s (*Report,* 1975). The latter was a particularly interesting model, featuring stages of increased association and involvement over time, as prisoners showed themselves ready to participate in new sets of activities with other prisoners. The envisaged sequence was one in which an assessment of the prisoner's level of skills and deficits that placed him at a "higher" stage would permit the prisoner to exercise new skills whose adequacy could then be assessed at the next stage of the game.

Unfortunately, these American and Canadian models quickly degenerated into stripped-down segregation settings in which a "control mentality" dominated. Vantour (1991) describes this development in Canada:

> In particular, inmates are routinely moved from cell to common-room to recreation yard individually with at least two officers accompanying them; interviews are conducted through grills; overhead catwalks are patrolled by armed officers. Yet despite all this, restraint equipment—handcuffs—have become the rule rather than the exception, whenever an inmate is in the presence of staff. The phases only exist on paper. Meaningful activities have been virtually non-existent. These are essentially non-contact prisons. The regime is a repressive one. Control has become the watchword. (p. 93)

Such experiences illustrate the importance of protecting prison innovations from outsiders or conservative staff members who become obsessed with security concerns, especially in relation to disruptive inmates.

DETENTION SETTINGS

By default, penal institutions have become residential mental health facilities. In the US, for example, 200,000 seriously mentally ill patients are incarcerated, while fewer than 70,000 reside in state mental hospitals (Cloud, 1999). Disturbed offenders in such situations may discover that they can receive services in confinement that are not otherwise available to them in the community.

> Unpleasant as jail and prison are, it is not terribly unusual to hear ex-inmates talk about jail or prison as having "saved their life." In fact, for some people with serious mental illness living on the streets, jail- or prison-based services may be the only mental health treatment they have received in years. (Barr, 1999, p. 37)

In a story about an addicted schizophrenic, the *New York Times* reports that in jail he "received care he would have been unlikely to find on the outside," and "because he was in jail, there was more time to adjust his medication, a luxury that rarely exists outside" (Winerap, 1999). The same story notes, however, that the jail (Rikers Island) had almost no beds "for mentally ill drug abusers, who make up a large proportion of the offenders."

Civilian services and prison mental health care are often experienced in tandem during an individual's career. In a study of disturbed violent offenders, we found that four of 10 offenders who had received mental health services before they were imprisoned continued to receive them in prison; 7% had to be hospitalized and 6% were repeatedly hospitalized. Fewer than 4% of violent offenders with no history of mental health services required services in prison; only one inmate out of a sample of 544 had to be sent to a hospital (Toch & Adams, 1994). There was also a striking relationship among severity of illness, seriousness of violence, and the need for mental health services in prison. We reported that

> Our findings are dramatic and consistent: Individuals who are disturbed in the prison after they offend tend to be disturbed before they offend, and when we look at the samples in more detail we discover that the most disturbed inmates have committed the most extreme violence and, mostly, the "craziest" violence. (p. 177)

These facts raised questions about the relative merits of mental health services delivered in mental hospitals and prisons. We pointed out that "the problems associated with mental health services in prisons may be serious, but one must recognize that mental hospitals have counterpart problems in dealing with serious violent offenders" (p. 181).

> Mental health staff who work in hospitals are apt to be intimidated by violence and may approach the offender uneasily and with fear. This creates problems for staff morale, but it can also affect patient care because staff apprehension leads to overmedication as a reassuring "management" tool. (p. 182)

While prisons are clearly not designed to accommodate the mentally ill, they are attuned to persons with behaviour problems. Moreover, prisons are arguably more "normalized" environments than hospitals, because they offer a panoply of vocational and educational programmes as well as a range of sub-environments (Toch, 1992). Prisons can also use the sorts of interdisciplinary approaches that are responsive to offenders with multiple problems:

The presumption is that they must be less monothematic than current strategies, using a wider range of interventions and expertise. The disturbed violent offender's needs are nonoptional in this regard because he or she demands interdisciplinary confluence, interagency collaboration, and teaming in delivering services. The necessity of experimenting with staff interface arrangements forces prisons to evolve flexible models for responding to multiproblem clients with multiservice approaches. This is an exciting frontier for experimentation and innovation. (Toch & Adams, 1994, p. 195)

PRISON SETTINGS

Mental health services in jails and prisons are frequently organized to make constructive collaborations with custody staff possible. Such arrangements have obvious advantages, which are in theory reciprocal. Jemelka, Rahman, and Trupin (1993) note that "it is evident that a joint venture might represent the 'best of both worlds' in that the advantages of correctional management and management by a mental health division would accrue" (p. 18).

Multi-problem prisoners—and especially disturbed disruptive inmates—have consistently invited the practice of "bus therapy," whereby troublesome clients are shuttled among institutions such as prisons and hospitals (Toch, 1982). Collaborative settings provide a means to replace this practice, which erodes the continuity of inmate assessment and treatment.

But a collaborative endeavour can interlink the insights or expertise of mental health staff and correctional officers only if the two parties respect and trust each other. Ideally, the clinicians and officers must have the shared objective of understanding the behaviour of disturbed disruptive prisoners, so that it can be modified. The officers involved in these collaborative studies experience a fruitful expansion or enrichment of their roles, and officers who find human-service work satisfying can become particularly effective. "There is evidence that positive effects can occur when front-line staff have combined treatment and security duties" (Rice & Harris, 1993, p. 109).

For correctional-mental health collaborative arrangements to evolve into close team efforts, the relationship must be one of unqualified reciprocity. This result cannot be achieved if mental health staff view correctional officers as sources of information about prisoners but do not provide information in return. If one presumes that all the staff in a programme share the goal of modifying inmate behaviour, it follows that they must jointly study and address the behaviour.

Confidentiality and Training Issues

One familiar obstacle to collaborative activity is the premise of confidentiality, which can be invoked to undergird the hoarding of clinical information. A relationship of equity instead implies that to the extent to which one party has access to another's observations and to the data recorded in their files, they should be obligated to reciprocate. This would especially hold if all the staff in a programme must think as a group about diverse information from a variety of sources.

Confidentiality provisions apply where prisoners are assured that what they say to mental health staff members is available only to mental health staff. If this elementary stricture is observed, the mental health staff can offer conclusions and recommendations but cannot reveal the documentation on which the inferences are based. This would mean that the inferences must be accepted on faith, and that joint thinking that involves non-mental health staff is precluded.

Fortunately, there is no reason why assurances of confidentiality cannot extend to members of a team, since they would all be engaged in treatment and would all presumptively have the interests of the prisoner in mind. In fact, restricting confidentiality to mental health staff would suggest to the prisoners that officers cannot be trusted or (even worse) might use information to the detriment of the prisoners.

Fred Cohen, a prominent student of prison mental health law, points out that "confidentiality of medical and mental health records is a veritable labyrinth of professional ethics, statutes, various judicial decisions in the context of tort litigation, and constitutional law" (Cohen, 1993, p. 56). He notes that there are situations in prison where exceptions to confidentiality norms clearly become desirable for the benefit of the inmates. For example, "there is a case to be made that some security staff should be aware of an inmate's psychotropic medication in order to monitor for compliance and deal with side effects. Suicide information should be shared as part of a preventive approach" (p. 57). By the same token, if officers refer a prisoner for examination, one can argue that they are entitled to feedback about the prisoner's condition. In the absence of feedback, the officers may be discouraged from making referrals. The re-evaluation of prescriptions is also made easier if officers feel that their comments and observations are valued.

There is consensus that officers who work with mental health staff in programmes for disturbed disruptive inmates must receive training related to issues of mental health. But this does not mean that such training need take the form of classroom instruction, which can become patronizing and "academic" in the worst sense of the word. The training of officers can instead focus on the problems the officers face—those presented by the prisoners with whom they interact. One modality of such training is case conferences, in which analysis is combined with planning and programming. Officers can also be supplied with supplementary reading material to help them understand specific issues that come up in reviewing the information about the prisoners. Knowledge of this kind is especially meaningful because it places observations in context, indicating how the behaviour of individual prisoners illustrates generalizable principles.

In experiments described by Quinsey (Quinsey, 1977, 1979; St. Thomas Psychiatric Hospital, 1976) front-line staff conducted research into violent incidents and designed training programmes and other interventions to prevent or reduce violence. In one setting, teams compiled psychological autopsies of critical incidents and a committee made policy recommendations based on the data. In another setting—a maximum security psychiatric unit—an "assault prevention task force" was constituted, made up of attendant staff, attendant supervisors, and a psychologist. This group made recommendations and achieved a reduction in staff victimizations (it did not reduce injury to patients).

Kevin Corcoran, a staff member of HMP Belmarsh in London, has underlined the importance of post-incident study and review:

> When it is all over nursing staff should try to find the reason for the distur-
> bance, try to reconstruct the situation in order to see if better observation
> might have allowed them to predict and so to prevent it. The nursing staff
> should try to be frank in their discussion of the causes of the outburst and
> should seriously examine their own actions in order to discover to what ex-
> tent they may have themselves unwillingly provoked it.... Other people's
> evaluations of the part each has played should be accepted. This should be
> done not in a spirit of criticism but in an attempt to coordinate the approach
> to the inmate and to prevent recurrence of the incident. (Corcoran, 1992,
> p. 5)

Rice, Harris, Varney, and Quinsey (1989) have outlined a training paradigm. The model can assist staff most especially in responding to the angry outbursts charac-teristic of manic episodes. The model contains detailed instructions for calming ex-cited patients and defusing their unfocused rage. Techniques of restraint are also described in the event that verbal approaches fail. The paradigm has been applied in a hospital but could easily benefit officers who work with disturbed prisoners.

Other types of training for officers could be specific to the involvements that are expected of them and can be delivered through mentoring, process reviews, and collateral reading. (Such training models have been developed in therapeutic com-munities for disturbed prisoners in which officers function as group leaders and co-therapists. We shall return to this subject later.)

INHOUSE CONSULTATION

Working with disturbed disruptive prisoners in any setting is a stressful and poten-tially thankless assignment. The prisoners' problems may look obdurate and unre-sponsive to intervention. One may even have arrived at a juncture where one feels that one has exercised every option one can think of with no discernible results. One may feel in need of fresh ideas or new perspectives, or reassurance and support.

Such a juncture may be independently reached by different staff at different lo-cations, who may all be struggling with comparable or intersecting dilemmas. Lovell and Rhodes (1997) observe that "inmates who engage in apparently irrational be-havior, regardless of diagnosis, pose problems that cross three traditional boundaries in prison organizations: between institutions, between mental illness and behavior disorder, and between custody and treatment" (p. 40). Beefing up lines of communi-cation among persons who must deal with different aspects of an obdurate problem can reduce feelings of isolation. Promoting dialogues among such persons can offer the benefit of pooled experiences and produce interdisciplinary cross-fertilization. At a minimum, exchanges can reduce barriers that arise when staff operate in isola-tion from each other. Lovell and Rhodes point out, for instance, that in the state of Washington "rigid definitions of the areas of custodial and mental health expertise left workers with scant means of helping each other with problems that crossed the boundaries" (pp. 40–41).

Communication is especially helpful during crises in which the solutions one has tried seem not to work and in which out-of-control prisoners appear refractory to intervention. At such junctures it is useful to be able to mobilize the expertise of colleagues elsewhere in the system and experts of a different discipline. The Mobile Consultation Team of the Washington Department of Corrections was an innovative experiment along these lines, designed in collaboration with the University of Washington in Seattle. Team members included four mental health professionals, two nurses, three programme supervisors, and six experienced, sophisticated corrections officers. A visiting team of four could be convoked on short notice to work with prison staff who requested a consultation. The team members had been trained to engage in joint problem solving with the local staff, after "review of records, visit to [the prisoner's] living unit, interviews with staff and [the] inmate, [and] behavioral observation if indicated" (Lovell & Rhodes, 1997, p. 41).

Inhouse consultation in a prison system can be combined with external consultation, such as with experts in psychopharmacology.[5] In Washington, the university on occasion arranged for specialists whose help was requested by the team and the local staff. The product of consultation visits would be an action plan, or proposal, for intervention. Some of the interventions could be implemented locally, while others might entail transfer of the prisoner to a different programme or institution.

Transfers among settings requires coordination, and should involve personal contacts between the sending and receiving facilities to ensure treatment continuity. Continuity of treatment can also be assured if the inmate has been assigned a case manager, which is especially desirable with prisoners who are living exemplars of comorbidity (Toch, 1995).

A source of resistance to consultation can be local prison management, which might pride itself on its self-sufficiency. There is also a need for periodic team meetings to keep the collaborative process alive, ensuring that consultants continue to see themselves as persons who think with their colleagues instead of assuming that they possess special expertise.

Therapeutic Communities

The therapeutic community—or TC, as it is known to its aficionados—has been introduced in Europe as a substitute for the custodial warehousing of disruptive prisoners. In the US no such development has occurred. The American prison TC tends to be narrowly aimed at the resocialization of substance abusers. Its technology is one derived from a tradition of religiously oriented confessional groups. This approach was first applied to moral transgressions, later to problems of alcoholism, and last to the rehabilitation of drug addicts. American prison TCs have emulated their predecessors in the community, used their graduates as paraprofessional staff, and cycled ex-prisoners into community TCs.

Among the attributes of the American type of TC is reliance on attack or confrontation of offenders in peer groups, modulated—in theory, at least—by caring and support. Another feature common to the TCs has been progression or sequencing of individual members from paternalistic regimentation to increasing levels of autonomy, congruent with presumptive personal maturation. Prison TCs also invariably attempt to create a culture among their residents that is antithetical to the convict or prisoner subculture.

A relatively recent development in the US are proposals to adapt the TC model for use with disturbed prisoners who are addicted.

> The recognized success of prison TCs provides an excellent opportunity to build upon an established technology by enhancing and expanding it to meet the psychiatric needs associated with substance abuse. It is reasonable to entertain the possibility that an enhanced prison TC model that also treats co-morbid psychiatric problems may significantly increase the effectiveness of the modality. (Wechsler, 1997, p. 174)

Wechsler (1997) reports that persons who run prison TCs are generally concerned about these proposals. They worry about the possibility of disturbed residents becoming addicted to psychoactive medication. There is also a fear that mental health staff in TCs may promote an "impersonal atmosphere" incompatible with "a cohesive and caring community environment." Wechsler argues that "it would probably be a mistake if a mental health orientation became dominant in any joint venture with the TC, because the effectiveness demonstrated by the TC approach might be compromised" (p. 176).

The concern about an anti-community bias of mental health staff is especially ironic, because in Europe TCs originated in democratized hospital wards and strongly emphasize community elements (Toch, 1980). Moreover, prison TCs in countries other than the US have preferentially targeted prisoners who have a history of mental illness or disruptive behaviour.

Such has been the case in Canada, where a distinctive treatment programme was created in the Social Therapy Unit at Oak Ridge, in the Penetang Psychiatric Hospital at Penetanguishene, Ontario. The prisoners who were residents in this unit had been convicted of a variety of very serious and violent offences. In the programme, disturbed violent offenders were trained to function as therapists for other violent offenders.

According to Elliott Barker, the founder of the treatment modality, a key requisite was that of matching inmates with "intersecting pathologies" who could neutralize each other in groups:

> Intelligent extroverts display great ability in observing details of behavior, correctly describing it, proposing practical alternatives, and organizing activities. The introverts offer much in terms of emotional support and empathy. For individuals, introvert or extrovert, this combination provides a multidimensional picture of their situation, and a wide range of resources within which to fulfill their needs. The program seems to be stabilized by this combination, which provides checks and balances, softening the raw practicality of the extrovert with the dreaminess of the introvert, introverted idealism with extroverted politics. (Barker, 1980, p. 80)

As another case in point, Barker and Mason (1968) observe that

> a schizophrenic will object to the slick solution to a problem adeptly flashed
> out by a psychopath. The psychopath will point with some justice to the
> woolliness and diffuse idealism of the schizophrenic. Or again no one can so
> unerringly highlight the subtle manipulations of a severely sick psychopath
> as one who is similarly crazy. No one can perceive the first crumblings of a
> schizophrenic disintegration more quickly than one who has once similarly
> collapsed himself. (p. 63)

In addition to attending twice-a-day community meetings, the residents at
Penetang worked with each other in dyads, triads, and small groups for a total of up
to 80 hours a week. The intricate operation not only was run by prisoner committees,
but prisoners devised much of the content of the programme. When a disturbed prisoner experienced a crisis, for example, fellow patients enacted a procedure that they
themselves invented involving physical support via handcuffs, which predictably
accelerated recovery.

The Penetanguishene Program, as it was called, was characterized by searching
analytic dialogues designed to make "what is unconscious, conscious," and by emotional intensity. Barker (1980) has written that the inmates could justifiably claim
that "the unit is in the business of upsetting people" because "the processes of anxiety arousal, recognition and change are central ones" (p. 76).

By coercing close cohabitation, Penetang promoted a climate of rarefied intimacy, to the extent of using "total-encounter capsules" in which small groups of
naked and sleep-deprived volunteers were isolated for intensive feedback sessions.
The programme also experimented with the administration of scopolomine and me-
thedrine, to reduce defences and induce mild psychotic episodes. Barker, Mason,
and Wilson (1969) assert that the medicated patients "emerge from the experience
with their aggressiveness considerably diluted." They also report:

> The immediately obvious "insanity" of the patient on scopola-
> mine-methedrine also defines unmedicated patients in clear helping roles.
> Close bonds of responsibility and affection are sometimes developed be-
> tween the "sane" patient therapists and the chemically "insane" patients. At
> times when four patients in the same unit are receiving the drugs simultane-
> ously, every member of the unit is involved in immediate physical interaction
> with one of them. It seems that much of the value of DDT lies in the active
> participation of patients in the process of caring for one another. (p. 358)

The peer-therapy orientation of Penetang included de-emphasis of staff involvement. Barker (1980) declared that officers "must be instructed not to participate in
programs" (p. 79), but some of the officers were encouraged to play stereotypical
roles. For example,

> I liked the fact that in the midst of the patients talking about matters psycho-
> dynamic, the guards could always come up with the comment, "you're still a
> goddamn rapist to me." Which is very therapeutic, and reflects the outside
> culture they would be going back to, so that they never left that base too far.
> (p. 127)

As for other staff, Barker (1980) contends that an abundance of professional staff makes programmes inoperable:

> Any (professional staff) in excess of the absolute minimum will fall back on their training and hunt out individual inmates to help. No more effective undermining of the system of inmate helping inmate can occur, since inmates often have the belief (probably delusional) that professional staff persons are better at helping people by virtue of their training. (p. 80)

I have listed some details of the Penetanguishene Program because an evaluation of this programme by Rice, Harris, and Cormier (1992) has produced some startling conclusions.[6] In analyzing outcome measures, the data in this study were disaggregated by psychopathy scale scores, and the authors report that

> psychopaths who participated in the therapeutic community exhibited higher rates of violent recidivism than did the psychopaths who did not. The opposite result was obtained for nonpsychopaths, and it should be noted that the nonpsychopath groups comprised both psychotic and nonpsychotic individuals. (p. 408)

They conclude that the Penetanguishene Program inculcated or reinforced interpersonal skills, which psychopathic offenders "put...to quite unintended uses" (p. 409). These authors also suggest that the study supports the use of therapeutic communities "for psychotic and nonpsychotic offenders as long as they are not psychopaths" (p. 409). The Penetang unit, however, is clearly far from a typical therapeutic community. It is plausible that a highly charged operation like Penetang works best for those of its residents who are the most psychologically disturbed. In particular, the application of Barker's strategy of engineering intersecting pathologies may produce asymmetrical benefits. In other words, the less disturbed inmates, referred to as "psychopaths," may help the more disturbed inmates, at some expense to themselves.

English TCs and Special Units

Therapeutic communities for disturbed or disruptive inmates were introduced in England in the early 1960s. The prison Grendon Underwood, located near London, is the flagship of this approach. It is an experimental psychiatric facility comprising five TCs of between 35 and 42 residents. The treatment process at these TCs centres on small groups with two co-therapists, one of whom is a corrections officer. Most of the staff in the prison are uniformed officers.

The residents of Grendon are referred from other prisons, usually by mental health staff and physicians; 40% are lifers, and most have had extensive problems adjusting to confinement. These problems at Grendon are regarded as grist for social learning. Eric Cullen explains that

> the behaviour...is not punished by conventional prison means but turned instead back into the therapeutic process. The prescription "take it to your

group" encourages both individual and collective responsibilities to be accountable and to change. (Cullen, 1997, p. 85)

An example of this approach to transgressions is the following vignette reported by Genders and Player (1995). The prisoner who is described by the authors "routinely tried the patience of wing staff." On one occasion the inmate was observed storming into an office in which mail was being sorted:

> When he was informed that the post was not yet ready to be distributed he hurled a tirade of abuse and accused the officer of dereliction of duty and gross incompetence. The officer concerned responded by calmly apologizing for the delay and politely informing him that, contrary to his expectations, the Prison Department had still not issued instructions to suspend all other duties in the interests of expediting the delivery of his copy of *The Australian.*
>
> Implicit in this was the recognition by the officer that it would be counter-productive to challenge this man's abusive manner there and then. Instead, the issue would be taken up for discussion on his group or during a community meeting. (p. 125)

One of the assumptions underlying the Grendon approach is that *ad seriatim* disciplining of inmates reinforces feelings of bitterness and resentment that motivate acting-out behaviour. Peter Lewis, who was director of therapy at Grendon, points out that

> the significant therapeutic task for staff is to try to understand the subtle danger of repeating such a destructive interpersonal re-enactment. It is all too easy in everyday interaction for inmate and officer to become engaged in such a non-productive repetition of unhelpful ingrained behaviour. (Lewis, 1997, p. 210)

The point is to avoid playing into expectations that undergird anti-authoritarian and destructive behaviour, but instead to subject such premises to review and analysis. Constructive responses foster a "corrective emotional experience," which can draw attention to the "defective emotional experience" that frequently has had its inception in "early years of rejection and inconsistency of care." The presumption is that the disconfirming experience of an environment that includes non-rejecting authority figures "frees the person to experiment with new styles of thought, feeling and behaviours in his psychological journey to personality reformation" (p. 210). In order to inculcate what is described as "an understanding of interdependence and trust that had previously been lacking," the staff at Grendon "model" constructive resolutions of interpersonal conflicts and problems that involve authority figures (p. 213).

The principal treatment modality at Grendon, group psychotherapy, requires that the officers who function as co-therapists learn a great deal about running groups. Grendon avoids referring to this process as "training." The professional development of the officers consists of mentoring them as they actually run groups, and of engaging in frequent, systematic process reviews of sessions, which are referred to as "feedback." Lewis (1997) notes that in the face of budget constraints "enhancement of time available for post group discussions is [considered] essential and a continuing development of the quality of such discussion is vital" (p. 217).

Though officers at Grendon are encouraged to read, their supervisors supply clinical and other theoretical constructs when the experiences to which the constructs apply arise in therapeutic encounters. There are also periodic staff meetings across the groups and wings in which techniques are discussed and analyses of therapy sessions take place. Outside courses are made available to all staff, including the officers.

Grendon inmates are expected to review their life stories—including their criminal involvements—in the groups, which mostly highlight violent acts. According to Cullen (1997), "the treatment premise is that the crime was a product, or consequence of the interpersonal conflict arising from the personality disorder" (p. 88). As in most therapeutic communities, there is emphasis on the here and now, and any observed "parallels between current behaviour and prior offending...are brought into the therapeutic process" (p. 80).

An end product of therapy at Grendon is the formulation of strategies by the inmate for responding to human encounters so as to avoid future misconduct. This goal is nicely described by Genders and Player (1995):

What Grendon attempts to do is to empower individuals to take control over that which is within their power: namely, their ability to make choices which alleviate their own and others' victimization, and to anticipate, and take responsibility for, the consequences of their actions. (p. 14)

Predictably, Grendon prisoners experience reintegration problems when they return to regular prisons. The way reintegration is dealt with by the prison to which the inmate is assigned makes a great deal of difference. According to Genders and Player (1995), those Grendon graduates who have been afforded "opportunities...to put into practice what they have learned" (p. 176) experience smooth transitions.

Among other prison settings in England that serve disruptive prisoners are so-called special units. One of these is C-Wing at Parkhurst, which provides treatment to former residents of segregation settings, under psychiatric supervision.

In England the prevalence of psychosis in prisons is reduced through transfer of seriously mentally ill inmates to forensic hospitals. Despite this fact, Coid (1991) reports that only 10% of disruptive prisoners in special units were found free of lifetime (Axis I) major mental disorders. He also reports that 20% of the unit residents "were suffering from serious mental illness when first interviewed" (p. 50).

One man padded the staircases and landings of a unit aimlessly, unable to engage in any meaningful activities whatsoever, and received the maximum recommended levels of several antipsychotic medications. He still regularly pleaded with prison staff to give more. He had wrecked the patients' social club in a special hospital and had promptly been returned to prison. (pp. 50–51)

Coid (1991) also makes an observation that duplicates my own experience, which is that "a significant proportion of [disruptive prisoners] showed features of mood disorder which did not amount to a diagnosis of mental illness but resulted in fluctuating symptoms of irritability, anxiety, tension and depression" (p. 51). He additionally reports encountering a good deal of paranoia among the inmates. In summarizing the impressions he gained in his research with residents of the special unit, Coid describes typical downhill careers of disturbed disruptive inmates:

> [Their] last period of imprisonment was characterised by increasing periods of segregation and movements from one prison to another. Hardened malignancy of attitude had now set in with ingrained, repetitive patterns of behavioural disorder. Repeated punishments within the prison setting and the increasingly negative attitudes of prison staff had further confirmed the process, with many men locked into a vicious spiral of punishment – resentment – retaliation – more punishment, from which neither side seemed able to find a way out. Features of mental illness now remained untreated as for some cases the avenue of psychiatric treatment had become closed to them. For others the behavioural disorder remained unchanged in spite of all attempts at psychiatric treatment. (p. 70)

Unsurprisingly, Coid (1991) observes in the conclusion to his study that "it remains unclear at this stage how effective the units will be with these men" (p. 70). At minimum, this suggests that most small units face a daunting and redoubtable challenge.

Scottish Special Units

Uncontestably, the most famous special unit established for disruptive prisons is the Barlinnie Special Unit (BSU) in Scotland. As David Cooke puts it, "the BSU became an ikon" (Cooke, 1997, p. 101). One reason for the singular stature of the BSU is that it represented the diametric opposite of the approach that had been previously used with its residents. Prisoners who had been serving extended time in supermaximum control units were taken out of dungeons and placed into a heavily democratic milieu. But the retooling of authoritarian milieus had ample precedent in Scotland, where Maxwell Jones—a Scot—co-invented the therapeutic community.

The period preceding the establishment of the BSU had featured a number of riots and incidents of hostage-taking. A working party convoked to study this proliferation of violence concluded that a small number of recidivistic prisoners were responsible for a lion's share of the problem. The group also observed that punitive responses seemed to have exacerbated the prisoners' destructiveness. Though some of the prisoners were arguably disturbed, their pathology was not deemed exculpatory and did not "bring them within the provisions of the Mental Health Act" (Light, 1985, p. 15).

The challenge was to create a setting that would break the observed redundant cycles linking disruptiveness and punitive confinement. In this setting, "an attempt was made to move from the traditional officer/prisoner relationship towards something approaching a nurse/patient relationship" (Cooke, 1997, p. 102). Other components of the TC were also emulated, including the use of community meetings and ad hoc therapeutic groups that could be convoked as problems or crises developed.

All BSU residents had been convicted of violent offences, and the majority were serving life sentences. Moreover, most had been tried for offences committed in prison. Prisoners on long-term medication regimens were, however, excluded from the unit, as were those deemed "unable to cope with the stressful regime" (Cooke, 1989, p. 130).

One of several unique features of the BSU was the fostering of creative talent among its residents. Jimmy Boyle, arguably the most violent prisoner in Scotland, became an established sculptor and writer. Another resident, Larry Winters, evolved into a well-regarded poet, and a third, Hugh Collins, also became a successful sculptor. None of these prisoners had shown prior evidence of artistic talents or aptitudes.

The psychological disconfirmation process described by Grendon staff was replicated among the prisoners at the BSU. Boyle (1997), in his first book, *A Sense of Freedom,* recalls that after he arrived at the unit he found the experience distressing:

> [T]here was a great amount of hatred in me for all screws, yet some of the unit staff would approach me in a way that was so natural and innocent it made it difficult to tell them to fuck off. Something inside me, in spite of all the pent-up hatred, would tell me there was something genuine within them. I knew I didn't really want to recognise this part of the screws. I preferred to see them all as bastards, this would have been so much easier for me...[but] they were so unlike the screws that I had known in the past. At nights I would lie in my bed tearing my guts out thinking intensely about this place and what it was all about, and often wishing I were back in solitary. (p. 237)

Boyle confesses that "finally, I decided that I had to get the fuck out of the place, and so I went to the Governor and told him...the only way for me to get any peace of mind was to...return to the solitary situation, as that was the method I could handle best" (p. 240). The experience that Boyle describes is one of incipient unfreezing of his customary frame of reference, which included accommodation to the punitive confinement settings in which he had spent much of his time. There was also the painful challenge of having to relinquish a militant warfare posture by reciprocating the disarming trust bids of the officers in the unit.

The BSU was established in 1973 and was closed in 1995. In an early evaluation, Cooke (1992) calculated that if a cohort of 25 unit residents had maintained their rates of assaultive behaviour in the unit they would have perpetrated 105 assaults during a period in which there were in fact only two. There were nine other disruptive incidents in the BSU, while the expected number was 154.

The unit's closure was not a response to a crisis situation or dramatic demonstration of failure. Rather, the decision resulted from the realization that the BSU over time had undergone stagnation or stultification. The Inspectorate of Prisons for Scotland (1993) pointed out that "in the normally accepted sense of the word, a regime does not exist in any structured or formal sense for prisoners in the unit" (p. 15). The inmates had become permanent fixtures, individually doing their time. In interviews, they "expressed themselves as content to remain where they were in the absence of any target to aim for" (p. 19). There was little interaction among the residents. Community meetings had become perfunctory; in the understated words of the Inspectorate, "these meetings would appear in recent times to have lost much of their impetus" (p. 32).

The Inspectorate outlined the need for drastic reforms, but a working party decided to close the BSU and start over with a set of contrasting units for different types of disruptive inmates (Wozniak, 1995). Common among the units would be a community emphasis and the use of groups for the resocialization of the prisoners.

Setting up a new set of units is a complex and difficult process, but several prescriptive implications follow from the recent Scottish experience. I shall record some of these implications, as I see them, by way of conclusion to this chapter.

The goal of prisoner rehabilitation must inform all programme decisions and activities. When a special programme is being planned, emphasis must centre on the treatment modality, rather than on restrictions, privileges, and other contextual concerns. If prisoners are involved in planning, along with the staff—which is desirable if it can be arranged—the discussion must be about details of the regime, rather than becoming an acrimonious negotiation of rules and perquisites. It must always remain clear that the focus of activities in the programme is on the examination and working through of problematic behaviour of the residents. A community meeting, for example, must not become a vehicle for the prisoners to grouse about unpopular actions of the staff. Any administrative matters that arise must be relegated to administrative channels, which can include committees and grievance mechanisms.

Activity is better than inactivity, but meaningful activity is vastly preferable to time-filling activity. "Meaning" can derive from the product or the process of an activity. A meaningful product would be one that is beneficial to others, such as the manufacture of toys for disadvantaged children. Meaning that is inherent in process can centre on team or collaborative activity—especially involving inmates with staff—and on the acquisition of skills. Activities can also provide opportunities to display or manifest one's personal or interpersonal difficulties, so that they can be discussed in groups.

Staff must come to understand the behaviour of prisoners. Each prisoner must have one assigned staff member to work with on a daily basis. However, there must be many opportunities for all the staff to review and discuss the behaviour of all the prisoners, starting with pre-induction reviews and culminating in pre-release assessments. Most of the staff discussions in a programme should be followed by feedback to the prisoner. By the same token, activities of staff (especially group sessions) should be followed by process reviews.

Staff training in programmes for difficult prisoners must be a valued benefit. Special programmes provide unique opportunities for the staff to learn and practise skills. If possible, all supervision, teaching, counselling, and evaluation of a programme should be in the hands of the programme staff. If staff members have special skills that can somehow be utilized in the programme, opportunities should be provided for their exercise. Training must be made available for the development of new skills and the acquisition of new knowledge that can be applied. Any training thus received must be utilized.

The rehabilitation process must be systematically sequenced and integrated and must be tailored to the needs of each prisoner. A programme can accommodate diverse treatment modalities, but ought to never become a patchwork quilt. The first task is to help prisoners who have been segregated to make the transition from solitary confinement to congregate living. Once the inmates have recaptured the rules of personal co-existence, they are ready to embark on the road of self-exploration and (it is hoped) of self-understanding. The final challenge is to increase prisoners' coping competence, so they can manage in a regular prison population. The outcome measure that demonstrates success is the inmate's ability to survive—without untoward incidents—in the prison at large.

A generic rehabilitative module of any kind—for instance, cognitive or interpersonal skills training—may be helpful during the orientation stage, but most subsequent experiences must address the prisoner's unique deficits and vulnerabilities. There are also benefits when the inmate participates in the recovery process of other residents in the programme, who may have problems different from his or her own.

While key programme components must address the prisoner's problems, there should be opportunities to develop and build on any aptitude, skill, or interest that the prisoner may manifest. Such involvements, however, must be considered ancillary to the treatment process, which is the core of the programme.

"Structure" is not a dirty word. Solitary confinement is an experience without psychological structure, involving extended periods of sleep and redundant ruminations. Structure is needed in programmes such as special units to dissipate the effects of this experience, which include secondary symptomatology as well as fantasy, disorientation, mood swings, and an undercurrent of fear and suspicion. Structure means knowing what to expect and what others expect one to do. A detailed compact or contractual arrangement before an inmate enters a programme may be helpful, and it is important that this document (if it is written) outline tasks and products expected of them. Wherever possible, the rationale underlying proposed activities ought to be specified or explained. The prisoner must also know the rules governing behaviour in the programme, and the reasons for them.

Community meetings can be democratic yet structured. Such meetings are useful for working out assignments and schedules, including responsibilities for maintenance tasks, membership in committees, and so forth. Schedules and rosters should be posted, and updated as required.

Criteria for the promotion or release of inmates must be tangible and specific. Many programmes have formal steps or stages, which provide increments of benefits and expanded responsibilities and obligations. Some programmes feature less formalized progression or advancement, and their residents also move from one set of experiences to another, contingent on the evaluation of performance.

In any sequence, it is important that the behavioural criteria, which form the basis for decisions, be specified in advance. Inmates must know what they have to demonstrate by way of accomplishments to move to the next rung of the programme ladder and to eventually graduate from the programme. They must know what is expected of them, and what information will be used to gauge their accomplishments. A projected timetable is also helpful, with provisions for more-or-less accelerated advancement.

Adherence to behavioural criteria is especially important in prisons, where fairness, equity, and justice are salient values and strongly felt concerns. Schedules and criteria are especially important, not only because release from a programme may expedite release from the prison, but also because longer-than-required tenure can mean wasting scarce resources that are needed for new programme candidates.

Where decisions of programme staff must be bureaucratically ratified, it must be emphasized to the inmate in advance that any process initiated by staff recommendations must run its organizational course, and that the staff will do their very best to expedite matters. No outcomes ought to be promised that cannot be delivered by the staff.

The proof of a good programme is not the absence of problems but the adequacy and ingenuity of solutions. When one works with difficult prisoners, it is inevitable that problematic incidents and critical situations will arise. A life free of crises, in fact, is arguably undesirable, because the difficulties one must face provide the impetus for learning and problem-solving. And since special units are laboratories, they are places where new knowledge and fresh insights are developed as experiences cumulate. Solutions to unanticipated problems—even unsuccessful solutions—are a legacy from which programme staff and others can learn. A record of such experiences also provides a basis for evaluating programmes, given the problems with which they had to deal. The record is useful on another count: It provides a vehicle for cross-fertilization and a scientific basis for improved mental health services and correctional reform. Cumulating experiences of experimental programmes for disturbed and disruptive inmates must be recorded and shared, because they can ultimately help to lay the foundation for an effective approach to the rehabilitation of the most difficult clients in stressful confinement settings.

Retrospect

Emotionally disturbed prisoners who behave disruptively tend to be responded to in compartmentalized fashion. Their misbehaviour inspires punitive dispositions, while their symptoms invite ameliorative ministrations. The composite is fragmented, uncoordinated, illogical, and arguably iatrogenic, especially where it entails extended periods of disciplinary segregation, which exacerbate mental health problems.

The most promising interventions that have addressed the problem have involved the creation of special units staffed by teams comprising mental health and custodial workers. In these units, group-based and community-based therapeutic modalities can be deployed to address the dysfunctional behaviour of the unit residents. The treatment modalities typically include cognitive and emotional learning components. The learning process requires systematic analysis of destructive and/or self-destructive behaviour patterns of the unit residents. Emotional learning is experiential and must focus on here-and-now interpersonal difficulties experienced in the prison, with opportunities to rehearse constructive and prosocial behaviour.

Therapeutic unit regimes must be constituted to provide opportunities for intensive, constructive feedback and for support of change. The design and operation of these types of regime is a challenging task, which presupposes delicate sequencing and admixtures of permissiveness and structure, self-governance and disciplined guided rehabilitative experiences. No recipe for such enterprises exists, and the prison staff members who operate units for disturbed disruptive prisoners at present continue to be innovators and pioneers in relatively unexplored terrain.

Notes

1. J. curves or J distributions were first described by social psychologists interested in institutional conformity and non-conformity. According to Katz and Schanck (1938), "the J distribution has the practical importance of furnishing a measure of institutional strength and stability.... The more the distribution approaches the J form, and the steeper the curve, the stronger the institution" (pp. 45–46). Comparisons of hospital J curves to prison misconduct distributions confirm that hospital behaviour control is more effective.
2. The modal career pattern for disruptive prisoners is one of early involvements followed by sustained improved behaviour throughout the remainder of the inmate's stay in the prison.
3. In other countries—such as in Britain under the *Mental Health Act*—disruptive prisoners who are certified as mentally ill can be removed to hospital settings. The *British Prison Discipline Manual* calls for a medical examination before a disciplinary hearing takes place. A spokesman for the Prison Service points out that "the medical officer is required to examine a prisoner to a sufficient degree to enable him to advise the adjudicator whether or not the prisoner is fit to attend the hearing and, if necessary, to undergo a punishment of cellular confinement.... However, the Prison Discipline Manual makes it clear that the final decision as to whether or not the prisoner is fit to proceed is the adjudicator's" (Watson, 1999).
4. Clinical studies of prisoners in long-term segregation units have described the development of significant psychiatric symptomatology among individuals with no pre-existing symptoms (Grassian, 1983; Kupers, 1999). Such symptomatology is sufficiently prevalent to qualify as an iatrogenic disorder, known as the SHU syndrome.
5. An experiment in telemedicine (telecommunications links with medical consultants) was recently instituted in the US federal prison system. An evaluation of this experiment found that six of 10 consultations (58% of visits) were psychiatric in nature (McDonald, Hassol, & Carlson, 1999).
6. Barker and Mason (1968) suggested a need for transitional "re-training" of Penetang graduates. They wrote: "It must be remembered that a man who has accustomed himself to speak with complete honesty about what he feels and thinks about himself and other people is regarded as something of a nut in our society" (p. 70).

References

Barker, E.T. (1980). The Penetanguishene Program: A personal review. In H. Toch (Ed.), *Therapeutic communities in corrections* (pp. 73–81). New York: Praeger.

Barker, E.T., & Mason, M.H. (1968). Buber behind bars. *Canadian Psychiatric Association Journal, 13,* 61–71.

Barker, E.T., Mason, M.H., & Wilson, J. (1969). Defense-disrupting therapy. *Canadian Psychiatric Association Journal, 14,* 355–359.

Barr, H. (1999). *Prisons and jails: Hospitals of last resort.* New York: Correctional Association of New York and Urban Justice Center.

Boyle, J. (1977). *A sense of freedom.* London: Pan Canongate.

Clines, F.X. (1994, October 14). A futuristic prison awaits the hard-core 400. *New York Times,* pp. A1, B10.

Cloud, J. (1999, June 7). Mental health reform: What it would really take. *Time,* pp. 54–55.

Cohen, F. (1993). The legal context for mental health services. In H.J. Steadman & J.J. Cocozza (Eds.), *Mental illness in America's prisons* (pp. 25–60). Seattle: National Coalition for the Mentally Ill in the Criminal Justice System.

Cohen, F. (1995). "Pelican Bay": Excessive force, mental and general health care so deficient as to show deliberate indifference. *Correctional Law Reporter, 5,* 81–93.

Coid, J. (1991). Psychiatric profiles of difficult/disruptive prisoners. In K. Bottomley & W. Hay (Eds.), *Special units for difficult prisoners* (pp. 44–71). Hull, UK: Centre of Criminology and Criminal Justice, University of Hull.

Cooke, D.J. (1989). Containing violent prisoners: An analysis of the Barlinnie Special Unit. *British Journal of Criminology, 29,* 129–143.

Cooke, D.J. (1992). Violence in prisons: A Scottish perspective. *Forum on Corrections Research, 4,* 23–30.

Cooke, D.J. (1997). The Barlinnie Special Unit: The rise and fall of a therapeutic experiment. In E. Cullen, L. Jones, & R. Woodward (Eds.), *Therapeutic communities for offenders* (pp. 101–120). Chichester: Wiley.

Corcoran, K. (1992, September). *Violence and the mentally ill in prisons.* Paper presented at the annual meeting of the Howard League for Penal Reform, Oxford, UK.

Cullen, E. (1997). Can a prison be a therapeutic community? The Grendon template. In E. Cullen, L. Jones, & R. Woodward (Eds.), *Therapeutic communities for offenders* (pp. 75–99). Chichester: Wiley.

Fox, V. (1958). Analysis of prison disciplinary problems. *Journal of Criminal Law, Criminology and Police Science, 49,* 321–326.

Genders, E., & Player, E. (1995). *Grendon: A study of a therapeutic prison.* Oxford: Clarendon.

Gonnerman, J. (1999, May 25). The supermax solution. *Village Voice,* pp. 38–45.

Grassian, S. (1983). Psychopathological effects of solitary confinement. *American Journal of Psychiatry, 11,* 1450–1454.

Hartstone, E., Steadman, H.J., Robbins, P.C., & Monahan, J. (1984). Identifying and treating the mentally disordered prison inmate. In L.A. Teplin (Ed.), *Mental health and criminal justice* (pp. 279–296). Beverly Hills, CA: Sage.

Hershberger, J.L. (1998). To the max: Supermax facilities provide prison administrators with more security options. *Corrections Today, 60,* 54–61.

Innes, C.A., & Verdeyen, D.V. (1997). Conceptualizing the management of violent inmates. *Corrections Management Quarterly, 1,* 1–9.

Inspectorate of Prisons for Scotland. (1993). *Report on HM Special Unit, Barlinnie.* Edinburgh: Scottish Office.

Jemelka, R.P., Rahman, S., & Trupin, E.W. (1993). Prison mental health: An overview. In H.J. Steadman & J.J. Cocozza (Eds.), *Mental illness in America's prisons* (pp. 9–24). Seattle: National Coalition for the Mentally Ill in the Criminal Justice System.

Judge details inmate abuse at state prison. (1995, January 13). *New York Times,* p. 12.

Katz, D., & Schanck, R.L. (1938). *Social psychology.* New York: Wiley.

Kozol, H.L., Boucher, R.J., & Garofalo, R.F. (1972). The diagnosis and treatment of dangerousness. *Crime and Delinquency, 18,* 371–392.

Kupers, T. (1999). *Prison madness: The mental health crisis behind bars and what we must do about it.* San Francisco: Jossey-Bass.

Lewis, P. (1997). Context for change (whilst consigned and confined): A challenge for systematic thinking. In E. Cullen, L. Jones, & R. Woodward (Eds.), *Therapeutic communities for offenders* (pp. 207–222). Chichester: Wiley.

Light, R. (1985). The Special Unit, Barlinnie Prison. *Prison Service Journal, 60,* 14–21.

Lovell, D., & Jemelka, R. (1998). *A profile of inmates identified as behaviorally disturbed. Washington Department of Corrections: A report.* Seattle: University of Washington.

Lovell, D., & Rhodes, L.A. (1997). Mobile consultation: Crossing correctional boundaries to cope with disturbed offenders. *Federal Probation, 61,* 40–45.

McDonald, D., Hassol, A., & Carlson, K. (1999). Can telemedicine reduce spending and improve prisoner health care? *National Institute of Justice Journal,* April, 20–25.

Ohio "super-max" diverts inmates with serious mental illness. (1998). *Mental Health Weekly, 8,* 1–6.

Ouimet, M. (1999). Remarkable rarity of violence toward staff in prisons. *Forum on Corrections Research, 11,* 25–28.

Quinsey, V.L. (1977). Studies in the reduction of assaults in a maximum security psychiatric institution. *Canada's Mental Health, 25,* 21–23.

Quinsey, V.L. (1979). Assessments of the dangerousness of mental patients held in maximum security. *International Journal of Law and Psychiatry, 2,* 389–406.

Report of the Study Group on Dissociation (J.A. Vantour, Chair). (1975). Ottawa: Solicitor General of Canada.

Rice, M.E., & Harris, G.T. (1993). Treatment for prisoners with mental disorder. In H.J. Steadman & J.J. Cocozza (Eds.), *Mental illness in America's prisons* (pp. 91–130). Seattle: National Coalition for the Mentally Ill in the Criminal Justice System.

Rice, M.E., Harris, G.T., & Cormier, C.A. (1992). An evaluation of a maximum security therapeutic community for psychopaths and other mentally disordered offenders. *Law and Human Behavior, 16,* 399–412.

Rice, M.E., Harris, G.T., Varney, G.W., & Quinsey, V.L. (1989). *Violence in institutions: Understanding, prevention and control.* Toronto: Hans Huber.

St. Thomas Psychiatric Hospital. (1976). A program for the prevention and management of disturbed behavior. *Hospital and Community Psychiatry, 27,* 724–727.

Toch, H. (1980). The therapeutic community as community. In H. Toch (Ed.), *Therapeutic communities in corrections* (pp. 3–20). New York: Praeger.

Toch, H. (1982). The disturbed disruptive inmate: Where does the bus stop? *Journal of Psychiatry and Law, 10,* 327–349.

Toch, H. (1992). *Living in prison: The ecology of survival.* Washington: American Psychological Association/APA Books.

Toch, H. (1995). Case managing multi-problem offenders. *Federal Probation, 59,* 41–47.

Toch, H. (1998). Psychopathy or antisocial personality in forensic settings. In T. Millon, E. Simonsen, M. Birket-Smith, & R.D. Davis (Eds.), *Psychopathy: Antisocial, criminal and violent behavior* (pp. 144–158). New York: Guilford.

Toch, H., & Adams, K. (1987). In the eye of the beholder? Assessments of psychopathology among prisoners by federal prison staff. *Journal of Research in Crime and Delinquency, 24,* 119–139.

Toch, H., & Adams, K. (1994). *The disturbed violent offender.* Washington: American Psychological Association/APA Books.

Toch, H., & Adams, K., with Grant, J.D. (1989). *Coping: Maladaptation in prisons.* New Brunswick, NJ: Transaction.

Vantour, J.A. (1991). Canadian experience: The special handling unit. In K. Bottomley & W. Hay (Eds.), *Special units for difficult prisoners* (pp. 89–98). Hull, UK: Centre for Criminology and Criminal Justice, University of Hull.

Watson, T. (1999, Winter). The Prison Service writes. *Inside Time,* p. 5.

Wechsler, H. (1997). Therapeutic communities in American prisons. In E. Cullen, L. Jones, & R. Woodward (Eds.), *Therapeutic communities for offenders* (pp. 165–179). Chichester: Wiley.

Winerap, M. (1999, June 3). After years adrift, treatment in jail. *New York Times,* pp. B1, B7.

Wozniak, E. (1995). The future of small units in the Scottish prison service. *Prison Service Journal,* 101, 14–18.

Hans Toch is associated with the School of Criminal Justice, State University of New York at Albany, Albany, New York, USA.

Author's Note

Comments or queries may be directed to Hans Toch, School of Criminal Justice, Nelson A. Rockefeller College of Public Affairs and Policy, State University of New York, 135 Western Avenue, Albany NY 12222 USA. Telephone: 518 442-5228. Fax: 518 442-5603.

Section V

PREVENTING VIOLENCE IN THE COMMUNITY

THE EFFICACY AND EFFECTIVENESS OF COMMUNITY TREATMENT PROGRAMMES IN PREVENTING CRIME AND VIOLENCE AMONG THOSE WITH SEVERE MENTAL ILLNESS IN THE COMMUNITY

KIRK HEILBRUN
LORI PETERS

There have recently been signs in the United States that treatment of mentally disordered offenders in the community will be influenced by laws and policies inclined towards longer-term incarceration and greater restriction on individual liberties. This represents a marked shift from the US tendency towards community-based treatment of mentally disordered offenders that has parallelled the deinstitutionalization movement for civilly committed patients over the past three decades. The 1997 US Supreme Court decision in *Kansas v. Hendricks* (1997), involving post-sentence commitment for sexual offenders who have completed a prison sentence, provides a good example of this trend. Public concern about mentally disordered offenders, as with criminal offenders more generally, will not only affect the programmes and interventions that can be offered in the community; it will also underscore the importance of crime and violence as outcome measures of the effectiveness of Community Based Forensic Treatment (CBFT) with this population.

For the purposes of this chapter, it is useful to distinguish between effectiveness studies, which focus on the impact of interventions made under usual conditions, and efficacy studies, which use controlled designs (such as clinical trials) to assess impact under ideal or "best practice" conditions (Wells, 1999). Our primary focus will be on effectiveness research in reviewing studies on the risk of violence and crime among those with severe mental disorders, in large part because there has been relatively little research using efficacy designs in this area. Some of the reasons for this will be addressed later in this chapter. Nevertheless, we will review the literature with the goal of facilitating empirically informed judgements about the impact of various interventions in preventing future violence and other crime by individuals who have received treatment services.

Issues of Definition

"Mentally disordered offender" has been used most often to designate an individual in one of five categories: (1) Incompetent to Stand Trial, (2) Not Guilty by Reason of Insanity (NGRI), (3) Mentally Disordered Sex Offender, or (4) Mentally Ill jail or prison inmate (Steadman, Monahan, Hartstone, Davis, & Robbins, 1982). In the

S. Hodgins (ed.), Violence among the Mentally Ill, 341–357.
© 2000 *Kluwer Academic Publishers. Printed in the Netherlands.*

community, the most applicable of these are (a) Parole or Probation, or (b) NGRI on conditional release (Heilbrun & Griffin, 1993, 1998). We will confine our focus to adults, since risk factors and relevant interventions may differ significantly with juveniles (Gordon, Arbuthnot, & Jurkovic, 1998). "Mental disorder" will include various forms of severe mental illness and co-occurring disorders such as substance abuse and personality disorder, but will not encompass individuals with substance abuse as the only diagnosis.

"Community-based" programmes and services will include halfway houses, outpatient clinics, crisis stabilization units, and inpatient psychiatric facilities that provide emergency or short-term mental health treatment in the community, but will not include jails. Those delivering such services will include not only psychiatrists, psychologists, social workers and nurses, but also case managers and parole and probation officers.

"Treatment services" will include psychotropic medication, case management, psychosocial rehabilitation, therapy and counselling, vocational training, and other forms of treatment. We will also include interventions designed for specific deficits (e.g., anger control difficulties or problem-solving deficits), as well as case management services.

Procedures

We identified articles published between January 1976 and January 2000 through the computerized databases PSYCHINFO, PSYCHALERT, Criminal Justice Periodical Index, Sociological Abstracts, MEDLINE, and EMBASE. Each empirical study so identified was categorized as having either: (1) an experimental or quasi-experimental design, with an intervention delivered to the experimental group, and a control group that received either a different intervention or simply the standard criminal justice conditions, with assignment to condition made randomly or participants matched across groups; or (2) a design in which a group was measured in terms of predictor and outcome variables, sometimes with a "comparison" group (neither matched nor randomly assigned) measured on the same predictors and outcomes.

Literature Review

META-ANALYSIS ON THE PREDICTION OF CRIMINAL AND VIOLENT RECIDIVISM AMONG MENTALLY DISORDERED OFFENDERS

A meta-analysis of studies published between 1959 and 1995 on the prediction of criminal and violent recidivism in mentally disordered offenders (Bonta, Law, & Hanson, 1998) is relevant for present purposes because this analysis permits the calculation of the predictive value of variables in several domains (demographic, criminal history, deviant lifestyle history, and clinical) for "general recidivism" (an arrest or rehospitalization for criminal behaviour) and "violent recidivism" (criminal re-offending involving an offence against persons). Since these studies do not address questions about the risk-reduction value of interventions, it is clear that its focus is on accuracy in *predicting* recidivism rather than gauging the impact of such interventions (see, for example, Heilbrun, 1997).

However, this meta-analysis does provide useful data on the empirical relationship between theoretically relevant risk factors and the outcomes of crime and violence. The strongest predictors of either form of recidivism for mentally disordered offenders were similar to those for offenders without mental disorder; criminal history (e.g., adult crime, juvenile delinquency, violence) was among the most powerful predictors, and clinical variables were among the weakest. Of particular relevance was the finding that the average effect size for "treatment history" as a predictor of general recidivism was nonsignificant. It is possible that this finding is attributable to the prevalence of mental health interventions that address deficits that are not risk-relevant or "criminogenic," and that interventions designed more specifically to reduce violence or crime would show a more favourable impact. This was the explanation offered by the authors (Bonta et al., 1998), and it certainly appears to merit research attention through the design and delivery of risk-relevant interventions and the measurement of their impact through appropriate outcome research.

REVIEWS OF COMMUNITY-BASED TREATMENT RELEVANT TO CRIME AND VIOLENCE

Several reviews of CBFT have focused on describing programmes and interventions for NGRI acquittees in the community (Heilbrun & Griffin, 1993) or NGRI acquittees and individuals with mental disorder on parole or probation (Heilbrun & Griffin, 1998), or have presented an overview of forensic treatment (Heilbrun & Griffin, 1999). These reviews suggest that most of the published information on CBFT is provided by a small number of sites; it is not clear how well their results can be generalized to sites and jurisdictions that do not publish such data. Also, few published accounts are empirical studies employing experimental or quasi-experimental designs, or performing inferential statistical analyses. Finally, even for the studies that are empirical and use inferential statistics, the majority have regression-based designs that are helpful in predicting an outcome (including crime or other behaviour that may result in rehospitalization, such as non-compliance with release conditions, but rarely on self-reported or collateral descriptions of violent behaviour). Very infrequently, however, are they designed to assess the impact of a particular intervention or programme.

TYPE 1 (EXPERIMENTAL OR QUASI-EXPERIMENTAL) STUDIES

In this section, we review studies having an experimental or quasi-experimental design in which one group received an intervention and a control group received either a different intervention or no intervention beyond the standard criminal justice conditions. Assignment to condition in Type 1 studies either was random or the control group was matched on relevant dimensions such as age, gender, race, criminal history, and mental disorder. Two studies met these criteria.

In a study involving NGRI acquittees ($N = 235$) from California (Wiederanders, 1992), one group was on conditional release in the community and a second group had been released into the community following hospitalization as NGRI but was not on conditional release. The group on conditional release had to meet requirements involving treatment compliance and other conditions. Individuals in the conditionally released group had a significantly lower arrest rate; they were also rehospitalized at a somewhat higher rate, although the latter difference was not statistically significant.

The second study (Cohen, Spodak, Silver, & Williams, 1998; Silver, Cohen, & Spodak, 1989) considered both hospital intervention and post-release community outcome. It included three groups: (1) NGRI acquittees ($N = 127$), (2) individuals convicted of felonies ($N = 127$), matched with the first group for age, race, length of incarceration, and type of offence, and (3) mentally disordered offenders transferred from prison to hospital for treatment ($N = 135$). Individuals in the first group had been acquitted by reason of insanity of felonies, released under a 5-year conditional release, and had lived in the community for an average of 10.5 years (ranging from 7 to 17 years). The outcomes of arrest, severity of offence, hospitalization, employment, and global functioning were assessed at three times: after 2.5 years, after 5 years, and over the entire follow-up period (up to 17 years). Rearrest rates after 5 years were as follows: NGRI acquittees 54%, convicted felon control group 65%, and hospitalized mentally disordered offenders 73%. Discriminant function analysis between arrested and not arrested sub-groups of NGRI acquittees showed that re-arrest was predicted by prior arrests, alcoholism, unemployment, type of offence, prior hospitalization for mental illness, hospital adjustment, and clinical assessment of hospital adjustment.

These studies demonstrate that it is possible to apply an efficacy design in studying an intervention such as conditional release with mentally disordered offenders in the community. Both were carried out by investigating a procedure that was already established, rather than assigned for the purpose of the study. While it is clearly more difficult to persuade officials to sanction a study that assigns conditions randomly for experimental purposes, even that task can be accomplished when appropriate safeguards are provided. For example, a group of Duke University researchers persuaded hospital and judicial authorities to allow the random assignment of outpatient commitment following hospitalization in order to assess its impact on rehospitalization (Swartz et al., 1999), in part because patients who were perceived as high risk were treated in a more controlled fashion than randomly assigned to condition. While such a design is more difficult to implement, it is particularly valuable because (as this section has clearly demonstrated) it is rare and because it provides much more specific data on the impact of particular interventions on outcomes of interest.

TYPE 2 (COMPARISON AND SINGLE GROUP) STUDIES

A larger number of studies used a design in which one group was measured in terms of predictor and outcome variables, with a "comparison" group (neither matched nor randomly assigned) also measured on these variables, or a single group in which predictor and outcome variables were analyzed using multiple regression. Such studies have examined the effect of (1) differences between jurisdictions, (2) diagnosis, (3) treatment/commitment, (4) type of release, and (5) type of case management.

One study considered insanity acquittees in three US states (California, New York, and Oregon), providing data on the rates of client contact, revocation of conditional release, re-offence, and rehospitalization for individuals over different periods (Oregon: 1978–86, N = 366; New York: 1980–87, N = 331; California: 1986–93, N = 888) (Wiederanders, Bromley, & Choate, 1997). California had the most frequent monthly outpatient service contacts, with Oregon reporting an intermediate number and New York the lowest. California also had the lowest "estimated annualized arrest rate" (3.4%), with Oregon at an intermediate level (5.8%) and New York at the highest (7.8%). This relationship between more service contacts and fewer arrests was seen most clearly for less serious offences, suggesting that intensive monitoring in the community (as provided through California's conditional release programme) might function to lower the risk of antisocial behaviour leading to arrest. Alternatively, it may be that minor acts of antisocial behaviour in California's programme were in some cases handled through means other than arrest.

An important programme of study was been carried out over more than a decade in Oregon. These studies addressed the impact of conditional release for individuals hospitalized as NGRI and subsequently returned from hospitalization into the community under the jurisdiction of the Oregon Psychiatric Security Review Board (PSRB) (Bigelow, Bloom, & Williams, 1990; Bloom & Bloom, 1981; Bloom, Bradford, & Kofoed, 1988; Bloom, Rogers, & Manson, 1982; Bloom, Rogers, Manson, & Williams, 1986; Bloom, Williams, & Bigelow, 1991, 1992; Bloom, Willliams, Rogers, & Barbur, 1986). This research used legislative changes in the forensic mental health system—implementation of the PSRB and conditional release—to assess the impact of conditional release and a review panel on outcomes such as rearrest and rehospitalization. A total of 971 NGRI acquittees were followed between 1978 and 1986 (Bloom et al., 1992). Findings suggest that conditional release is associated with a lower rate of criminal offending while the individual is under Review Board jurisdiction in the community. In one study (Bloom, Rogers, et al., 1986), the lifetime police contacts (including arrests and subarrest encounters) were compared for patients prior to, during, and following PSRB jurisdiction. The rate of police contacts per patient per year was 0.78 prior to conditional release, 0.20 while on conditional release under PSRB jurisdiction, and 0.54 following release from PSRB jurisdiction. When only patients with schizophrenia were studied (Bloom et al., 1992), a similar pattern was observed. Of 381 individuals, only 57 had criminal justice contacts while under PSRB jurisdiction. Following discharge from PSRB jurisdiction, subjects had significantly fewer criminal justice contacts (0.41 contacts per year) than they had before PSRB jurisdiction (0.69 per year). The Oregon studies point to the importance of conditional release, careful monitoring, centralized and rapid decision-making, and treatment interventions to address needs associated with symptoms, life skills, housing, and work in reducing the risk of criminal arrest.

Two types of release from secure hospitalization into the community for NGRI acquittees have been studied: (1) conditional release directly from the programme into the community, and (2) conditional release from the programme to a regional hospital, and then to the community (Silver et al., 1989; Tellefsen, Cohen, Silver, & Dougherty, 1992). Four outcomes were measured 5 years after release: (1) rearrest, (2) overall functioning in the community, (3) rehospitalization for mental illness, and (4) successful completion (non-revocation) of the conditional release. Discriminant analysis classified these four outcomes with an overall accuracy rate between 69% and 83% for the directly released patients and between 88% and 96% for the regionally released individuals. Such findings suggest that these groups can be distinguished at better than chance levels, although there was no cross-validation. The regionally released group was arrested more frequently (63% vs. 47%) and more quickly, and committed more serious offences, than the directly released group. No difference in the rate of rehospitalization was observed, but there was a difference in duration of rehospitalization: the regionally released group was rehospitalized for a longer period. Since there was no random assignment to release type, we cannot conclude that the "regional release" process was causally related to poorer outcome.

A study of the NGRI conditional release process in New York State communities (McGreevy, Steadman, Dvoskin, & Dollard, 1991) reviewed all NGRI acquittees on conditional release in New York State between 1980 and 1987 ($N = 331$) over an average outcome period of 3.8 years. During this period, a total of 22% of the individuals were arrested, and 5% were recommitted, with most rearrests and recommitments occurring during the first year in the community. Several "key features" of a successful conditional release programme were identified: centralized responsibility, a uniform system of treatment and supervision, and a network of community services.

Three studies focused on the characteristics of case management services. First, the impact of "assertive case management" was compared with that of standard case management,[1] by tracking individuals with chronic mental disorders ($N = 26$) who received case management services. Over a period of 36 months, they were compared with similar individuals ($N = 33$) who did not receive case management services (Wilson, Tien, & Eaves, 1995). Criminal justice contacts for both groups were recorded at 6, 12, and 18 months before incarceration and again at 6, 12, and 18 months after release. No significant differences between these groups were found in the average number of days spent in jail *before* incarceration. *Following* incarceration, however, the group receiving case management services spent fewer days in correctional institutions, and more days in the community ($M = 270.0$ days vs. $M = 119.6$ days), before coming into contact with the criminal justice system. These findings, although limited in their generalizability by both the research design and the small number of participants, are consistent with the assertion of a second pair of investigators (Dvoskin & Steadman, 1994), that intensive case management can reduce the risk of violence and criminality by mentally disordered offenders in the community.

The third study compared styles of case management provided as part of a randomized clinical trial for seriously mentally ill people who were homeless and leaving a large urban jail system (Solomon & Draine, 1995; Solomon, Draine, & Meyerson, 1994). A total of 60 individuals were assigned to the Assertive Community Treatment (ACT) team of case managers, 60 to individual case managers at community mental health centres, and 80 to the usual aftercare conditions of local mental health centres. A total of 41% of the clients were returned to jail, with significant differences reported among clients served by the ACT team (56%), assigned to individual case managers (22%), and referred to mental health centres (36%). The use of intensive case management in this study (unlike in the California study of conditional release; see Wiederanders, 1992) was *more* likely to result in reincarceration, which ACT case managers tended to seek even for relatively minor offences and technical violations. The contrasting results of these studies (Wiederanders, 1992, vs. Solomon & Draine; Solomon et al.) might suggest that the common features of conditional release and ACT yield more frequent contact with clients; whether such increased contact results in a different risk of incarceration probably depends on the policies of the larger programme and the experience and styles of individual case managers in the face of minor antisocial behaviour by clients.

A Swedish study (Belfrage, 1991) addressed the impact of mandatory psychiatric hospital treatment, compared with prison, on two groups: (1) offenders judged to have treatment needs equivalent to those of insanity acquittees ($N = 298$), and (2) offenders who did not have equivalent treatment needs ($N = 256$). The two groups were similar in age, gender, having previous criminal arrests, and the types of crime of which they were convicted, although not equivalent in the distribution of mental health diagnoses, with diagnoses of "borderline," "psychosis," "mental retardation," and "brain damage" observed in the first group but not in the second. Neither the treatment needs nor the interventions (mandatory psychiatric treatment and prison, respectively) for these groups were equivalent, so the relative impact of each intervention cannot be determined. Interestingly, however, violent offenders in the first group (psychiatric treatment) released to the community re-offended at a lower rate during the 3-year outcome period than those who had been imprisoned for violent offences. However, property offenders from the two groups re-offended at comparable rates, suggesting that community interventions for individuals with mental disorders might be more effective in reducing the risk of violent offending than property crimes.

Another study focused on the impact of specialized community treatment of mentally disordered offenders in Germany who are sentenced to hospital as an alternative to prison, meeting the criteria for either (a) diminished or absent criminal responsibility, or (b) high risk for future serious offending (Müller-Isberner, 1996). While on conditional release, one group ($N = 56$) were treated in a specialized forensic psychiatric clinic in the community, while another group ($N = 67$) did not receive that form of treatment. In the second group, about one third had no aftercare and the remainder received services through non-forensic outpatient institutions such as homes for the mentally ill, rehabilitation centres, and psychiatrists in private practice. More patients in the first group (specialized clinic) had initial offences involving violent crime or arson (89%) than those in the group not receiving services from the clinic (76%). This result notwithstanding, the percentage of clinic patients who were detected for another violent offence, or arson, was lower than the percentage of non-clinic patients (5% vs. 12%, over 32 and 31 months, respectively). The finding of a lower recidivism rate in a possibly higher-risk group is consistent with other findings discussed in this section on the potential risk-reducing impact of specialized forensic community intervention, although the absence of random assignment or matching in this study means that this can be considered only as suggestive.

Several studies have examined the influence of psychopathology on criminal recidivism. One study (Rice & Harris, 1992) considered individuals diagnosed with schizophrenia who had been treated in a maximum security facility and subsequently released ($N = 96$), and compared them with a matched sample of non-schizophrenic individuals who had been evaluated but not treated at the same facility ($N = 96$). Over an outcome period that ranged from initial contact (between 1975 and 1981) to final rating (1988), individuals with schizophrenia showed a significantly lower rate of criminal recidivism than individuals without this disorder (35% vs. 53%), and a somewhat lower rate of violent recidivism (16% vs. 24%). The difference in violent recidivism between these two groups was not statistically significant, however. These findings underscore the importance of the nature of the comparison group in determining how a certain variable may relate to an outcome such as crime or violence. In the Rice and Harris study, individuals with schizophrenia were compared with another group that contained individuals at relatively high risk for re-offending (such as psychopaths), so schizophrenia was associated with a lower risk for offending. However, if individuals with schizophrenia or other forms of severe mental disorder were compared with members of the general population without mental disorder, these mental disorders might be associated with higher rates of violent behaviour.[2]

In another study on mental illness as a risk factor for crime (Feder, 1991), offenders who were hospitalized for psychiatric reasons during prison incarceration ($N = 147$) were compared with those who were not ($N = 400$) over an 18-month period following release. Age and prior criminal record were associated with rearrest risk for both groups. No significant differences were found between these two groups in the rates or types of rearrest, except for drug offences (12% of the non-mentally ill group was arrested for drug offences, while 5% of the mentally ill group was arrested for such offences).

Diagnosis as a risk factor for re-offending was addressed (Hodgins & Gaston, 1989) by comparing five groups of individuals (total $N = 181$) adjudicated Incompetent to Stand Trial or NGRI in Quebec between 1973 and 1975. Using discriminant function analysis, the following groups were distinguished: (1) career criminals, (2) chronic schizophrenics, (3) violent psychotics, (4) violent middle-class individuals, and (5) intellectually handicapped individuals (see Hodgins, 1983, for a more complete description). When followed for an average of 6.1 years in the community following hospital discharge, these groups differed in the severity of their offending and the length of their sentences, but not in the frequency of their rehospitalization. "Career criminals" committed the fewest violent crimes, intellectually handicapped individuals the most.[3] The authors caution that the latter finding needs replication and should not be accepted uncritically.

Another study considered the relationship between (a) diagnostic and demographic characteristics, and (b) future criminal behaviour in 611 young adults who received public inpatient, outpatient, and community residential care in Missouri (Holcomb & Ahr, 1988). Substance abuse and organic brain syndrome were most strongly associated with offending during the 1-year outcome period; schizophrenia, major affective disorder, and personality disorder were associated with lower overall rates of offending. There were no differences between these groups in their respective rates of violent re-offending, however. Younger age, minority group membership, more lifetime felony arrests, and a younger age at which public mental health services were first received were also associated with higher overall re-offence risk.

Psychopathy as a risk factor for re-offending in mentally disordered offenders ($N = 169$) released from maximum security psychiatric hospitalization in Canada and followed over an average outcome period of 10 years has been addressed (Harris, Rice, & Cormier, 1991). Psychopathy was measured using the Psychopathy Checklist (completed on a "file only" basis). Psychopathy was a strong risk factor for violent re-offending; 77% of psychopaths but only 40% of the total sample committed a violent offence during the outcome period. These differences in violent re-offending were observed even for individuals over 40 years old.

Three groups of NGRI acquittees ($N = 61$) in Oklahoma—those released at an initial court review, those who completed the NGRI treatment programme, and those who escaped from secure hospitalization—indicated that those who had escaped during hospitalization had significantly more previous and subsequent arrests (over an outcome period that averaged more than 2.5 years) than those who had been discharged from treatment (Nicholson, Norwood, & Enyart, 1991). During this period, 16.6% of patients were rearrested, 16.6% were rehospitalized, and 16.6% were both rearrested and rehospitalized.

Finally, several studies are important because they identify risk factors for violence and crime in the community in similar populations with severe mental disorders. In a large-scale study of community violence among individuals with mental disorder (Steadman et al., 1998), a total of 1,136 male and female patients between the ages of 18 and 40 were monitored for violence towards others every 10 weeks during the year following discharge from psychiatric hospitalization. These results were compared with violence towards others by a comparison group ($N = 519$) that had been randomly sampled from the same census tracts as the patient group. Aggression was divided into two categories of seriousness: (1) serious acts of violence (battery resulting in physical injury, sexual assaults, and threats with a weapon), and (2) other aggressive acts (battery that did not result in physical injury and threats without a weapon). Information was obtained at 10-week intervals from self-report and collateral report (an observer who had been nominated by the participant at the beginning of the study), and through agency records reflecting arrest or rehospitalization. Several of their important findings include (1) the co-occurrence of a substance-abuse diagnosis with major mental disorders in 40–50% of cases; (2) the significant addition of self-report and collateral report to the identified frequency of violence and other aggressive acts beyond the frequency reflected in official records, raising this rate from 4.5% to 27.5% for violence and from 8.8% to 56.1% for other aggressive acts during the index period; (3) substance abuse was associated with increased frequency of both serious violence and other aggressive acts; (4) the patient group without substance abuse did not differ from the community control group without substance abuse in the frequency of either violence or other aggressive acts; (5) patients had symptoms of substance abuse more often than community controls; and (6) the patient group showed a greater risk of violence and other aggressive acts than community controls when both experienced symptoms of substance abuse, particularly during the period immediately following hospital discharge.

This study strongly suggests that patients with co-occurring psychotic and substance abuse disorders should be considered at higher risk (consistent with other recent European studies; see Modestin & Ammann, 1995; Raesaenen et al., 1998; Tiihonen, Isohanni, Raesaenen, Koiranen, & Moring, 1997), although it did not address the impact of a particular intervention. It also emphasizes the value of the use of collateral information in estimating the frequency at which violence occurs. One of the particular weaknesses of research on violence and aggression has been insensitive outcome measures (Monahan & Steadman, 1994). It is likely that studies using only rearrest and rehospitalization as outcome measures of crime or violence will significantly underestimate the incidence of relevant behaviour during the follow-up period. The addition of self-report and collateral report, as in this study (Steadman et al., 1998) and others (e.g., Lidz, Mulvey, & Gardner, 1993), is very likely to improve sensitivity in the detection of violence and result in a more accurate way of determining the accuracy of predictions or the impact of risk-reduction interventions.

The Efficacy and Effectiveness of Community Treatment Programmes in Preventing Crime and Violence

The literature provides limited empirical research that is relevant and well designed to address the impact of specific programmes or particular interventions in reducing the risk of non-violent crime or violent behaviour in mentally disordered offenders in the community. Most of the relevant research has used either single groups or two groups in a non-experimental design. It would require a major shift in research strategies to yield a sufficient number of studies to allow empirically based conclusions regarding effect sizes for interventions. This is the kind of information that would be most useful to programmes and treatment providers involved in risk-reducing rehabilitation for mentally disordered offenders in hospital and community settings, however.

This caution notwithstanding, it is possible to summarize several considerations that are empirically supported in designing community programmes and delivering interventions to reduce violence and criminality. First, the programme must identify the prevention of violence and criminality as among its most important goals, and communicate this priority to staff, clients, and others. Conditional release, increased intensity of outpatient case management, specialized programming designed for skills-based training among the severely mentally ill and delivered by those experienced with forensic populations, the delivery of a range of services including housing support and vocational assistance as well as clinical treatment, and a particular focus on rehabilitating and preventing substance abuse (whether it occurs as a primary diagnosis or co-occurs with a major mental disorder) can serve as tools to reduce the risk of violence. When programmes incorporate these services and conditions to the greatest extent possible, they are guided by the best empirical literature now available.

Another important step involves the assessment of risk for individual clients. A plan designed to minimize the risk for crime and violence in the community would consider relevant risk factors and determine which apply to the individual. Relevant risk factors include static variables (those that do not change through planned intervention, such as age, gender, and criminal history) and dynamic variables (those than have the potential to change through intervention, such as substance abuse and medication non-compliance). The two-stage process of assessing risk that may be seen in some of the recent risk-assessment tools such as the HCR-20 (Webster, Eaves, Douglas, & Wintrup, 1995) allows both a priori classification of risk, based primarily on static risk factors combined actuarially, and a section on dynamic risk factors that are relevant to risk-reduction intervention planning. When both stages are administered to an individual in a community programme, there are resulting implications for the intensity of the interventions and monitoring (higher for higher-risk individuals) and the nature of the interventions (delivered to address the individual's relevant risk factors). Given the emerging evidence on the value of the HCR-20 in relevant populations (Douglas, Ogloff, Nicholls, & Grant, 1999; Douglas & Webster, 1999), its use must be seriously considered in this context. It should be added, however, that a tool such as the Violence Risk Appraisal Guide (VRAG; see Harris, Rice, & Quinsey, 1993) would also be useful if the purpose were to obtain an empirically supported prediction of long-term re-offence risk (Quinsey, Harris, Rice, & Cormier, 1998), which could be combined with the assessment of dynamic risk factors in a comparable two-step process. This kind of approach focuses planning and service delivery in areas that are "criminogenic" (risk-reducing) and functions to divert individuals from further criminal behaviour, helping them build the skills that will allow them to lead responsible lives.

Implications

PRACTICE

Community programmes can prevent crime and violence by functioning effectively, and heeding what is currently available from the literature in the form of empirical guidance. Certain principles of effective community-based forensic treatment programmes have been described (Griffin, Steadman, & Heilbrun, 1991; Heilbrun & Griffin, 1998), and others can be added (Heilbrun & Peters, 2000) based on the current review:

1. Use conditional release, parole, or probation as a mechanism for designing and implementing treatment and monitoring compliance.
2. Communication encompassing both criminal justice and mental health personnel is essential for success.
3. Clarify the legal requirements in areas such as confidentiality and duty to protect, specific reporting demands (e.g., child abuse), and malpractice.
4. There must be an explicit balance between individual rights, the need for treatment, and public safety.
5. Set, practice, and monitor sound "risk management" procedures, including risk assessment and intervention planning, obtaining records, questioning clients re-

garding violent thoughts and acts, and communicating such information as indicated.

6. It is important to know the range of supervision and treatment needs of clients who will be served in the community, particularly "criminogenic" factors such as anger control, vocational skills, co-occurring disorders, and housing support.
7. Treat and monitor high-risk clients more intensely.
8. Allow clients to demonstrate increasing degrees of responsibility through progressively less intense levels of monitoring and greater levels of privilege.
9. Overall programme planning should include the delivery of interventions for common risk factors for mentally disordered offenders, including substance abuse, anger/impulse control, medication compliance, job skills, living circumstances, problem-solving skills, and social support.
10. Practise principles that promote health-care compliance (such as behavioural contracting), including specification of the conditions and expectations for treatment and the consequences of violating these conditions.
11. Develop a uniform system of treatment and supervision, to be applied within a network of community services.
12. Careful monitoring can provide information useful for a variety of purposes, including treatment planning, programme evaluation, and research on intervention effectiveness.

RESEARCH

It should be clear that the most important priority for research into reducing the risk for violence and crime by mentally disordered offenders in the community is the area of the impact of interventions on subsequent risk. Such interventions could be broad (e.g., conditional release), specific to a programme (e.g., one designed for individuals with co-occurring severe mental disorder and substance abuse on parole, incorporating case management, substance-abuse treatment, housing support, vocational training, and relapse prevention), and even more specific interventions (e.g., training in problem-solving skills) on the behavioural outcomes of crime and violence. These implications may be summarized as follows:

1. More controlled study of treatment interventions, specifically designed to address criminogenic deficits and strengthen protective factors, is needed. This could be accomplished in the community through the introduction of small pilot treatment programmes that could be contrasted with the outcomes obtained using the conditions of standard parole or conditional release. Since such programmes would be small, it might be possible to select participants on a random basis and obtain a clearer view of the impact of the programme itself.

2. Increased collaboration between external researchers and programmes, or research by programme staff, would help to facilitate such research. For example, some community treatment programmes for mentally disordered offenders have been developed as part of a collaboration between an agency or board and external researchers from a nearby university. This is an efficient form of collaboration in that it benefits both participants, and results in better research as a consequence.

3. Research in this area can be facilitated through the use of naturally occurring "experiments." Changes in law or policy, or policy that mandates some participants will be under jurisdiction for only a limited period of time, provide useful opportunities to examine the influence of important considerations such as the intensity of treatment and monitoring, the form of coercion (formal vs. informal), the durability of reduction in offending across changes in legal circumstances, and the "survival times" for outcomes such as substance-abuse relapse, medication non-compliance, and other risk factors relevant to offending.

4. Attention to both internal and external validity is important. More sensitive measurement of the outcomes of crime and violence is necessary, for example. Unless researchers can be confident that they have detected most relevant behaviour that has occurred, data on the impact of interventions cannot be meaningful. This is particularly true if there is some systematic bias in underreporting of violence on the part of certain kinds of clients. The use of self-report and collateral observer contact, in addition to official records, has yielded a more accurate estimate of the prevalence of violent behaviour in the community. This kind of enhanced sensitivity in outcome reporting can use features that are already in place in many systems and programmes treating mentally disordered offenders in the community. Likewise, there must be consideration of internal validity. Researchers must be confident that interventions purporting to deliver treatment in the area of relapse prevention, for example, actually do so consistently. The importance of treatment integrity is clear, and may be facilitated by the application of manualized interventions in some areas.

5. Research is needed on the relative impact of interventions for clients at different risk levels. Several promising research tools for assessing the risk of violence and crime in mentally disordered offenders have been introduced within the last 8 years. Such tools can be used in the attempt to discriminate sub-groups that may respond favourably to risk-reducing interventions from those that do not. When this is better understood, additional risk tools that are sensitive to treatment response and change in risk status can be added to the measures currently available, enhancing the accuracy of empirically informed planning and decision-making.

Notes

1. Standard case management services involve assistance to clients in areas such as housing, vocational or public assistance, transportation, substance abuse, mental health, and others as indicated. Assertive or intensive case management involves the additional feature of smaller caseloads for the case manager, permitting more frequent contacts and possibly additional services.
2. A re-analysis of data from the Epidemiologic Catchment Area study found that the presence of obsessive compulsive disorder, panic disorder, major depression, major depression with grief, mania or bipolar disorder, or schizophrenia or schizophreniform disorder raised

the frequency of self-reported violent behaviour during the preceding year from 2% (without these disorders) to 10–12%. Drug abuse was a stronger risk factor, raising the self-reported violence rate to 19% (cannabis), 25% (alcohol), and 35% (other drug) (Swanson, Holzer, Ganju, & Jono, 1990). This study is not included among those formally reviewed in this chapter, because the participants were not in the groups on which we have focused in the present discussion.

3. For a more complete discussion of patterns of criminal behaviour among mentally retarded persons, when compared with those without mental retardation, see Crocker and Hodgins (1997).

References

Belfrage, H. (1991). The crime preventive effect of psychiatric treatment on mentally disordered offenders in Sweden. *International Journal of Law and Psychiatry, 14,* 237–243.

Bigelow, D.A., Bloom, J.D., & Williams, M.H. (1990). Costs of managing insanity acquittees under a psychiatric security review board system. *Hospital and Community Psychiatry, 41,* 613–614.

Bloom, J.D., Bradford, J.M., & Kofoed, L. (1988). An overview of psychiatric treatment approaches to three offender groups. *Hospital and Community Psychiatry, 39,* 151–158.

Bloom, J.D., Rogers, J., & Manson, S. (1982). After Oregon's insanity defense: A comparison of conditional release and hospitalization. *International Journal of Law and Psychiatry, 5,* 391–402.

Bloom, J.D., Rogers, J., Manson, S., & Williams, M. (1986). Lifetime police contacts of discharged Psychiatric Security Review Board clients. *International Journal of Law and Psychiatry, 8,* 189–202.

Bloom, J.D., Williams, M.H., & Bigelow, D.A. (1991). Monitored conditional release of persons found Not Guilty by Reason of Insanity. *American Journal of Psychiatry, 148,* 444–448.

Bloom, J.D., Williams, M.H., & Bigelow, D.A. (1992). The involvement of schizophrenic insanity acquittees in the mental health and criminal justice systems. *Psychiatric Clinics of North America, 15,* 591–604.

Bloom, J.D., Williams, M., Rogers, J., & Barbur, P. (1986). Evaluation and treatment of insanity acquittees in the community. *Bulletin of the American Academy of Psychiatry and the Law, 14,* 231–244.

Bloom, J.L., & Bloom, J.D. (1981). Disposition of insanity defenses in Oregon. *Bulletin of the American Academy of Psychiatry and the Law, 9,* 93–100.

Bonta, J., Law, M., & Hanson, K. (1998). The prediction of criminal and violent recidivism among mentally disordered offenders: A meta-analysis. *Psychological Bulletin, 123,* 123–142.

Cohen, M.I., Spodak, M.K., Silver, S.B., & Williams, K. (1988). Predicting outcome of insanity acquittees released to the community. *Behavioral Sciences and the Law, 6,* 515–530.

Crocker, A.G., & Hodgins, S. (1997). The criminality of noninstitutionalized mentally retarded persons: Evidence from a birth cohort followed to age 30. *Criminal Justice and Behavior, 24,* 432–454.

Douglas, K., Ogloff, J.R.P., Nicholls, T., & Grant, I. (1999). Assessing risk for violence among psychiatric patients: The HCR-20 violence risk assessment scheme and the Psychopathy Checklist, Screening Version. *Journal of Consulting and Clinical Psychology, 67,* 917–930.

Douglas, K., & Webster, C. (1999). The HCR-20 violence risk assessment scheme: Concurrent validity in a sample of incarcerated offenders. *Criminal Justice and Behavior, 26,* 3–19.

Dvoskin, J., & Steadman, H.J. (1994). Using intensive case management to reduce violence by mentally ill persons in the community. *Hospital and Community Psychiatry, 45,* 679–684.

Feder, L. (1991). A comparison of the community adjustment of mentally ill offenders with those from the general prison population. *Law and Human Behavior, 15,* 477–493.

Gordon, D., Arbuthnot, J., & Jurkovic, G. (1998). Treatment of the juvenile offender. In R. Wettstein (Ed.), *Treatment of offenders with mental disorders* (pp. 365–428). New York: Guilford.

Griffin, P., Steadman, H.J., & Heilbrun, K. (1991). Designing conditional release systems for insanity acquittees. *Journal of Mental Health Administration, 18,* 231–241.

Harris, G.T., Rice, M.E., & Cormier, C.A. (1991). Psychopathy and violent recidivism. *Law and Human Behavior, 15,* 625–637.

Harris, G.T., Rice, M.E., & Quinsey, V.L. (1993). Violent recidivism of mentally disordered offenders: The development of a statistical prediction instrument. *Criminal Justice and Behavior, 20,* 315–335.

Heilbrun, K. (1997). Prediction vs. management models relevant to risk assessment: The importance of legal decision-making context. *Law and Human Behavior, 21,* 347–359.

Heilbrun, K., & Griffin, P. (1993). Community-based forensic treatment of insanity acquittees. *International Journal of Law and Psychiatry, 16,* 133–150.

Heilbrun, K., & Griffin, P. (1998). Community-based forensic treatment. In R. Wettstein (Ed.), *Treatment of offenders with mental disorders* (pp. 168–210). New York: Guilford.

Heilbrun, K., & Griffin, P. (1999). Forensic treatment: A review of programs and research. In R. Roesch, S. Hart, & J. Ogloff (Eds.), *Law and psychology: The state of the discipline* (pp. 242–274). New York: Kluwer/Plenum.

Heilbrun, K., & Peters, L. (2000). Community-based treatment programs. In S. Hodgins & R. Müller-Isberner (Eds.), *Violence, crime, and mentally disordered offenders.* New York: Wiley.

Hodgins, S. (1983). A follow-up study of persons found incompetent to stand trial and/or not guilty by reason of insanity in Quebec. *International Journal of Law and Psychiatry, 6,* 399–411.

Hodgins, S., & Gaston, L. (1989). Patterns of recidivism and relapse among groups of mentally disordered offenders. *Behavioral Sciences and the Law, 7,* 551–558.

Holcomb, W.R., & Ahr, P.R. (1988). Arrest rates among young adult psychiatric patients treated in inpatient and outpatient settings. *Hospital and Community Psychiatry, 39,* 52–57.

Kansas v. Hendricks. (1997). 117 U.S. 2072.

Lidz, C.W., Mulvey, E.P., & Gardner, W. (1993). The accuracy of predictions of violence to others. *Journal of the American Medical Association, 269,* 1007–1011.

McGreevy, M.A., Steadman, H.J., Dvoskin, J.A., & Dollard, N. (1991). New York State's system of managing insanity acquittees in the community. *Hospital and Community Psychiatry, 42,* 512–517.

Modestin, J., & Ammann, R. (1995). Mental disorders and criminal behaviour. *British Journal of Psychiatry, 166,* 667–675.

Monahan, J., & Steadman, H. (Eds.). (1994). *Violence and mental disorder: Developments in risk assessment.* Chicago: University of Chicago Press.

Müller-Isberner, J.R. (1996). Forensic psychiatric aftercare following hospital order treatment. *International Journal of Law and Psychiatry, 19,* 81–86.

Nicholson, R.A., Norwood, S., & Enyart, C. (1991). Characteristics and outcomes of insanity acquittees in Oklahoma. *Behavioral Sciences and the Law, 9,* 487–500.

Quinsey, V., Harris, G., Rice, M., & Cormier, C. (1998). *Violent offenders: Appraising and managing risk.* Washington: American Psychological Association.

Raesaenen, P., Tiihonen, J., Isohanni, M., Rantakallio, P., Lehtonen, J., & Moring, J. (1998). Schizophrenia, alcohol abuse, and violent behavior: A 26-year followup study of an unselected birth cohort. *Schizophrenia Bulletin, 24,* 437–441.

Rice, M.E., & Harris, G.T. (1992). A comparison of criminal recidivism among schizophrenic and nonschizophrenic offenders. *International Journal of Law and Psychiatry, 15,* 397–408.

Silver, S.B., Cohen, M., & Spodak, M. (1989). Follow-up after release of insanity acquittees, mentally disordered offenders, and convicted felons. *Bulletin of the American Academy of Psychiatry and the Law, 17,* 387–400.

Solomon, P., & Draine, J. (1995). One-year outcomes of a randomized trial of case management with seriously mentally ill clients leaving jail. *Evaluation Review, 19,* 256–273.

Solomon, P., Draine, J., & Meyerson, A. (1994). Jail recidivism and receipt of community mental health services. *Hospital and Community Psychiatry, 45,* 793–797.

Steadman, H.J., Monahan, J., Hartstone, E., Davis, S., & Robbins, P.C. (1982). Mentally disordered offenders: A national survey of patients and facilities. *Law and Human Behavior, 6,* 31–38.

Steadman, H.J., Mulvey, E., Monahan, J., Robbins, P., Appelbaum, P., Grisso, T., Roth, L., & Silver, E. (1998). Violence by people discharged from acute psychiatric inpatient facilities and by others in the same neighborhoods. *Archives of General Psychiatry, 55,* 1–9.

Swanson, J., Holzer, C., Ganju, V., & Jono, R. (1990). Violence and psychiatric disorder in the community: Evidence from the Epidemiologic Catchment Area surveys. *Hospital and Community Psychiatry, 41,* 761–770.

Swartz, M., Swanson, J., Wagner, H.R., Burns, B., Hiday, V., & Borum, R. (1999). Can outpatient commitment reduce hospital recidivism? Findings from a randomized trial in severely mentally ill individuals. *American Journal of Psychiatry, 156,* 1968–1975.

Tellefsen, C., Cohen, M.I., Silver, S.B., & Dougherty, C. (1992). Predicting success on conditional release for insanity acquittees: Regionalized versus nonregionalized hospital patients. *Bulletin of the American Academy of Psychiatry and Law, 20,* 87–100.

Tiihonen, J., Isohanni, M., Raesaenen, P., Koiranen, M., & Moring, J. (1997). Specific major mental disorders and criminality: A 26-year prospective study of the 1996 Northern Finland Birth Cohort. *American Journal of Psychiatry, 154,* 840–845.

Webster, C.D., Eaves, D., Douglas, K., & Wintrup, A. (1995). *The HCR-20 Scheme: The assessment of dangerousness and risk.* Burnaby, BC: Simon Fraser University and Forensic Psychiatric Services Commission of British Columbia.

Wells, K. (1999). Treatment research at the crossroads: The scientific interface of clinical trials and effectiveness research. *American Journal of Psychiatry, 156,* 5–10.

Wiederanders, M. (1992). Recidivism of disordered offenders who were conditionally vs. unconditionally released. *Behavioral Sciences and the Law, 10,* 141–148.

Wiederanders, M.R., Bromley, D.L., & Choate, P.A. (1997). Forensic conditional release programs and outcomes in three states. *International Journal of Law and Psychiatry, 20,* 249–257.

Wilson, D., Tien, G., & Eaves, D. (1995). Increasing the community tenure of mentally disordered offenders: An assertive case management program. *International Journal of Law and Psychiatry, 18,* 61–69.

Kirk Heilbrun and Lori Peters are associated with the Law and Psychology Program, Department of Clinical and Health Psychology, MCP Hahnemann University and Villanova School of Law, Philadelphia, Pennsylvania, USA.

Authors' Note

A chapter similar in some respects, but with greater emphasis on the implications of research findings for practice and policy, appears as: Heilbrun, K., & Peters, L. (2000). Community-based treatment programmes. In S. Hodgins & R. Müller-Isberner (Eds.), *Violence, crime, and mentally disordered offenders*. New York: Wiley.

We are grateful to Joseph Bloom, Patricia Griffin, Sheilagh Hodgins, John Monahan, Kim Mueser, and Hank Steadman for their helpful comments.

Comments or queries may be directed to Kirk Heilbrun, Department of Psychology, MCP Hahnemann University, MS 626, 245 North 15th Street, Philadelphia PA 19102-1192 USA. Telephone: 215 762-3634. Fax: 215 762-8625. E-mail: <Kirk.Heilbrun@drexel.edu>.

COMMENTARY

Heilbrun and Peters, "The Efficacy and Effectiveness of Community Treatment Programmes in Preventing Crime and Violence Among Those with Severe Mental Illness in the Community"

JAMES MCGUIRE

Some years ago when Professor Mednick, one of the distinguished contributors to the Advanced Study Institute, was carrying out research on creativity, he developed a measure known as the Remote Associations Test. It entailed providing respondents with two apparently unrelated words and asking them to generate ideas concerning possible connections between them. In making this response I feel as if I have a task of that kind: to attempt to identify links between two large areas of research which have remained surprisingly separate and are rarely considered conjointly—the treatment of, respectively, mentally disordered and non-disordered offenders. In what follows I hope to demonstrate that these areas are far from remote and that there is much to be gained by conceptualizing them in an interrelated, indeed integrated, way.

Warm thanks are due to Drs. Heilbrun and Peters for the excellent work they have done in preparing their paper and presentation. It was by no means an easy task to address this topic, primarily due to the shortage of relevant research studies and the sparsity of comparable and usable findings on which to base any conclusions. In surveying the work they have reviewed, it must be acknowledged immediately that research in this field presents some forbidding difficulties.

First, in almost any kind of research on interventions with offenders, locating appropriate comparison groups is problematic. Controlled trials are uncommon, quasi-experiments are much more typical, and many studies fall below this standard. Second, with mentally disordered client groups, evaluation of the efficacy of interventions requires an extensive follow-up period. Third, the "target behaviours" of concern are acts of violence and other forms of antisocial conduct which generally occur at a low frequency and may do so only at widely dispersed intervals, but which when they do transpire are catastrophic in their impact. Finally, ethical issues arise with possibly greater potency here than in many other spheres of research.

Drs. Heilbrun and Peters have conducted a review of evaluative studies on the effectiveness of community-based interventions with mentally disordered offenders. They have undertaken this important task in a thorough and systematic way. They

359

S. Hodgins (ed.), Violence among the Mentally Ill, 359–366.
© 2000 *Kluwer Academic Publishers. Printed in the Netherlands.*

commenced sensibly by defining their terms and clarifying the population with whom they wanted to deal, avoiding some of the potential confusions in the field. They proceeded by scanning the appropriate databases and then divided the documents and reports they obtained into three methodological subcategories: a group of four studies in which experimental and quasi-experimental designs were employed; a larger number of unmatched, non-randomized group comparisons and single-group studies; and a small number of descriptive studies.

It is regrettable but unavoidable that, due to limitations of the available literature in this area, it was not feasible to conduct a meta-analysis as the authors had originally intended. Even had this been technically viable in terms of study designs, it would have remained difficult to detect trends and draw conclusions as a consequence of other differences among the study samples that were employed. Such interpretational difficulties arise, for example, from the paper by Tellefsen, Cohen, Silver, and Dougherty (1992). Another major issue in this regard is the comparison of samples managed by different criminal justice or mental health jurisdictions. In such circumstances it can be difficult to discern whether decisions concerning rehospitalization, revocation of parole or of conditional release, and so on are being made on equivalent grounds. Outcome data may be a simple function of variations in discretionary practices among different groups of supervisory staff. This occurred in respect of the study by Wiederanders (1992). Some other findings reviewed could be a byproduct of the actions of case managers themselves. From what might be called the "mainstream" criminological literature, one can cite a large-scale study by Petersilia and Turner (1993) of intensive-supervision probation programmes. There, it became clear that with enhanced monitoring there is a commensurate increase in rates of technical violation which may lead to revocation of parole. Similar findings were obtained in the study by Solomon, Draine, and Meyerson (1994) reviewed here. The authors recognize all these limitations and are appropriately cautious in making interpretations and drawing conclusions.

Prediction of Recidivism and Treatment-Outcome Research

Early in their paper the present authors discuss a recent meta-analytic review by Bonta, Law, and Hansen (1998) on the prediction of general and violent recidivism amongst mentally disordered offenders. I agree with their important point that an integrative review of studies focused on the question of *prediction* does not of course tell us a great deal, if indeed it tells us anything, about reducing the frequency or severity of the target outcome variables. However, I see the findings of this review as having greater relevance and carrying significantly more weight than do the present authors and wonder if they could have pushed its conclusions further. An important implication of the Bonta et al. review is that programmes with the goal of reducing criminal and violent behaviour deploy the strategy of targeting specific dynamic risk factors *(criminogenic needs)* that show a positive relationship with risk of future recidivism. This point helps to forge a vital connection between the field of research being discussed and the general offender treatment-outcome literature. It is that link on which I wish to focus in these comments.

There are two reasons for developing this line of argument. First, the principal conclusion of Bonta et al. (1998) is that the predictor variables for recidivism isolated with respect to mentally disordered offenders are very similar to those obtained with non-mentally disordered offender populations. Second, the literature concerning the latter shows targeting of criminogenic needs to be extremely important in influencing outcome. Bonta et al. found clinical variables to be the poorest predictors of recidivism, calling into question our ready reliance on these categories as valid pieces of information for this purpose—at least as ingredients of an *actuarial* scale, a point to which I will return below.

Another advantage these findings may afford is in providing further justification for combining our thinking about mentally disordered offenders with the broader social psychological approach to crime outlined in the works of, for example, Andrews and Bonta (1998), Blackburn (1993), or Farrington (1996). We could also benefit from study of integrative models of the development of aggression proposed by, for example, Patterson and Yoerger (1993; and see McGuire, 1997).

The disappointment of Drs. Heilbrun and Peters that there was not a stronger effect size for treatment in the Bonta et al. (1998) review is wholly understandable. Treatment effects are probably not evidenced for the reasons they identify, namely that in the majority of studies non-criminogenic risk factors were targeted, so yielding negative effect sizes, while the number of studies focusing on criminogenic factors was too small to reverse this trend.

Overall, Bonta et al. (1998) found only 14 studies that included treatment as an independent variable. But if more parallels can be drawn between this area of research and the general offender treatment-outcome literature than have thus far been appreciated, then perhaps that literature can be surveyed for its potential usefulness and help to compensate for the paucity of treatment studies in this field.

Problems of interpretation remain, however—especially when outcomes are expressed in terms of comparisons among legal categories or across different jurisdictions. Fortunately, there are also many published studies with experimental designs of a sufficiently high standard to allow meta-analyses to be conducted, whilst incorporating a measure of design quality as an independent variable. Review of this research also enables us to peruse the nature of interventions. In any well-reported study the nature and content of interventions should be specified in some detail (and the extent to which this is so can also be coded as an independent variable in meta-analysis). This means that problems such as those noted by Heilbrun and Peters concerning the Wiederanders, Bromley, and Choate (1997) study can be avoided. What was the precise nature of the contact with clients in that study? The objectives, types, and quality of interactions involved in Assertive Case Management itself should be depicted in detail. For example, in evaluations of criminal justice services, associations have been found between recidivism outcome and hours of contact with supervisory staff (Whitehead & Lab, 1989) and also with staff supervision styles (Gendreau, Paparozzi, Little, & Goddard, 1993).

Another fundamental issue which Heilbrun and Peters touch upon is the importance of developing treatment plans based on individual offenders' problem profiles, rather than diagnostic category or offence type. This is a point which I wholeheartedly endorse, and the value of such an approach is surely beyond dispute. Expanding upon this, it may be that we need many more in-depth clinical research studies employing small-*n* time-series designs. Large-scale studies employing randomized controlled trial designs are accurately perceived as essential for hypothesis-testing purposes and multivariate analysis, but by themselves they leave a number of significant gaps in our understanding.

One such gap is the perennial problem of extrapolating from aggregate data to the single case. This underlies a number of clinical and ethical dilemmas concerning risk assessment and prediction. While such a task must have its foundations in an actuarial approach, the latter inevitably has limitations when applied in clinical practice. The gap also appears with regard to design and delivery of interventions. The voluminous literature on treatment-outcome effects with psychological therapies (Chambliss & Hollon, 1998; Lambert & Bergin, 1994; Lipsey & Wilson, 1993; Nathan & Gorman, 1998; Roth & Fonagy, 1996) has been criticized on these grounds. Objectors (e.g., Persons & Silberschatz, 1998) have stated that "manualized" treatments neglect within-group variance, are not tailored to individual symptom patterns or problem profiles, and do not correspond to the manner of provision of therapy in most clinical services. As an alternative, the use of functional analysis of problem behaviour and clinical case formulation has been advocated. For mentally disordered offenders, an understanding of the relationships between symptoms and antisocial behaviours, and between both of these and antecedent factors (proximal and distal), could yield improvement in terms of both individualized risk assessments and treatment programmes. Attention could be directed to short-term fluctuations in dynamic risk factors such as delusional states or anger. Here the potential of *clinical* predictors might come to the fore.

A recently published study by Zamble and Quinsey (1997) has a close bearing on this. These authors followed up 311 discharged prisoners who re-offended, and compared them with a much smaller sample (*n* = 36) who did not. Recidivists reported more problems in the period after release and had fewer or less effective skills for coping with their problems. Recidivists more often experienced, and had poorer strategies for managing, negative emotional states such as anger, anxiety, and depression. They also thought more frequently about substance abuse and possible crimes, and less about employment and about the future in an optimistic light. They experienced increased fluctuation in emotional states in the 48 hours preceding a re-offence.

Crime-Prevention Strategies

Interventions designed to reduce crime are sometimes depicted in terms of three levels: primary, secondary, and tertiary. The first, also called "developmental prevention," entails provision of services to families and children in environments such as socioeconomically deprived neighbourhoods, with the aim of reducing long-term difficulties, including delinquency but also mental health problems and substance abuse. Secondary prevention is focused on known at-risk groups—for example, individuals who have conduct disorders or residents of child-care facilities in an attempt to avert subsequent involvement in juvenile offending. Tertiary prevention is addressed to adjudicated offenders—those already convicted of crimes—with the objective of reducing rates of recidivism.

Evidence concerning this third category (sometimes, following Martinson's [1974] paper, referred to as research on "what works") is drawn from a series of large-scale systematic reviews, cumulatively encompassing approximately 2,000 outcome studies, employing the statistical techniques of meta-analysis (Cooper & Hedges, 1994; Durlak & Lipsey, 1991). The reviews show, first, that there is strong evidence of the possibility of reducing recidivism rates amongst persistent offenders (Harland 1996; Lipsey, 1995; Lipton, Pearson, Cleland, & Yee, 1997; Lösel, 1995; McGuire, 1995; Redondo, Garrido, & Sánchez-Meca, 1997; Sherman et al., 1997). Second, the probability of achieving this outcome can be maximized by combining a number of elements in offender programmes. Third, these components are distinct from the legal sanction or sentence imposed on individuals (McGuire, in press). On balance, community-based interventions have larger effect sizes than those delivered in institutions (Andrews et al., 1990; Lipsey & Wilson, 1998). On the basis of the available reviews, a consensus has emerged regarding guidelines for intervention programmes designed to reduce recidivism. The following features have been identified as likely to contribute to the success of an intervention:

- Programmes and services are founded on an explicit and well-articulated model of the causes of crime and criminal acts, one which is conceptually clear and which is drawn from an empirically sound knowledge base in psychology, criminology, and allied social sciences.
- Weight is given to assessment of risk of re-offending, based on criminal history and other variables, and allocation to different levels of supervision or service in accordance with this information.
- Procedures are in place for assessment of "criminogenic needs" or dynamic risk factors such as antisocial attitudes, influence of criminal associates, skills deficits, substance abuse, or self-control problems which are known to be linked to offending behaviour and which change over time.
- Intervention methods correspond to the active, focused, and participatory learning and change styles found in many offenders, alongside an acknowledged need to adapt services to individual differences in this respect.
- Application of intervention methods is characterized by clear objectives and by skilled and structured engagement on the part of staff in tasks which are readily accepted as relevant to the needs of individual offenders.
- A "cognitive-behavioural" approach is taken, comprising a collection of theoretically interrelated methods which focus on the interplay of an individual's thoughts, feelings, and behaviour at the time of an offence. (The most consistently effective services have been found to take this approach.)
- Service managers ensure that all of these functions are fulfilled by appropriately trained and resourced staff who adhere to their appointed objectives, adopt suitable methods, and undertake systematic evaluation of each individual's progress and of the outcomes of their services overall.

When these features are present in combination, the impact on future recidivism may be very substantial. Andrews et al. (1990) show that incorporating these ingredients into an offender programme can lead to reductions in recidivism greater than

50%; in some more recently published primary studies, still better outcomes have occasionally been obtained (e.g., Borduin, Mann, Cone, & Henggeler, 1995).

Possibilities

Arising from the above comments, and building on the review reported by Drs. Heilbrun and Peters, some suggestions can be made about possible future directions in this field. One useful departure might be to compile a directory of the "good practice" programmes to which the authors refer. Why are they so perceived, and what might other practitioners, and also researchers, learn from them? Second, there is an evident need for research towards validation of procedures for assessment of, respectively, "static" and "dynamic" risk factors. Third, expanding on the points raised by Heilbrun and Peters, it would be advantageous to see more use made of functional analysis and clinical case formulation, and reporting of small-scale research which might help to bridge the gap between controlled trials and everyday clinical practice.

On an organizational level, much is currently being done within some criminal justice services to establish mechanisms for quality control of planned interventions, through procedures for accreditation of programmes and services. In the United Kingdom to date, this has occurred primarily in prison settings. In the more complex environment of community services, where parallel developments are now taking place, steps should be taken to ensure that those measures which involve increased monitoring of clients are linked to mobilization of supports rather than triggering of sanctions. Where controlled trials of interventions and treatments are conducted, the inclusion of "significant others" as an added variable should be considered by clinical researchers.

Finally, whilst these comments have been concerned with the interlinking of the research fields of crime prevention and, respectively, mentally disordered and non-disordered offenders, there is yet another, adjacent, area with which links ought to be built. This is the study of substance abuse, which numerous studies link to both severe mental health problems and persistent criminality (e.g., Hodgins, 1993). It should perhaps be a priority of researchers to focus in detail on the connections between these problems and on the identification of effective treatments. This could possibly be the theme of a future ASI as well.

References

Andrews, D.A., & Bonta, J. (1998). *The psychology of criminal conduct.* Cincinnati: Anderson.

Andrews, D.A., Zinger, I., Hoge, R.D., Bonta, J., Gendreau, P., & Cullen, F.T. (1990). Does correctional treatment work? A clinically relevant and psychologically informed meta-analysis. *Criminology, 28,* 369–404.

Blackburn, R. (1993). *The psychology of criminal conduct.* Chichester: Wiley.

Bonta, J., Law, M., & Hansen, K. (1998). The prediction of criminal and violent recidivism amongst mentally disordered offenders: A meta-analysis. *Psychological Bulletin, 123,* 123–142.

Borduin, C.M., Mann, B.J., Cone, L.T., & Henggeler, S.W. (1995). Multi-systemic treatment of serious juvenile offenders: Long-term prevention of criminality and violence. *Journal of Consulting and Clinical Psychology, 63,* 569–578.

Chambless, D.L., & Hollon, S.D. (1998). Defining empirically supported therapies. *Journal of Consulting and Clinical Psychology, 66,* 7–18.

Cooper, H., & Hedges, L.V. (Eds.). (1994). *Handbook of research synthesis.* New York: Russell Sage Foundation.

Durlak, J.A., & Lipsey, M.W. (1991). A practitioner's guide to meta-analysis. *American Journal of Community Psychology, 19,* 291–333.

Farrington, D.P. (1996). The explanation and prevention of youthful offending. In J.D. Hawkins (Ed.), *Delinquency and crime: Current theories* (pp. 68–148). Cambridge: Cambridge University Press.

Gendreau, P., Paparozzi, M., Little, T., & Goddard, M. (1993). Does "Punishing Smarter" work? An assessment of the new generation of alternative sanctions in probation. *Forum on Corrections Research, 5,* 31–34.

Harland, A.T. (Ed.). (1996). *Choosing correctional options that work: Defining the demand and evaluating the supply.* Thousand Oaks, CA: Sage.

Hodgins, S. (1993). The criminality of mentally disordered persons. In S. Hodgins (Ed.), *Mental disorder and crime.* Newbury Park, CA: Sage.

Lambert, M.J., & Bergin, A.E. (1994). The effectiveness of psychotherapy. In A.E. Bergin & S.L. Garfield (Eds.), *Handbook of psychotherapy and behavior change* (pp. 143–189). New York: Wiley.

Lipsey, M.W. (1995). What do we learn from 400 studies on the effectiveness of treatment with juvenile delinquents? In J. McGuire (Ed.), *What works: Reducing reoffending: Guidelines from research and practice* (pp. 63–78). Chichester: Wiley.

Lipsey, M.W., & Wilson, D.B. (1993). The efficacy of psychological, educational, and behavioral treatment: Confirmation from meta-analysis. *American Psychologist, 48,* 1181–1209.

Lipsey, M.W., & Wilson, D.B. (1998). Effective intervention for serious juvenile offenders: A synthesis of research. In R. Loeber & D.P. Farrington (Eds.), *Serious and violent juvenile offenders: Risk factors and successful interventions* (pp. 313–345). Thousand Oaks, CA: Sage.

Lipton, D.S., Pearson, F.S., Cleland, C., & Yee, D. (1997, July). *Synthesizing correctional treatment outcomes: Preliminary CDATE findings.* Paper presented at the 5th annual National Institute of Justice Conference on Research and Evaluation in Criminal Justice, Washington, DC.

Lösel, F. (1995). The efficacy of correctional treatment: A review and synthesis of meta-evaluations. In J. McGuire (Ed.), *What works: Reducing re-offending: Guidelines from research and practice* (pp. 79–111). Chichester: Wiley.

Martinson, R. (1974). What works? Questions and answers about prison reform. *Public Interest, 10,* 22–54.

McGuire, J. (Ed.). (1995). *What works: Reducing re-offending: Guidelines from research and practice.* Chichester: Wiley.

McGuire, J. (1997). Psycho-social approaches to understanding and reducing violence in young people. In V. Varma (Ed.), *Violence in children and adolescents* (pp. 65–83). London: Jessica Kingsley.

McGuire, J. (in press). Criminal sanctions versus psychologically-based interventions with offenders: A comparative and empirically-based review. *Psychology, Crime and Law.*

Nathan, P.E., & Gorman, J.M. (Eds.). (1998). *A guide to treatments that work.* New York: Oxford University Press.

Patterson, G.R., & Yoerger, K. (1993). Developmental models for delinquent behavior. In S. Hodgins (Ed.), *Mental disorder and crime* (pp. 140–172). Newbury Park, CA: Sage.

Persons, J.B., & Silberschatz, G. (1998). Are results of randomized controlled trials useful to psychotherapists? *Journal of Consulting and Clinical Psychology, 66,* 126–135.

Petersilia, J., & Turner, S. (1993). Intensive probation and parole. *Crime and Justice, 17,* 281–335.

Redondo, S., Garrido, V., & Sánchez-Meca, J. (1997). What works in correctional rehabilitation in Europe: A meta-analytical review. In S. Redondo, V. Garrido, J. Pérez, & R. Barberet (Eds.), *Advances in psychology and law* (pp. 499–523). Berlin: De Gruyter.

Roth, A., & Fonagy, P. (1996). *What works for whom? A critical review of psychotherapy research.* New York: Guilford.

Sherman, L.W., Gottfredson, D., MacKenzie, D., Eck, J., Reuter, P., & Bushway, S. (1997). *Preventing crime: What works, what doesn't, what's promising.* Washington: Office of Justice Programs.

Solomon, P., Draine, J., & Meyerson, A. (1994). Jail recidivism and receipt of community mental health services. *Hospital and Community Psychiatry, 45,* 793–797.

Tellefsen, C., Cohen, M.I., Silver, S.B., & Dougherty, C. (1992). Predicting success on conditional release for insanity acquittees: Regionalized versus nonregionalized hospital patients. *Bulletin of the American Academy of Psychiatry and Law, 20,* 87–100.

Whitehead, J.T., & Lab, S.P. (1989). A meta-analysis of juvenile correctional treatment. *Journal of Research in Crime and Delinquency, 26,* 276–295.

Wiederanders, M. (1992). Recidivism of disordered offenders who were conditionally versus unconditionally released. *Behavioral Sciences and the Law, 10,* 141–148.

Wiederanders, M., Bromley, D.L., & Choate, P.A. (1997). Forensic conditional release programs and outcomes in three states. *International Journal of Law and Psychiatry, 20,* 249–257.

Zamble, E., & Quinsey, V.L. (1997). *The criminal recidivism process.* Cambridge: Cambridge University Press.

James McGuire is Course Director of the Doctorate in Clinical Psychology, University of Liverpool, UK.

Author's Note

Comments or queries may be directed to James McGuire, PhD, Department of Clinical Psychology, University of Liverpool, Ground Floor, Whelan Building, Liverpool L69 3BX UK. Telephone: 44 151 794 5530/5534. Fax: 44 151 794 5537. E-mail: <merc@liverpool.ac.uk>.

SOCIAL SERVICES NECESSARY FOR COMMUNITY TREATMENT PROGRAMMES DESIGNED TO PREVENT CRIME AND VIOLENCE AMONG PERSONS WITH MAJOR MENTAL DISORDERS

GEORG HØYER

Introduction

Treatment programmes designed to prevent crime and violence among persons with major mental disorders should result in reduced crime rates and violent episodes among patients in these programmes, compared to those in other programmes or in none at all. The relationship among crime rates, violence, and specific programmes is problematic for a number of reasons, primary among them the almost endless number of factors that contribute to the outcome in a given case. Problems related to the design of studies in this field also seriously limit our ability to draw firm conclusions about the effects of specific programmes or interventions. This chapter will focus on some of the theoretical and methodological problems that arise when the effectiveness of specially designed treatment programmes is examined. It will then review, in the light of this theoretical framework, some of the studies that have looked at the role of social services in outpatient rehabilitation programmes.

Theoretical Considerations

The title suggests that some community treatment programmes are explicitly designed to prevent violence and crime among persons with major mental disorders. However, literature reviews have not identified a single study or programme whose sole or main purpose was stated as violence or crime reduction. It seems to be presumed that treatment programmes are always beneficial to the patient *and,* at the same time, effective in reducing crime. From a theoretical point of view, this is not necessarily so. Repressive programmes may prove to be anti-therapeutic or even harmful, even if they are successful in reducing crime rates, while programmes that are effective in relieving psychiatric symptoms may prove to have little impact on criminal behaviour. The appropriateness or effectiveness of an outpatient programme must be evaluated in relation to its purpose. It is thus important that the rationale for implementing a programme be clear. Surprisingly few programmes described in the literature had an explicit purpose; in most cases it was expressed in

S. Hodgins (ed.), Violence among the Mentally Ill, 367–382.
© 2000 *Kluwer Academic Publishers. Printed in the Netherlands.*

global and rather vague terms. It is always difficult to choose proper end-points when measuring the effectiveness of interventions, and lack of clarity in the expressed purpose of a programme adds to the problem.

Lack of Programme Standardization

Another problem with intervention programmes is lack of standardization. Even if one looks only at outpatient or community treatment programmes designed for persons with severe mental illnesses, the most striking feature is heterogeneity. Few if any programmes comprise the same elements, and even elements that appear similar at first glance often differ in content (psychotherapy, for instance, can be a common denominator for interventions that are very different). Perhaps little can be done about this problem. Experimental designs and controlled studies are likely not feasible at all, considering the organizational and contextual characteristics of community-based rehabilitation programmes. Research activity in the field has consequently been based on outcome evaluation of different programmes in their natural settings. This dearth of experimental studies, combined with poor standardization of treatment interventions, makes comparison and generalization of results rather problematic. Nevertheless, many randomized controlled studies comparing outpatient treatment programmes have been published (Burns & Santos, 1995; Marshall, Gray, Lockwood, & Green, 1998; Marshall & Lockwood, 1998), even if the quality of these studies does vary. In the Cochrane review of assertive community treatment trials conducted by Marshall and Lockwood, only 20 of a total of 75 randomized trials survived the Cochrane base quality criteria, and only one of the eight papers reviewed by Burns and Santos was among those 20 studies.

This proves how difficult it is to apply strict research standards in natural settings, especially when violent crime and serious mental disorders are involved. In addition to those problems related to lack of standardization and study design, there are problems with recruitment of subjects. For example, it is sometimes necessary, for security reasons, to exclude potentially dangerous patients from the randomization process (Dickey et al., 1996). Another difficulty is that ethical review boards usually allow patients to participate in studies only if they are capable of giving informed consent. For this reason, patients with major mental disorders are often excluded. Thus the most disturbed and those believed to be the most dangerous—in other words the patients most interesting to study from a violence prevention perspective —are in most cases not eligible for inclusion in scientific studies.

In addition, patients enrolled in outpatient treatment programmes have different backgrounds, in terms of both criminal and mental health careers.

Different legislation, different diversion policies, and other differences in the organization of health and social services result in selection of patients into different programmes (Brabbins & Travers, 1994; Davis, 1994; Steadman, Barbera, & Dennis, 1994). These mechanisms explain, for instance, why the proportion of prisoners with a major mental disorder varies greatly from one country to another and over time (Belfrage, 1992; Brabbins & Travers; Geddes, Newton, Bailey, Freeman, & Young, 1996; Grossman, Haywood, Cavanough, Davis, & Lewis, 1995; Prins,

1994; Wormith & McKeague, 1996). Teplin (1990) has demonstrated an extreme variance of severe mental disorders among inmates, ranging from 3 to 75%. The result of diversion policies, often, is that community treatment programmes exclusively serve patients recruited from either the criminal justice system or the mental health care system (or other referring agencies, depending on the organizational or administrative structure). The outcome of this recruitment procedure is different goals: Programmes for patients without a criminal record are more therapeutically oriented, while those for mentally disordered offenders focus on surveillance and compliance with the conditions for release into the community. The rationality of these differences in programme profiles is open to question. The needs of patients with major mental disorders living in the community are probably very similar, regardless of their prior criminal record. If it is true that crime and violence committed by persons with severe mental disorders are products of the mental illness itself, and if the ultimate goal is prevention of violence, it seems reasonable that mentally disordered offenders should be subjected to the same procedures as non-criminal patients.

Research Implications

The great variance in aftercare and rehabilitation programmes, in terms of both the kind of patients who enter the programmes and the purpose and content of the programmes, is obviously problematic from a research point of view, especially if the researcher intends to look at the specific effects of social services. Because social services are always more or less integrated into community treatment programmes, it is difficult to distinguish their effects from the effects of other elements of the programme. An interesting question in this respect is whether social services has the potential to improve the mental condition or to modify behaviour in itself, or if it is merely a supplement to medical and psychological treatment. Answering this question would require an operational definition of social services, yet social services differ from country to country and even within countries. Legal frameworks, organization of services, and the professional backgrounds of service providers might all be different, and the tasks assigned to social services in different cultures and countries might be markedly different. It is almost impossible to define social services, simply because it means different things in different parts of the world.

What Do Social Services Comprise?

In spite of the almost impossible task of defining social services, most people (at least those in Western societies) probably have a common understanding of what constitutes the core elements of social services. They might agree that the main functions of social services are to provide shelter, food, and clothing to those people unable to provide these basic needs themselves. However, although descriptive studies have demonstrated over and over again that persons with chronic mental disorders, substance abusers, and ex-prisoners lack housing, employment, education, health insurance, and social welfare much more than other members of society (Callahan & Silver, 1998; Cohen, 1993; Dennis, Buckner, Lipton, & Levine, 1991; Dixon, Friedman, & Lehman, 1993; Drake, Osher, & Wallach, 1991; Goldman, Morrissey, Ridgely, & Frank, 1992; Jeffreys et al., 1997; Marrone, Balzell, & Gold, 1995; Nordentoft, 1994), the *consequences* of doing without these basic needs have not been studied according to strict scientific standards. The reason for their not being studied is probably simple: Everybody knows that it is better to be rich and healthy than poor and ill, and a study exploring whether it is better to have a place to live than not to have one will be regarded a waste of time and money.

Nevertheless, there is a point worth considering when discussing the impact of social services on violence prevention programmes for the seriously mentally disordered. Because we take it for granted that housing, employment, and so on are always beneficial, we know little about *how* important they are. Nor do we know much about the *relative* importance of these basic elements of social life. This kind of knowledge could prove to be important when it comes to setting priorities for rehabilitation programmes.

If we consider only housing, locating secure and decent housing is commonly described as one of the greatest problems for rehabilitation programmes (Dennis et al., 1991; Dixon, Krauss, Kernan, Lehman, & DeForge, 1995). It is most likely also the most expensive basic need (Hallam, Beecham, Knapp, & Fenyo, 1994). If we do not know exactly what effect the lack of access to decent housing will have on resocialization, should we still give priority to housing? Put another way, if we do not know how important accommodation is, and if we do not know the relative importance of housing compared to psychological and psychiatric treatment, how can we use restricted resources in the best possible way? And how can we construct the most efficient treatment and rehabilitation programmes? It is interesting to observe that, in interviews, mental health professionals and social workers tend to attribute the effectiveness of programmes to psychological treatment interventions, while patients underline the importance of more material factors like occupation and housing (MacDonald & Sheldon, 1997; Wormith & McKeague, 1996).

Availability and Coordination of Services

When evaluating the impact of community treatment or rehabilitation programmes, it is not enough to determine whether all the required services are in place. One should also look at cooperation among services and the way in which the services are organized. For instance, although it is reasonable to assume that availability of services is important, studies seldom take this into consideration. Availability comprises factors like location, whether the services are provided free of charge, opening hours, and whether appointments are taken on a drop-in basis or if patients must follow procedures in order to see therapists or other service providers. But even before availability becomes relevant, there is a basic precondition for efficient utilization of the various services: *knowledge* of their existence. Further, patients must not only know that the services exist; for the system to function properly, they must also know their rights and entitlements. There are some reports indicating that underprivileged patients lack both information about relevant services (Cohen, 1993; Dennis et al., 1991; Hanoa, 1997; Krogstrup & Stenbak, 1993) and knowledge of their legal rights (Høyer, 1986; Molven & Vetvik, 1985; Saltnes, 1980). This may explain the reported under-use of social services by marginal groups (Druss & Rosenheck, 1998; Geddes et al., 1996). Attitudes of care providers and interaction between clients and providers are also important, as is the ability to respond in emergencies. All the above factors are of great importance in any discussion of the effectiveness of services.

The large number of services that make up community treatment packages are often organized in different sectors, making coordination of services an issue (Diamond, 1996; Hadley & Goldman, 1995; McFarland & Blair, 1995; Shepherd, Muijen, Hadley, & Goldman, 1996). Hallam et al. (1994) report that some long-stay mental patients received more than 40 different services after discharge. The obvious need for coordination of services in aftercare programmes was perhaps the main reason for the case management strategies that emerged in many Western countries some 20 to 30 years ago. The World Health Organization recognizes the importance of inter-agency coordination in rehabilitation programmes, pointing out, in its report on community rehabilitation, that these programmes must include services from more than one sector and that coordination is crucial (World Health Organization, 1994). The basic idea of case management is that one person be given total responsibility for community follow-up and delivery of services. Apart from the recognized need for coordination and integration of services, in some countries case management is motivated by the idea that persons with multiple problems—such as those with chronic mental disorders, substance abuse problems, and social maladjustment—represent a heavy workload for many agencies, and case management is a way to reduce over-use of services and thus costs (Corrado, Doherty, & Glackman, 1989; Wilson, Tien, & Eaves 1995). The empirical evidence supporting the over-use of services by these patients is not convincing, however. On the contrary, many studies have found that this group of patients are under-users (Cohen, 1993; Dennis et al., 1991; Druss & Rosenheck, 1998; Geddes et al., 1996). This seemingly conflicting evidence on service use may be a result of the differences in service organization and quality discussed above, and may also explain why cost analyses of case management programmes produce conflicting results (Corrado et al.; Ford et al., 1997; Morse et al., 1997; Wolff et al., 1997).

Case management programmes take many forms. The most comprehensive are often called "assertive case management" or "intensive case management." Differences among programmes centre on matters like number of clients per case manager, whether case managers service geographically defined areas, the professional training and background of case managers, and whether case managers should be recruited from a single agency. Another question is whether one agency should be given the leadership role in a programme, and which agency is best qualified for this role (general practitioners, parole officers, social workers). These questions may be dealt with in different ways, but all must be taken into consideration in any evaluation of the efficiency of case management programmes.

Case management programmes are often confused with assertive community treatment (ACT) programmes, but there are important distinctions. ACT programmes, first described by Test and colleagues (Marx, Test, & Stein, 1973; Stein & Test, 1980), are managed by a team that provides all the necessary services. They work according to extensive outreach principles and offer 24-hour services to their clients. ACT teams seem to be more compliant with programme procedures than case managers, who may choose whatever they think is beneficial on a pragmatic basis. This difference is important, as ACT programmes appear to be more effective than case management ones (Lafave, Souza, & Gerber, 1996; Marshall et al., 1998; Marshall & Lockwood, 1998). The content and quality of ACT programmes do, however, vary substantially. A review of all ACT programmes in the United States found that only one third fulfilled the defined quality criteria for ACT (Deci, Santos, Hiott, Schoenwald, & Dias, 1995).

The Importance of Context in the Functioning of Social Services

The various services offered to clients in comprehensive treatment or rehabilitation programmes do not exist in a vacuum. Any evaluation of the effectiveness of social services and specific treatment programmes should consider factors not directly related to patient care. For instance, how do national insurance programmes function in different countries? If they provide reasonable economic security for everybody, regardless of ability to pay, then the absence of financial support within a programme may not be a flaw, whereas in a country with inadequate national insurance it could represent a serious shortcoming (Cohen, 1993; Dennis et al., 1991; Lurigio & Lewis, 1989). The same considerations apply to national policies on housing, employment, and so on. Also, culturally based phenomena like tolerance, coherence, and solidarity in the general population, as well as ethical standards and how the mass media portray persons with mental disorders, can influence the functioning of treatment and rehabilitation programmes in different parts of the world. It is interesting to note that Raja, Azzoni, and Lubich (1997) found an extremely low prevalence of inpatient violence in Rome, Italy, and concluded that this was mainly a result of cultural and ideological factors.

Epidemiological Considerations

When the phenomenon of crime and violence perpetrated by persons with major mental disorders is approached from an epidemiological point of view, it soon becomes apparent that the potential to influence the overall rate of violence in the society is rather limited. Though prevalence figures vary around the world, the point prevalence figure is 1% or less in the total population of persons with major mental disorders (Jablensky, 1995). Very few of these patients commit acts of violence (Wallace et al., 1998), and of those who do, a large proportion are not in contact with any service providers at the time of the crime, either because they suffer from a first-episode psychosis or because they have, for various reasons, terminated treatment or aftercare. For example, a review was recently conducted of all persons in Norway in 1994–96 charged with murder or attempted murder and found not criminally responsible because they were suffering from a major mental disorder at the time of the crime. It was found that only 15.4% had a history of previous violent crime and approximately 62% had no contact with the mental health care system at the time of the crime (Sosial- og Helsedepartementet, 1998). Luettgen, Chrapko, and Reddon (1998) correspondingly report that 65% of mentally disordered offenders were not receiving mental health services at the time of their offence. The significance of these figures is obvious: Treatment programmes can be offered only to those who are known to care providers or the criminal justice system. These circumstances, combined with the fact that violent acts are rare in themselves—and the more serious the act the rarer it is—leave us with a scenario in which even successful violence prevention programmes for seriously mentally disordered patients will have only a marginal impact on the total rates of violence in the society.

It must also be remembered that those suffering from chronic major mental disorders differ demographically from the general population. They are single (i.e., have never married or cohabited) to a much higher degree than the population at large, have low social status, are seldom part of the workforce, and have unstable housing patterns (Dixon et al., 1995; Lafave, Pinkney, & Gerber, 1993; Lamb & Weinberger, 1998; Marshall, Lockwood, & Gath, 1995; McGilloway & Donelly, 1998; Morse, Calsyn, Allan, Tempelhof, & Smith, 1992; Rog et al., 1995). This situation has implications for the social networks of these patients; their networks are fragile or non-existent, and they are often dependent on relatives (Estroff, Zimmer, Lachicotte, & Benoit, 1994).

The Role of Alcohol and Drug Abuse

In no discussion of violence and crime prevention can the role of substance abuse be avoided. In addition to the demographic characteristics of the chronically mentally ill, a striking feature of mentally disordered offenders is the high prevalence of substance abuse. Rates vary from a low of 38% (Brooke, Taylor, Gunn, & Maden, 1996) to a high of 90% (McFarland & Blair, 1995; Wilson et al., 1995), while most studies report prevalence rates of between 40 and 60% (Belfrage, 1991; Brems & Johnson, 1997; Dennis et al., 1991; Lehman, Myers, Dixon, & Johnsen, 1994; Luettgen et al., 1998). Many studies are not explicit about how substance abuse is recorded, and it is sometimes unclear whether figures include a primary diagnosis of substance abuse only, dual or concurrent diagnosis, secondary diagnosis, or a combination of these. Furthermore, comparisons between incidents committed by those with major mental disorders and those with substance abuse do not always take account of dual diagnosis among the severe mentally ill, and thus perhaps underestimate the effect of substance abuse. Two recently published studies on violence among mentally disordered patients found that mentally disordered persons without substance abuse were no more likely to be violent than community controls (Steadman et al., 1998; Wallace et al., 1998). This finding is inconsistent with those of previously published studies on the relation between mental disorder and dangerousness, many of them concluding that patients with schizophrenia are more violent than persons without mental disorders (Gottlieb, Gabrielsen, & Kramp,

1987; Lindqvist, 1989; Lindqvist & Allebeck, 1990; Swanson, Holzer, Ganju, & Jono, 1990). On the other hand, many studies of re-arrests have not been able to find a link between diagnosis and re-arrest rate (Harris & Koepsell, 1996; Marshall, Nehring, Taylor, & Gath, 1994; Satsumi, Inada, & Yamauchi, 1998; Swartz et al., 1998).

Under all circumstances, there is little doubt that substance abuse represents the single most important predictor of violent behaviour and violent crime. Throughout history there have been instances of reduced violent crime accompanying restricted availability of alcohol. In Ireland, serious crime dropped to 1/16th of prior rates when a religious temperance crusade reached its peak in 1913. In Scandinavia, violence has been substantially reduced during periods of liquor-store strikes. In Poland, rioting was observed to be greatly reduced during a temporary alcohol prohibition in 1980. Finally, in the former Soviet Union during a period of alcohol restriction, the age-standardized homicide rate for Russian men dropped by 40%, from 19.5% in 1984 to 11.5% in 1987 (all events cited from Graham et al., 1998).

In our context, the question is whether, in order to be effective in preventing violence, community treatment programmes (including social services) should target primarily persons with substance abuse (including those with a concurrent major mental disorder). At the very least it must be questioned whether the practice, found in many countries, of separating health services from services for substance abuse should be reconsidered in the interests of providing more homogeneous and coordinated services to persons with dual diagnosis. These are probably the persons who present the greatest risk for future violence. At the same time, persons with substance abuse have the lowest rate of aftercare compliance (Callahan & Silver, 1998; Dixon et al., 1993; Harris & Koepsell, 1996; Marshall et al., 1994; Swartz et al., 1998; Wolpe, Gorton, Serota, & Sanford, 1993).

Persons with substance abuse and mental disorders are probably also the group most in need of social services. They usually subsist at a poverty level, with unstable, poor housing (if any), are mostly unemployed, and are poorly educated (Cohen, 1993; Dennis et al., 1991; Hylton, 1995). The key factor in this respect is most likely housing. Maintaining sobriety may be impossible without adequate housing (Drake et al., 1991; Teague, Drake, & Ackerson, 1995; Wittman, 1989). McLellan et al. (1998) report increased treatment compliance when social services were added to traditional substance abuse programmes. It has also been demonstrated that drug treatment programmes can be successfully integrated with ACT programmes (Dennis et al.; Teague et al.).

Do Social Services Play a Preventative Role?

What do we know about the role of social services in preventing violence and crime among persons with major mental disorders? This question can be answered in a single word: nothing—at least as far as empirical evidence is concerned. As stated above, our regard for social services is based mainly on common sense: It has always been taken for granted that social services are beneficial in one way or another. In addition, social services are interwoven with treatment programmes in such a way that it is difficult to demonstrate their effectiveness. The lack of identification of effectiveness of individual elements in different programmes has been pointed out by others (Dennis et al., 1991; Essock & Kontos, 1995). In evaluating the impact of social services, therefore, we must rely on studies of comprehensive treatment programmes of which social services are an integral part. Furthermore, as our focus is prevention of violence and crime, and as violence is not usually recorded as an outcome measure in studies of non-forensic patient populations, we must concentrate on follow-up studies of *mentally disordered offenders.*

Of particular interest are outcome measures in terms of jail recidivism, inpatient psychiatric services, and frequency of violent behaviour.

Outcome of Selected Community Treatment Programmes

Of nine studies exploring the impact of comprehensive outpatient programmes on re-institutionalization and prevalence of disruptive behaviour, three concluded that patients receiving the perceived best follow-up were re-incarcerated more frequently than controls (McFarland & Blair, 1995; McGrew, Bond, Dietzen, McKasson, & Miller, 1995; Solomon, Draine, & Meyerson, 1994), three reached the opposite conclusion (Lafave et al., 1993; Ventura, Cassel, Jacoby, & Huang, 1998; Wilson et al., 1995), and three found no significant differences in outcome measures on mental health and social functioning between an intensive-care programme and standard aftercare (Ford et al., 1997; Holloway & Carson, 1998; Marshall et al., 1995). All these programmes had a more or less explicit mandate to increase community tenure, and it must be questioned why the results contrast so widely. Why do some ACT or intensive managed care programmes succeed and others fail?

The differences in outcome can most likely be explained by cultural, ideological, organizational, and, to some extent, financial factors. It has been pointed out that ACT programmes may deteriorate into surveillance regimes (Albonetti & Hepburn, 1997; Essock & Kontos, 1995; McFarland & Blair, 1995; Solomon et al., 1994), and this may be the reason why some studies have found an increased re-imprisonment rate following assertive care. Organizational issues may also contribute to the outcome of a programme. McFarland and Blair found significant inter-agency ideological conflicts and hold that these were responsible for poor outcome. Similar problematic relationships between social services and health services have been reported from the United Kingdom (Hadley & Goldman, 1995; Shepherd et al., 1996). Conflicts over leadership also undermine the efficiency of programmes: Not surprisingly, parole officers argue they are best suited for this role (Smith, 1997); social workers are convinced they should take the lead (MacDonald & Sheldon, 1997); and general practitioners find that they do a better job as case mangers than the other parties involved (Shepherd et al.). A publication of the British Home Office gives some support to the superiority of general practitioners over the other two groups (Home Office, 1995). Others have recommended the introduction of police officers in case management (Dvoskin & Steadman, 1994; Lamb & Weinberger, 1998). It is natural to believe that this would increase the surveillance potential of community programmes, which has been described as a failure of ACT programmes. Whether it would prove effective in preventing violence is another matter.

Concerning the organization of services, Goldman et al. (1992) and Teague et al. (1995) stress the importance of uniform organization, avoiding a combination of services run by different government departments, as well as the importance of administrative support and clarity in programme administration.

It may be that some of the problems related to aftercare and follow-up in the community can be solved by improving the planning of such services before the patient is released from institutional care. In Scotland, a written aftercare plan is now required before a prisoner can be released on parole, and this is regarded as a key factor in the effectiveness of aftercare programmes (Paterson, 1998). Lack of cooperation between institutional and community care providers represents a major problem for rehabilitation programmes, as pointed out by Zapf, Roesch, and Hart (1996). It has been suggested that Norway's new mental health act include mandatory collaboration between primary health care providers and mental health professionals, in order to draw up an effective community treatment plan, but it remains to be seen whether cooperation can be achieved by legal statute.

The success of programmes that actually met the stated goals of reducing crime recidivism and increasing community tenure (Lafave et al., 1993; Ventura et al., 1998; Wilson et al., 1995) can be explained by the fact that they apparently avoided the above pitfalls. In addition, they stressed the importance of identifying patient needs and the role of patient advocacy on the treatment teams. This has been underlined by other authors (Dennis et al., 1991; MacDonald & Sheldon, 1997), while Dixon et al. (1995) describe how specially designed "mini-teams" were particularly effective in serving the severely mentally ill in the community.

While some programmes resulted in a parallel decrease in re-incarceration and re-hospitalization, others resulted in an increase in re-hospitalization but an decrease in re-imprisonment (Luettgen et al., 1998; Marshall et al., 1998; Wiederanders, Bromley, & Choate, 1997). This latter pattern raises interesting questions. Can low-threshold inpatient services prevent crime? Is deliberate use of inpatient services an acceptable strategy for controlling potentially violent behaviour? In general terms, these questions concern the revolving-door policy, which has mainly been looked upon as proof of failure. It may be that this policy is an effective instrument for avoiding criminalization of the severe mentally ill. At present there is no clear answer to these questions.

In the overall analysis of Marshall and co-workers for the Cochrane Library, the main findings were that ACT programmes improved accommodation status, increased employment rates, and increased patient satisfaction compared to standard community treatment (Marshall & Lockwood, 1998). When ACT was compared to hospital-based aftercare, improvement was also found with regard to programme compliance and length of inpatient stays. The review of assertive case management, however, did not demonstrate the same positive results. Except for increased compliance, no advantages were found in case management over standard community aftercare. On the contrary, case management was found to increase re-hospitalization rates (Marshall et al., 1998). The conclusion of Dvoskin and Steadman (1994), that case management is the key to managing the risk of violence among people with mental illness in the community, has not been confirmed by the Cochrane review. Another interesting finding of the Cochrane ACT review is that the higher the quality of the study, the less difference in outcome found between ACT and standard treatment. This finding probably reflects the difficult research problems involved in evaluating comprehensive outpatient programmes, as discussed earlier in this chapter.

Conclusions

Social services have limited potential to reduce the rates of crime and violence among persons with major mental disorders, because the majority of persons with major mental disorders who commit violent crimes are previously unknown to providers of health and social services. The low base rate of violent crimes, when combined with the low prevalence of persons with major mental disorders living in the community, in itself limits the potential for reduced crime and violence through the introduction of social services.

Most treatment and rehabilitation programmes offer some social services as an integral part of the programme. Lack of cooperation among service providers and lack of coordination of services are identified as the most serious hindrances to the provision of effective social services to persons with major mental disorders in the community.

A large proportion of persons with major mental disorders who commit violent crimes have a concurrent diagnosis of substance abuse. This makes cooperation between mental health care providers and substance abuse rehabilitation programmes vital. In many countries those services are poorly integrated and are administered under different government departments.

Many studies have found that offenders with major mental disorders require particularly intensive case management or assertive team-based treatment when they live in the community, in order to prevent recidivism. There is conflicting evidence, however, on the effectiveness of intensive community treatment programmes, both in terms of cost-effectiveness, improvement in the mental disorder, and relapse and in terms of re-admissions and re-offending.

The opinions of providers and users concerning the importance of different kinds of social services are not always identical. In this respect, more attention should be paid to the opinion of the patients.

References

Albonetti, C.A., & Hepburn, J.R. (1997). Probation revocation: A proportional hazard model of the conditioning effects of social disadvantage. *Social problems, 44*, 124–138.

Belfrage, H. (1991). The crime preventive effect of psychiatric treatment on mentally disordered offenders in Sweden. *International Journal of Law and Psychiatry, 14*, 237–243.

Belfrage, H. (1992). Den økande andelen psykisk störda brotslinger i fängelserna [The increased proportion of mentally disordered offenders among prisoners]. *Nordisk Tidsskrift for Kriminalvidenskab, 79*, 214–221.

Brabbins, C.J., & Travers, R.F. (1994). Mental disorder amongst defendants in Liverpool Magistrates' Court. *Medicine, Science and the Law, 34,* 279–283.

Brems, C., & Johnson, M.E. (1997). Clinical implications of the co-occurrence of substance use and other psychiatric disorders. *Professional Psychology: Research and Practice, 28,* 437–447.

Brooke, D., Taylor, C., Gunn, J., & Maden, A. (1996). Point prevalence of mental disorder in unconvicted male prisoners in England and Wales. *British Medical Journal, 313,* 1524–1527.

Burns, B.J., & Santos, A.B. (1995). Assertive community treatment: An update on randomized trials. *Psychiatric Services, 46,* 669–675.

Callahan, L.A., & Silver, E. (1998). Revocation of conditional release. *International Journal of Law and Psychiatry, 21,* 177–186.

Cohen, C. (1993). Poverty and the course of schizophrenia. *Hospital and Community Psychiatry, 44,* 951–957.

Corrado, R.R., Doherty, D., & Glackman, W. (1989). A demonstration program for chronic recidivists of criminal justice, health, and social service agencies. *International Journal of Law and Psychiatry, 12,* 211–229.

Davis, S. (1994). Factors associated with the diversion of mentally disordered offenders. *Bulletin of the American Academy of Psychiatry and the Law, 22,* 389–397.

Deci, P.A., Santos, A.B., Hiott, D.W., Schoenwald, S., & Dias, J.K. (1995). Dissemination of assertive community treatment programs. *Psychiatric Services, 46,* 676–678.

Dennis, D.L., Buckner, J.C., Lipton, F.R., & Levine, I.S. (1991). A decade of research and services for homeless mentally ill persons: Where do we stand? *American Psychologist, 46,* 1129–1138.

Diamond, R.J. (1996). Coercion and tenacious treatment in the community: Applications to the real world. In D.L. Dennis & J. Monahan (Eds.), *Coercion and aggressive community treatment: A new frontier in mental health law.* New York: Plenum.

Dickey, B., Gonzalez, O., Latimer, E., Latimer, E., Powers, K., Schutt, R., & Goldfinger, S. (1996). Use of mental health services by formerly homeless adults residing in group and independent housing. *Psychiatric Services, 47,* 152–158.

Dixon, L., Friedman, N., & Lehman, A. (1993). Housing patterns of homeless mentally ill persons receiving assertive treatment services. *Hospital and Community Psychiatry, 44,* 286–288.

Dixon, L., Krauss, N., Kernan, E., Lehman, A.F., & DeForge, B.R. (1995). Modifying the PACT model to serve homeless persons with severe mental illness. *Psychiatric Services, 46,* 684–688.

Drake, R.E., Osher, F.C., & Wallach, M.A. (1991). Homelessness and dual diagnosis. *American Psychologist, 46,* 1149–1158.

Druss, B.G., & Rosenheck, R.A. (1998). Mental disorders and access to medical care in the United States. *American Journal of Psychiatry, 155,* 1775–1777.

Dvoskin, J.A., & Steadman, H.J. (1994). Using intensive case management to reduce violence by mentally ill persons in the community. *Hospital and Community Psychiatry, 45,* 679–684.

Essock, S.M., & Kontos, N. (1995. Implementing assertive community treatment. *Psychiatric Services, 46,* 679–683.

Estroff, S.E., Zimmer, C., Lachicotte, S., & Benoit, J. (1994). The influence of social networks and social support on violence by persons with serious mental illness. *Hospital and Community Psychiatry, 45,* 669–679.

Ford, R., Raftery, J., Ryan, A., Beadsmoore, A., Craig, T., & Muijen, M. (1997). Intensive case management for people with serious mental illness. *Journal of Mental Health (UK)*, *6*, 191–199.

Geddes, J.R., Newton, J.R., Bailey, S., Freeman, C., & Young, G. (1996). Prevalence of psychiatric disorders, cognitive impairment and functional disability among homeless people resident in hostels. *Health Bulletin, 54*, 276–279.

Goldman, H.H., Morrissey, J.P., Ridgely, M.S., & Frank, R.G. (1992). Lesson from the program on chronic mental illness. *Health Affairs, 11*, 55–68.

Gottlieb, P., Gabrielsen, G., & Kramp, P. (1987). Psychotic homicides in Copenhagen from 1959–1983. *Acta Psychiatrica Scandinavica, 76*, 285–292.

Graham, K., Leonard, K.E., Room, R., Wild, C.T., Pihl, R.O., Bois, C., & Single, E. (1998). Current directions in research on understanding and preventing intoxicated aggression. *Addiction, 93*, 659–677.

Grossman, L.S., Haywood, T.W., & Cavanough, J.L., Davis, J.M., & Lewis, D.A. (1995). State psychiatric hospital patients with past arrests for violent crimes. *Psychiatric Services, 46*, 790–795.

Hadley, T.R., & Goldman, H. (1995). Effect of recent health and social service policy reforms on Britain's mental health system. *British Medical Journal, 311*, 1556–1558.

Hallam, A., Beecham, J., Knapp, M., & Fenyo, A. (1994). The costs of accommodation and care: Community provision for former long-stay psychiatric hospital patients. *European Archives of Psychiatry and Clinical Neuroscience, 243*, 304–310.

Hanoa, R. (1997). *Sosialmedisinske behov og uførhet i et saneringsstrøk i Oslo* [Needs of social medicine and disability in an inner-city area of Oslo]. Oslo: Gyldendal.

Harris, G.T., & Koepsell, T.D. (1996). Criminal recidivism in mentally ill offenders. *Bulletin of the American Academy of Psychiatry and the Law, 24*, 177–186.

Holloway, F., & Carson, J. (1998). Intensive case management for the severely mentally ill. *British Journal of Psychiatry, 174*, 19–22.

Home Office. (1995). *The supervision of restricted patients in the community.* London: Home Office Research and Statistics Department, Research Findings #19.

Høyer, G. (1986). Compulsory admitted patients' ability to make use of their legal rights. *International Journal of Law and Psychiatry, 8*, 413–422.

Hylton, J.H. (1995). Health or criminal justice options for the long-term seriously mentally ill in a Canadian province. *International Journal of Law and Psychiatry, 18*, 45–59.

Jablensky, A. (Ed.). (1995). Epidemiological psychiatry. *Clinical Psychiatry: International Practice and Research, 1*(2), Balliére Tindall.

Jeffreys, S.E., Harvey, C.A., McNaught, A.S., Quale, A.S., King, M.B., & Bird, A.S. (1997). The Hampstead Schizophrenia Survey 1991. I: Prevalence and service use comparison in an inner London health authority, 1986–1991. *British Journal of Psychiatry, 170*, 301–306.

Krogstrup, H.K., & Stenbak, E. (1993). *Fra udstødning til deltagelse* [From exclusion to participation]. Copenhagen: Socialministeriet.

Lafave, H., Souza, H.R., & Gerber, G.J. (1996). Assertive community treatment of severe mental illness: A Canadian experience. *Psychiatric Services, 47*, 757–759.

Lafave, H.G., Pinkney, A.A., & Gerber, G.J. (1993). Criminal activity by psychiatric clients after hospital discharge. *Hospital and Community Psychiatry, 44*, 180–181.

Lamb, H.R., & Weinberger, L.E. (1998). Persons with severe mental illness in jails and prisons: A review. *Psychiatric Services, 49*, 483–492.

Lehman, A.F., Myers, P., Dixon, L., & Johnsen, J.L. (1994). Defining subgroups of dual diagnosis patients for service planning. *Hospital and Community Psychiatry, 45*, 556–561.

Lindqvist, P. (1989). *Violence against a person: The role of mental disorder and abuse.* Umeå: Umeå University Medical Dissertations.

Lindqvist, P., & Allebeck, P. (1990). Schizophrenia and crime: A longitudinal follow-up of 644 schizophrenics in Stockholm. *British Journal of Psychiatry, 157,* 345–350.

Luettgen, J., Chrapko, W.E., & Reddon, J.R. (1998). Preventing violent re-offending in not criminally responsible patients: An evaluation of a continuity of treatment program. *International Journal of Law and Psychiatry, 21,* 89–98.

Lurigio, A.J., & Lewis, D.A. (1989). Worlds that fail: A longitudinal study of urban mental patients. *Journal of Social issues, 45,* 79–90.

MacDonald, G., & Sheldon, B. (1997). Community care services for the mentally ill: Consumers' views. *International Journal of Social Psychiatry, 43,* 35–55.

Marrone, J., Balzell, A., & Gold, M. (1995). Employment supports for people with mental illness. *Psychiatric Services, 46,* 707–711.

Marshall, M., Gray, A., Lockwood, A., & Green, R. (1998*). Case management for people with severe mental disorders.* Cochrane Library, Issue 3. Oxford: Update Software.

Marshall, M., & Lockwood, A. (1998*). Assertive community treatment for people with severe mental disorders.* Cochrane Library, Issue 3. Oxford: Update Software.

Marshall, M., Lockwood, A., & Gath, D. (1995). Social services case-management for long-term mental disorders: A randomised controlled trial. *Lancet, 345,* 409–412.

Marshall, M., Nehring, J., Taylor, C., & Gath, D. (1994). Characteristics of homeless mentally ill people who lose contact with caring agencies. *Irish Journal of Psychological Medicine, 11,* 160–163.

Marx, A.J., Test, M.A., & Stein, L.I. (1973). Extrahospital management of severe mental illness. *Archives of General Psychiatry, 29,* 505–511.

McFarland, B.H., & Blair, G. (1995). Delivering comprehensive services to homeless mentally ill offenders. *Psychiatric Services, 46,* 179–181.

McGilloway, S., & Donelly, M. (1998). Service utilization by former long stay psychiatric patients in Northern Ireland. *International Journal of Social Psychiatry, 44,* 12–21.

McGrew, J.H., Bond, G.R., Dietzen, L., McKasson, M., & Miller, L.D. (1995). A multisite study of client outcomes in assertive community treatment. *Psychiatric Services, 46,* 696–701.

McLellan, A.T., Hagan, T.A., Levine, M., Gould, F., Meyers, K., Bencivengo, M., & Durell, J. (1998). Supplemental social services improve outlook in public addiction treatment. *Addiction, 93,* 1489–1501.

Molven, O., & Vetvik, E. (1985). *Publikums kjennskap til forvaltningens praktisering og forvaltningsloven* [The public's knowledge about administration and administrative law]. Oslo: Delrapport.

Morse, G.A., Calsyn, R.J., Allan, G., Tempelhof, B., & Smith, R. (1992). Experimental comparison of the effects of three treatment programs for homeless mentally ill people. *Hospital and Community Psychiatry, 43,* 1005–1010.

Morse, G.A., Calsyn, R.J., Klinkenberg, W.D., Trusty, M.L., Gerber, F., Smith, R., Tempelhof, B., & Ahmad, L. (1997). An experimental comparison of three types of case management for homeless mentally ill persons. *Psychiatric Services, 48,* 497–503.

Nordentoft, M. (1994). Hjemløse i Københavns gader [Homeless in the streets of Copenhagen]. *Ugeskrift for Læger, 156,* 3032–3039.

Paterson, F. (1998). Reducing offending: Towards more effective practice in Scotland. In *Kriminalvårdsstyrelsen. What works?* Norrköping.

Prins, H. (1994). Is diversion just a diversion? *Medicine, Science and the Law, 34,* 137–147.

Raja, M., Azzoni, A., & Lubich, L. (1997). Aggressive and violent behavior in a population of psychiatric inpatients. *Social Psychiatry and Psychiatric Epidemiology, 32,* 428–434.

Rog, D.J., McCombs, T., Kimberly, L., Mongelli, G., Ariana, M., Brito, M., & Conseuelo, E. (1995). Implementation of the homeless family program. 2: Characteristics, strengths and needs of participants families. *American Journal of Orthospsychiatry, 65,* 514–528.

Saltnes, K. (1980). *Rettighetsinformasjon til foreldre/foresatte med funksjonshemmede førskolebarn i Møre og Romsdal* [Information concerning the legal rights of parents/guardians of handicapped preschool children]. Molde, Norway: Høyskolen i Molde.

Satsumi, Y., Inada, T., & Yamauchi, T. (1998). Criminal offenses among discharged mentally ill individuals. *International Journal of Law and Psychiatry, 21,* 197–207.

Shepherd, G., Muijen, M., Hadley, T.R., & Goldman, H. (1996). Effects of mental health services reform on clinical practice in the United Kingdom. *Psychiatric Services, 47,* 1351–1355.

Solomon, P., Draine, J., & Meyerson, A. (1994). Jail recidivism and rejection of community mental health services. *Hospital and Community Psychiatry, 45,* 793–797.

Sosial- og Helsedepartementet. (1998). *Innstilling til det kgl Sosial- og helsedepartementet fra Rasmussenutvalget* [Report to the Department of Social Affairs and Health from the Rasmussen Committee]. Oslo: Department of Social Affairs and Health.

Smith, G. (1997). Risk assessment and management at the interface between the probation service and psychiatric practice. *International Review of Psychiatry, 9,* 283–288.

Steadman, H.J., Barbera, S.S., & Dennis, D.L. (1994). A national survey of jail diversion programs for mentally ill detainees. *Hospital and Community Psychiatry, 45,* 1109–1113.

Steadman, H.J., Mulvey, E.P., Monahan, J., Clark Robbins, P., Appelbaum, P.S., Grisso, T., Roth, L.H., & Silver, E. (1998). Violence by people discharged from acute psychiatric inpatient facilities and by others in the same neighborhoods. *Archives of General Psychiatry, 55,* 393–401.

Stein, L.I., & Test, M.A. (1980). Alternative to mental hospital treatment. I: Conceptual model, treatment program and clinical evaluation. *Archives of General Psychiatry, 37,* 392–397.

Swanson, J.W., Holzer, C.E., Ganju, V.K., & Jono, R.T. (1990). Violence and psychiatric disorder in the community: Evidence from the Epidemiological Catchment Area surveys. *Hospital and Community Psychiatry, 41,* 761–770.

Swartz, M.S., Swanson, J.W., Hiday, V.A., Borum, R., Wagner, H.R., & Burns, B.J. (1998). Violence and severe mental illness: The effect of substance abuse and nonadherence to medication. *American Journal of Psychiatry, 155,* 226–231.

Teague, G.B., Drake, R.E., & Ackerson, T.H. (1995). Evaluating use of continuous treatment for persons with mental illness and substance abuse. *Psychiatric Services, 46,* 689–695.

Teplin, L. (1990). The prevalence of severe mental disorder among male urban jail detainees: Comparison with the Epidemiological Catchment Area program. *American Journal of Public Health, 80,* 663–669.

Ventura, L.A., Cassel, C.A., Jacoby, J.A., & Huang, B. (1998). Case management of mentally ill persons released from jail. *Psychiatric Services, 49,* 1330–1337.

Wallace, C., Mullen, P., Burgess, A., Palmer, S., Ruschena, D., & Browne, C. (1998). Serious criminal offending and mental disorder: Case linkage study. *British Journal of Psychiatry, 172,* 477–484.

Wiederanders, M.R., Bromley, D.L., & Choate, P.A. (1997). Forensic conditional release programs and outcomes in three states. *International Journal of Law and Psychiatry, 20,* 249–257.

Wilson, D., Tien, G., & Eaves, D. (1995). Increasing the community tenure of mentally disordered offenders: An assertive case management program. *International Journal of Law and Psychiatry, 18,* 61–69.

Wittman, F.D. (1989). Housing models for alcohol programs serving homeless people. *Contemporary Drug Problems, 16,* 483–504.

Wolff, N., Helminiak, T.W., Morse, G.A., Calsyn, R.J., Klinkenberg, W.D., & Trusty, M.L. (1997). Cost-effectiveness evaluation of three approaches to case management for homeless mentally ill clients. *American Journal of Psychiatry, 154,* 341–348.

Wolpe, P.R., Gorton, G., Serota, R., & Sanford, B. (1993). Predicting compliance of dual diagnosis inpatients with aftercare treatment. *Hospital and Community Psychiatry, 44,* 45–49.

World Health Organization. (1994). *Community-based rehabilitation and the health care referral services.* Geneva: Author.

Wormith, J.S., & McKeague, F. (1996). A mental health survey of community correctional clients in Canada. *Criminal Behaviour and Mental Health, 6,* 49–72.

Zapf, P.A., Roesch, R., & Hart, S.D. (1996). An examination of the relationship of homelessness to mental disorder, criminal behavior and health care in a pretrial jail population. *Canadian Journal of Psychiatry, 41,* 435–440.

Georg Høyer is associated with the Institute of Community Medicine, University of Tromsø, Norway.

Author's Note

Comments or queries may be directed to Georg Høyer, Institute of Community Medicine, Department of Social Medicine, University of Tromsø, 9037 Tromsø, Norway. Telephone: 47 77 64 48 16. Fax: 47 77 64 48 31. E-mail: <Georg.Hoyer @ism.uit.no>.

SOCIAL AND COMMUNITY SERVICES AND THE RISK FOR VIOLENCE AMONG PEOPLE WITH SERIOUS PSYCHIATRIC DISORDERS

In Search of Mechanisms

SUE E. ESTROFF

Høyer's review of the empirical findings on the role of social services in preventing violence by persons with serious psychiatric disorders is insightful and analytically keen. He concludes that there is insufficient evidence from randomized controlled trials to make a claim about the influence of these resources *qua* interventions in decreasing the incidence of violent acts and threats in this diverse population. It is clear, nonetheless, that uncoordinated, inaccessible, inadequate, and inhospitable services—arguably the norm in many public mental health systems in the United States—have no detectable impact on the risks for and incidence of violence, except perhaps to increase them.

There are some promising, if inconclusive, findings concerning community-based service interventions that are associated with reduced risk for violence among people with serious psychiatric disorders. Dvoskin and Steadman (1997) report unpublished findings from New York and Texas where intensive case management was associated with lowered rates of violence and reduced recidivism among patients with a history of violence. Ventura, Cassel, Jacoby, and Huang (1998) found that community case management significantly lowered re-arrest rates in mentally ill persons released from jail in Toledo, Ohio. In our collaborative work (Estroff, Swanson, Lachicotte, Swartz, & Bolduc, 1998; Swanson et al., 1997), we found that research participants who listed mental health professionals as key members of their social networks had lower risk for violence, and that people with more than 50 visits over 18 months had a lower risk for violence than people with the fewest mental health visits. On the other hand, Segal, Akutsu, and Watson (1998) found that community services had no impact on involuntary psychiatric treatment recidivism based on dangerousness in the San Francisco Bay area during a 12-month period. Johnson et al. (1998) found that intensive mental health and social services in a United Kingdom health sector with a high rate of adverse events (including violent ones) did not reduce the incidence of those events; even after the intensive services had been provided, this sector showed a higher rate of homicides, violence, and suicides in comparison to a health sector with lower risk at the outset and a standard (less intensive) intervention.

S. Hodgins (ed.), Violence among the Mentally Ill, 383–387.
© 2000 *Kluwer Academic Publishers. Printed in the Netherlands.*

In view of these mixed and preliminary findings, it may be useful to engage in this topic from a more basic perspective and level of inquiry. After all, the conclusion that social services *could* have an effect on violence and criminality rests on a series of assumptions that require examination. What mechanisms would produce such an effect? More specifically, we will examine the following related questions:

1. What rationale, set of assumptions, or sense of optimism leads us to expect that participation in community mental health and social services will have an appreciable impact on the frequency and severity of violent acts and threats by (and perhaps towards) persons with serious psychiatric disorders?

2. Why would (or do) community mental health and social services decrease the need and opportunity (Estroff et al., 1998) for violent acts and threats by persons with serious psychiatric disorders?

3. How do community mental health and social services directly or indirectly address known risk factors for violent acts and threats by persons with serious psychiatric disorders?

In order to address these questions, we must identify and define "community mental health and social services." Høyer's definition (this volume) is accurate and informative at one level. Yet we must take the discussion further if we are to examine the mechanisms—what services do and how they are provided—that might have an impact on the incidence of violent acts and threats. Ware, Tugenberg, Dickey, and McHorney (1999) provide a comprehensive description well suited to this discussion. According to these authors, care mechanisms in the community consist of the following actions:

* *Pinch-hitting:* stepping outside prescribed role to undertake tasks usually performed by someone else
* *Trouble-shooting:* anticipating and addressing potential problems before they develop
* *Smoothing transitions:* avoiding gaps in service; minimizing disruptions in routine; fostering familiarity; creating overlaps in people, knowledge, and services
* *Creating flexibility:* adapting services and routines to meet the needs of individual clients; for example, scheduling to honour client preferences
* *Speeding up the system:* monitoring, coordinating, reminding segments of the system to keep moving; building and using networks of providers
* *Contextualizing:* using biographical information to interpret needs and circumstances; constructing a time frame so that improvements and progressions are visible.

Ware et al. (1999) describe how optimal community care would be delivered—that is, by flexible, imaginative, resourceful providers who are engaged in ongoing relationships with their clientele. Such relationships and activities are central to almost every model of assertive community treatment and prescription for effective case management. However, Rapp (1998) points out that workable models are based on small case loads of 20:1 or less, 24-hour-a-day, seven-day-a-week availability, and the locating of authority in the case manager-client relationship. In essence, community mental health and social services should offer their clients enduring relationships with skilled providers, including instrumental and affective support in whatever domain of treatment and daily living each particular client requires. The next task is to consider how this ideal could or would have a preventive impact on violence by persons with serious psychiatric disorders.

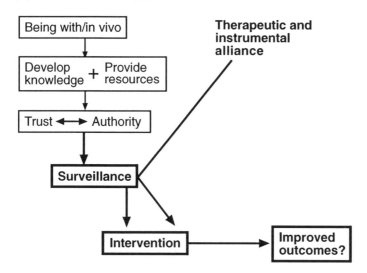

Figure 1. How services might decrease need and opportunity for violence

Services and Need and Opportunity for Violence

Figure 1 is a graphic representation of mechanisms by which community services might reduce or prevent violence by persons with serious psychiatric disorders. I suggest that services might function as follows:

- Ongoing assertive outreach *(being with)* and *in vivo* contact constitute *surveillance,* which can lead to *intervention* by: (a) alerting of potential targets; (b) intervening with respondent and target (mediating disputes, advocating for respondent, etc.); (c) alerting other potential interveners (police, family, other mental health professionals); and/or (d) hospitalizing or removing respondent from contact with target or source of provocation.
- An enduring relationship across the life domains of the respondent (described above) leads to a climate of *authority* and *trust* between provider and client; information is exchanged; provider has *knowledge* of individual risk factors and triggers. Based on this foundation, the provider can: (a) provide empathy, support, and guidance during a period of threatening behaviour or fearfulness; (b) recognize early signs of agitation, threat, or hostility and work with the respondent to alleviate them; be present and allay fears; and/or (c) play the role of trusted ally.
- Multidisciplinary resources and components provide *diversions* or *alternatives to violence, material resources,* and other means of expressing anger or releasing fear. Mental health and social service systems could: (a) provide a place for the respondent to visit or reside during high-risk periods; (b) help to provide opportunities for work or productive activity; (c) help the respondent to access money,

recreation, social activity, and amicable relationships; and/or (d) provide alternatives to interaction with law-enforcement personnel.

- Clinical expertise and medication can effectively *treat symptoms* of psychosis, agitation, and depression.
- Affiliations, relationships, and access to a social network could help to *decrease isolation* and the client could experience dignity, autonomy, and a sense of optimism.

With these resources, relationships, and services in place, we might expect to make a measurable impact on the incidence of violence among persons with serious psychiatric disorders. Surveillance alone, conducted by various means and in various ways (see McGuire, this volume), may account for most of the reduction in violence, but this speculation awaits rigorous testing. No doubt there are systems in place that meet the criteria set out above, and we need outcome data on their ability to reduce violence. It is perhaps more feasible to carefully collect outcome data from existing programmes that put these elements into practice than to rely exclusively on randomized controlled trials. When we have developed a more precise understanding of the impact of surveillance compared with medication adherence, for example, controlled trials will provide invaluable information for the next generation of practice.

Services and Known Risk Factors

The evidence is not encouraging regarding the direct impact of services on many known risk factors for violence in this population (Question 3, above). Services cannot, of course, alter demographics such as age, gender, or marital status. Diagnosis—e.g., schizophrenia—is also unaltered by services, clearly, although accurate diagnosis and subsequent effective/appropriate treatment may result from high-quality services. Medication adherence is one area in which high-quality services may have a substantial impact on violence, but adherence is problematic for many consumers and service providers, particularly where psychiatrists' time is limited and turnover of personnel is high, as is the case in many US public mental health systems. The evidence is overwhelming that substance use among the seriously mentally ill population is under-diagnosed and under- and mistreated. There is every reason to expect that increased and improved attention to substance abuse and addiction will have a measurable impact on violence within the target group.

Conclusions

The next generation of studies on reducing the incidence of and risk for violence by persons with psychiatric disorders will have to take account of the requirements of translation between clinical research and services research (Wells, 1999). Policymakers will need more than clinical trials and hypothetical scenarios to improve services and outcomes—rigorous findings from extant programmes that seem to be effective may be as persuasive as expensive clinically controlled experiments. Therapeutic and instrumental alliances that lead to relationships of trust and authority between providers and clients, which in turn lead to a decrease in need and opportunities for violence and an increase in opportunities to intervene, could then lead to improved outcomes. These mechanisms deserve further attention, refinement, and testing—in both everyday and experimental settings—if we are to determine how services affect community-based violent acts and threats.

References

Dvoskin, J., & Steadman, H. (1997). Using intensive case management to reduce violence by mentally ill persons in the community. *Psychiatric Services, 45,* 697–684.

Estroff, S., Swanson, E.J.W., Lachicotte, W.S., Swartz, M., & Bolduc, M. (1998). Risk reconsidered: Targets of violence in the social networks of people with serious psychiatric disorders. *Social Psychiatry and Psychiatric Epidemiology, 33*(Suppl 1), 95–101.

Johnson, S., Leese, M., Brooks, L., Clarkson, P., Guite, H., Thornicroft, G., Holloway, F., & Wykes, T. (1998). Frequency and predictors of adverse events: PriSM Psychosis Study 3. *British Journal of Psychiatry, 173,* 376–384.

Rapp, C.A. (1998). The active ingredients of effective case management: A research synthesis. *Community Mental Health Journal, 34*(4), 363–380.

Segal, S.P., Akutsu, P., & Watson, M. (1998). Factors associated with involuntary return to a psychiatric emergency service within 12 months. *Psychiatric Services, 49,* 1212–1217.

Swanson, J.W., Estroff, S.E., Swartz, M., Borum, R., Lachicotte, W., Zimmer, C., & Wagner, R. (1997). Violence and severe mental disorder in clinical and community populations: The effects of psychotic symptoms, comorbidity, and disaffiliation from treatment. *Psychiatry, 60*(1), 1–22.

Ventura, L.A., Cassel, C., Jacoby, J.E., & Huang, B. (1998). Case management and recidivism of mentally ill persons released from jail. *Psychiatric Services, 49,* 1330–1337.

Ware, N.C., Tugenberg, T., Dickey, B., & McHorney, C.A. (1999). An ethnographic study of the meaning of continuity of care in mental health services. *Psychiatric Services, 50*(3), 395–400.

Wells, K.B. (1999). Treatment research at the crossroads: The scientific interface of clinical trials and effectiveness research. *American Journal of Psychiatry, 156*(1), 5–10.

Sue E. Estroff is associated with the Department of Social Medicine, University of North Carolina at Chapel Hill, Chapel Hill, North Carolina, USA.

Author's Note

Comments or queries may be directed to Sue E. Estroff, PhD, Department of Social Medicine, School of Medicine, CB 7240, Wing D, University of North Carolina, Chapel Hill NC 27599-7240 USA. Telephone: 919 843-8076. Fax: 919 966-7499. E-mail: <Sue_Estroff@med.unc.edu>.

COMMUNITY TREATMENT PROGRAMMES IN EUROPE AND THE UNITED KINGDOM THAT HAVE PROVEN EFFECTIVE IN PREVENTING VIOLENCE BY THE MENTALLY ILL IN THE COMMUNITY

Administrative, Organizational, Legal, and Clinical Aspects

ROBERT FERRIS

Introduction

The complexity involved in any analysis of community treatment programmes is demonstrated by the need to include four aspects—administrative, organizational, legal, and clinical—in the above subtitle.

Clinicians are used to dealing with the complex interplay of forces operating at these various levels and influencing their decision-making in relation to individual patients, even if much of the material is second nature or operating virtually at an unconscious level—for example, knowledge of mental health legislation in the clinician's local area.

Figure 1 illustrates this complex interplay. It is taken from an English homicide inquiry report (Richardson, Chiswick, & Nutting, 1997) and shows all of the agencies which had been involved in the care and treatment of a patient who killed a mother and her two children in 1995 by burning down their house, in which he had been a lodger.

The patient did not move around a great deal in the 2 years before the homicide, so the number of agencies involved cannot be explained by a wandering lifestyle. He lived in two places about 40 miles apart and was at various times an inpatient in three psychiatric hospitals. The letters HA stand for Health Authority and the letters SSD for Social Services Department, reflecting the split between health and social services which is characteristic of the scene in the United Kingdom, from the centre down.

The patient was living in the community for about 15 months before the homicides, and the relevance of the figure is that it demonstrates the large number of agencies and, by inference, mental health professionals and other professionals involved in the care of just one patient. It is also important to remember that for any individual patient moving back and forth between the hospital and the community it may not make much sense to separate inpatient from outpatient or community care.

389

S. Hodgins (ed.), Violence among the Mentally Ill, 389–408.
© 2000 *Kluwer Academic Publishers. Printed in the Netherlands.*

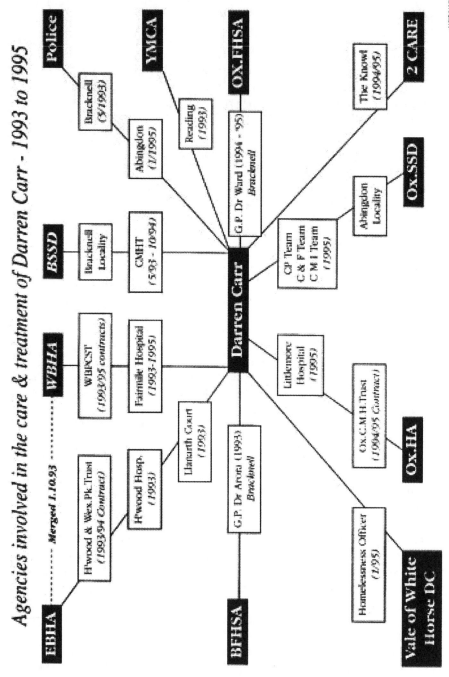

Figure 1. Agencies involved in the care and treatment of Darren Carr—1993 to 1995
(reprinted from Richardson et al., 1997)

When it comes to the question of research into programmes of community care and the measurement of violence or crime committed by patients as an outcome, a comment attributed to the United States Secretary of Defense, Robert McNamara, during the Vietnam war may be relevant. Annoyed by the endless flow of statistics relating to the supposed enemy dead—the "body count"—put to him as an indication of the success of the US military operation, McNamara suggested that what was needed was a way of making the important measurable instead of making the measurable important. If violence and criminal behaviour by mentally ill patients being cared for in the community are outcomes which are important to measure, then no one in the UK has yet succeeded in showing directly that particular community treatment programmes can reduce such behaviour. There is a small amount of direct evidence from elsewhere in Europe pointing to this conclusion, as well as a larger body of indirect evidence, but it falls well short of proof.

The scope and main divisions of this chapter are as follows: (1) empirical research findings, (2) legal aspects, (3) administrative and organizational aspects, and (4) conclusions, incorporating possible attributes of an "ideal" community treatment programme.

In relation to empirical research and administrative and organizational aspects, the focus will be mainly, but not exclusively, on the UK. Discussion of legislation and legal frameworks will have a more genuinely European perspective.

It seems important to emphasise that in relation to research and the general body of relevant literature, two theoretically and administratively distinct populations of patients are being considered, and frequently confused. The first is the large overall group of patients suffering from serious mental illness; the second is the much smaller sub-population formally designated as "forensic" patients or, possibly, "mentally disordered offenders." Although specialist (forensic) community services and programmes for mentally disordered offenders exist, it is wrong to assume that mentally disordered offenders will be dealt with exclusively by them. Indeed it has been estimated that at any given time approximately 70% of mentally disordered offenders are in the care of general psychiatric services (H. Guite, personal communication, 1997).

The literature on treatment of forensic or offender populations is understandably concerned with violence and criminal behaviour as an outcome: the literature relating to the treatment—at least in the community—of "ordinary patients" with serious mental illness has been concerned hardly at all with such behaviour. It is important to remember the distinction when attempting to survey the relevant research.

Relevant Research in the United Kingdom and Europe

Several systematic reviews have been done by workers at the Cochrane Collaboration in Oxford (Marshall, Gray, Lockwood, & Green, 1999; Marshall & Lockwood, 1999; Tyrer, Coid, Simmonds, Joseph, & Marriott, 1999), but before examining them it is worthwhile reviewing the various models of community treatment described in the research literature. Mueser, Bond, Drake, and Resnick (1998) reviewed a total of 75 studies relating to case management of persons with severe mental illness in the community and referred to the following six models of case management: (1) broker service model, (2) clinical case management model, (3) assertive community treatment (ACT) model, (4) intensive case management (ICM) model, (5) strengths model, and (6) rehabilitation model.

It is not necessary here to examine all of the features of each model. The broker case management, the original from which others evolved or were derived, had the following key features: (1) assessment, (2) planning, (3) linking to services, (4) monitoring, and (5) advocacy.

By contrast, the essential features of the ACT model, which dates back to the work of Stein and Test in Madison first published in 1980, the Programme for Assertive Community Treatment (PACT), are as follows: (1) low patient-to-staff ratios (e.g., 10:1), (2) most services provided in the community rather than in the office or clinic, (3) case load shared across clinicians, rather than individual case loads, (4) 24-hour coverage, (5) most services provided directly by the ACT team rather than brokered out, and (6) time-unlimited service (Stein & Test, 1980).

The intensive case management (ICM) model has many features in common with the ACT model. One distinction is that case loads are not shared in the ICM model; however, some descriptions of ICM models do refer to shared case loads (e.g., Aberg-Wistedt, Cressell, Lidberg, Liljenberg, & Osby, 1995; Degen, Cole, Tamaye, & Dzerovych, 1990).

In their review, Mueser et al. (1998) included ACT as one of the six case management models and chose to refer to ICM models that incorporated shared case loads as ACT models. This approach contrasts with that taken in three separate systematic reviews by the Cochrane Collaboration workers (Marshall et al., 1999; Marshall & Lockwood, 1999; Tyrer et al., 1999).

COCHRANE COLLABORATION SYSTEMATIC REVIEWS

Each of the Cochrane Collaboration systematic reviews drew together patient data from selected randomized controlled trials (RCTs) carried out worldwide, in order to conduct a meta-analysis. It is important to note that these workers drew a sharp distinction between ACT and case management, to the extent of reviewing them separately. They considered the crucial distinction to be that the ACT model emphasises team work and team responsibility, with the vital link being that between the team and the client group rather than that between individual team members and particular clients. By contrast, case management emphasises professional autonomy and individual responsibility, with the vital link being that between a single case manager and his or her case load of clients, this being true even for ICM, which can therefore (by and large) be distinguished from ACT.

The importance of the distinction is confirmed by the results of the reviews, which essentially demonstrate a positive outcome so far as ACT is concerned and a negative outcome for case management. The authors accept, however, that the method used to draw the distinction between ACT and case management, namely the label the trialists used to describe the intervention, is open to criticism. They perceive a need for a more systematic way of classifying ACT and case management in future trials—for example, by way of a validated ACT fidelity scale such as proposed by McGrew, Bond, Dietzen, and Salyers (1994).

The first review compared case management and standard care, selecting 11 RCTs from a total of 67 in the pool. Of these, three were from London and one from Oxford (Conway, 1995; Ford et al., 1995; Ford, Rafferty, et al., 1997; Ford, Ryan, Beadsmoore, Craig, & Muijen, 1997; Lear, 1993; Marshall, Lockwood, & Gath, 1995; McCrone, Beecham, & Knapp, 1994; Muijen, Cooney, Strathdee, Bell, & Hudson, 1994; Tyrer et al., 1995).

Essentially, the reviewers found that case management was more effective than standard care in keeping patients in contact with services, with a number needed to treat (NNT) of 15. Case management doubled the rate of hospital admissions relative to standard care, and four out of six trials suggested that it increased the duration of hospital admissions. It was considered unlikely that case management had been shown to produce substantial improvement in clinical or social outcome, except that one trial found a significant increase in compliance with medication.

The only outcome variable featured which was directly relevant to violent or criminal behaviour was rate of imprisonment. The authors concluded that it was not clear whether or not case management affected rates of imprisonment.

The second review (Marshall & Lockwood, 1999) compared ACT with three alternatives: standard community care, traditional hospital-based rehabilitation, and case management.

For each comparison the main outcome indices were: (1) remaining in contact with psychiatric services, (2) the extent of psychiatric hospital admissions, (3) clinical and social outcome, and (4) costs. Again, in some but not all of the studies, imprisonment, police contacts, and arrests were included under the heading of clinical and social outcomes.

Of 75 trials gathered originally, 17 met inclusion criteria for the comparison with standard care, three for comparison with hospital-based rehabilitation, and six for comparison with case management (Aberg-Wistedt et al., 1995; Audini, Marks, Lawrence, Connolly, & Watts, 1994; Bond et al., 1990; Bond, Miller, Krumwied, & Ward, 1988; Bush, Langford, Rosen, & Gott, 1990; Chandler, Meisel, McGowen, Mintz, & Madison, 1996; Cohen, Test, & Brown, 1991; De Cangas, 1994; Essock & Kontos, 1995; Herinckx, Kinney, Clarke, & Paulson, 1997; Kuhlman, 1992; Lafave, deSouza, & Gerber, 1996; Lehman, Dixon, Kernan, & Deforge, 1995; Marx, Stein, & Test, 1973; Morse et al., 1997; Morse, Calsyn, Allen, Tempelhoff, & Smith, 1992; Quinlivan et al., 1995; Rosenheck, Neale, & Gallup, 1993; Rosenheck, Neale, Leaf, Milstein, & Frisman, 1995; Solomon, Draine, & Meyerson, 1994; Test et al., 1991; Wolff et al., 1997). Of these 26 trials, only two were European, one from Stockholm (Aberg-Wistedt et al.) and one from London (Audini et al.).

The imprisonment, arrest, and police contact data may be considered separately from the other elements of clinical and social outcome. When ACT was compared to standard care there was no clear difference in rates of imprisonment, arrest, or police contact. When it was compared to hospital rehabilitation there was a statistically significant difference, with ACT showing a lower rate of imprisonment, but this arose from only one study, in Quebec (De Cangas, 1994), and was therefore not considered to be a robust finding. Similarly, in the trials comparing ACT and case management there were no significant differences.

The overall conclusion is that ACT is an effective way of caring for severely ill people in the community, maintaining contact with them, dramatically reducing the use of inpatient care, and improving some aspects of outcome. However, it should be reiterated that none of the trials reviewed contained any direct measure of violence and there was no conclusive evidence that ACT reduced imprisonment, arrest rates, or rates of police contact, by comparison with the other three treatment modalities.

Other researchers in the UK do not agree with the Cochrane reviewers' attempts to draw such a sharp distinction between ACT and case management, especially ICM. Some consider that when the services being delivered are thoroughly scrutinized the differences between ICM, certainly as it is practised in Europe, and ACT, as it has evolved in the US, tend to blur and disappear (T. Burns, personal communication, 1999).

A further review worthy of brief examination surveyed the effectiveness of Community Mental Health Teams (CMHTs) in managing patients with severe mental illnesses and disordered personalities (Tyrer et al., 1999). Because trials which related to ACT or case management were deliberately excluded, only five studies, three of which came from London (UK) (Burns, Beadsmoore, Bhat, & Oliver, 1993; Burns, Raftery, Beadsmoore, McGuigan, & Dickson, 1993; Merson et al., 1992; Tyrer et al., 1998; Tyrer, Merson, Onyett, & Johnson, 1994), were finally included. The standard or usual care to which a CMHT was being compared was whatever was the norm in the area concerned.

The results of this third review can be summarized as follows: CMHT management may help reduce suicide and be more acceptable to those with mental illness than a non-team standard-care approach. It is also more likely that a person managed by a CMHT will avoid hospital admission and spend less time as an inpatient, but there are no substantial data either supporting or refuting the use of CMHT management with respect to mental state, social functioning, or family burden. None of the studies recorded violence to others, though two recorded police contacts (Merson et al., 1992; Tyrer et al., 1994, 1998). The 1998 study of Tyrer et al. showed no significant difference between the CMHT clients and the clients of a hospital-based care programme (after discharge from inpatient care).

OTHER RESEARCH

The range of results or outcome measures used in the 75 studies reviewed by Mueser et al. (1998) were as follows: time in hospital, housing stability, jail/arrests, medication compliance, symptoms, substance abuse, social adjustment, vocational functioning, quality of life, and patient satisfaction and relative satisfaction.

The only measure that related directly to violent or criminal behaviour was jail/arrests. Some of the others might be expected to be correlates of violent or criminal behaviour, but it is arguably almost arbitrary as to how they would be prioritized. This writer would rank substance misuse, medication compliance, and symptoms in descending order of importance, but housing stability, vocational functioning, and social adjustment might also be considered. The reviewers have divided the studies into random assignment community-care studies and non-controlled community-care studies. Nearly all came from North America but the random assignment studies included four from Europe—three from London (Marx et al., 1994; Merson et al., 1992; Muijen et al., 1994) and one from Stockholm (Aberg-Wistedt et al., 1995)—and the non-controlled studies included one from Mannheim in Germany (Rossler, Loffler, Fatkenheuer, & Riecher-Rossler, 1992). None of these five European studies, two of which were included in one or the other of the previously discussed Cochrane reviews, recorded any findings for the outcomes of jail/arrests, substance abuse, medication compliance, or vocational functioning.

It is worth noting, apropos the distinction between forensic or mentally disordered offender populations and "ordinary patients" referred to earlier, that, although not a European study, the only controlled study located which involved a forensic population was that of Solomon and Draine (1995) carried out in 1995 in Philadelphia. This study examined ACT for homeless persons with severe mental illness recently released from jail, comparing ACT with both forensic case management and standard case management. The researchers found that ACT was not superior to the other two forms of management on any outcome measure, including jail time and arrest rates. These results might be thought to indicate that ACT is not suitable or effective for this group of patients. However, one other quasi-experimental study, conducted by Wilson et al. in Vancouver in 1995 (Wilson, Tien, & Eaves, 1995), compared ACT in 26 subjects with standard care in 33 subjects also being released from jail. The ACT group were engaged in treatment 3 to 4 weeks before release. The authors found that the ACT group spent 60% fewer days in prison and were on average twice as long in the community as controls before being reconvicted.

At this point mention can also be made of research currently proceeding in the UK (Creed et al., 1999). The UK 700 group have carried out a four-site trial comparing intensive and standard case management in Manchester and three other urban sites, all in London. Analysis of the initial results concerning the outcome time spent in hospital showed the presence of a group of 12 statistical outliers who were skewing the data. Of a total of 200 subjects, nearly all came within the range of 10–90 days spent in hospital over a 2-year follow-up period, but the 12 outliers had spent 18 months or more of the 2 years in hospital. All the members of this group were young male schizophrenic patients with a forensic profile who stood out dramatically from the other 95% of subjects. One of the researchers speculated that in other places—for example, the US—this small group of patients would more likely be kept very long-term in state hospitals, whereas in the UK they are more likely to be mixed in with general services and to be a group for whom ICM or ACT is not appropriate (T. Burns, personal communication, 1999). These results might be seen once again to draw attention to the differences between the "ordinary" community patient and the "forensic" subgroup.

Overall, this review of the research involving both random assignment community-care studies and non-controlled community-care studies points to the conclusion that little firm evidence has so far emerged either that the models of care being studied can achieve significant reductions in levels of violent or criminal behaviour by "ordinary" (non-offender) patients or that they cannot. Direct measurement of violent behaviour is rare, and even proxy measures such as jail and arrest rates are seldom employed. As would be expected, in the small number of studies focusing on offender patients, violent and criminal behaviour has received more attention, and there is some evidence indicating that forensic treatment programmes can have a beneficial effect.

Legal Aspects

The principal focus here is on the legal powers provided in different places to coerce patients in the community into receiving treatment or supervision. No mention will be made of legislation that relates primarily to the detention of patients in hospital. While the focus is mainly on the UK, mention can also be made of other individual European countries.

Two pieces of legislation are of particular relevance in England and Wales. One exists and the other does not. The first is a Restriction Order made out under the English Mental Health Act. The second is a Community Treatment Order (CTO), which does not exist in the UK but has been discussed often over the last 15 years and is being very much debated at present. Such an order would be equivalent in some respects to involuntary outpatient commitment, which is found in various guises in about 30 US states (Swartz et al., 1995).

RESTRICTION ORDER

The Restriction Order can be issued only by a judge, at the point when he or she sends the patient involuntarily to hospital under the Mental Health Act, essentially after conviction for a (serious) criminal offence and as an alternative to imprisonment. The Restriction Order therefore applies only to a forensic population of usually serious offenders who are being sent to hospital by the court—and mostly to secure hospitals. Its relevance to this discussion is that it provides—eventually, when the patient is judged ready to leave hospital—for a conditional discharge (release) into the community.

A conditionally discharged patient typically is obliged to accept psychiatric and social supervision (the latter from either a probation officer or a social worker) and, often, to reside in a particular place. Failure to comply with treatment and to meet the conditions renders the patient liable to administrative recall to hospital. This situation persists indefinitely for conditionally discharged patients in the community (because nearly all Restriction Orders are without limit of time) unless or until the patient is granted an absolute discharge by either a Mental Health Review Tribunal or the relevant government minister. For patients coming out of special hospital (high security), the average length of time they remain conditionally discharged in the community before achieving an absolute discharge—provided they are not recalled to hospital—is about 5 years. At any given time, in a country with a population of some 60 million, there are about 2,500 restricted patients—1,500 in hospital and 1,000 on conditional discharge. Approximately 150 patients are made subject to new Restriction Orders each year and a similar number achieve conditional discharge (Dent, 1997).

Thus this legislation provides a good deal of coercive power over a highly selected group of mentally disordered (serious) offenders. A study of the reasons for recall in a group of 183 conditionally discharged patients recalled to hospital found that re-offending (or "public danger") was the reason for recall in only 26% of cases, while in a further 26% "cause for concern" was the reason for recall and in 17% it was "uncooperative behaviour" (Hedderman, 1995). It might be argued intuitively that in this group of obviously high-risk patients the pre-emptive exercise of the power to recall helps prevent further violent or criminal behaviour in some. Certainly the majority of forensic psychiatrists in England and Wales would agree with this proposition and would also assert that conditional discharge sometimes facilitates the safe release from hospital of patients who otherwise would have to remain there.

In scrutinizing a cohort of English special hospital (high-security) patients, it should be noted that not all patients made the subject of a Restriction Order are admitted to high security, and of those who are so admitted some are eventually absolutely discharged rather than conditionally discharged into the community. In 1992 Bailey and McCulloch (1992) followed up a special hospital cohort of discharged patients and examined re-offending rates. They found that absolute rather than conditional discharge correlated with a higher rate of post-discharge criminal conviction for a serious offence, providing some evidence that a conditional discharge via a Restriction Order reduces violence in the overall group. Of course allocation to absolutely discharged rather than conditionally discharged categories is not random and would be extremely difficult to randomize.

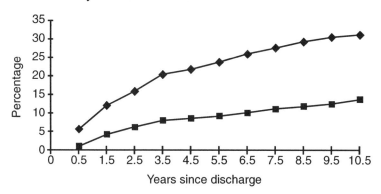

Figure 2. Proportion of patients discharged from special hospital who had
been convicted of any offence (◆) and a serious offence
(■), by years since discharge (source: Buchanan, 1998)

More recently, Buchanan (1998) looked at criminal conviction over a 10.5-year period after discharge from special hospital in a cohort of 425 patients. Buchanan did not find that reconviction rates were affected by whether or not a patient was conditionally discharged. Rather, he found that age, a legal category of psychopathic disorder (i.e., personality disorder) rather than mental illness, and prior criminal record had a significant but small predictive effect. Figure 2 shows the proportion of patients discharged from special hospital who were convicted, firstly, of any offence, and secondly, of a serious offence. Ten years after discharge more than 10% of the patients had been convicted of a serious offence—that is, any of the following: murder, attempted murder, conspiracy to murder, manslaughter, wounding, grievous bodily harm, actual bodily harm (multiple), child stealing, buggery, attempted buggery, rape, indecent assault, incest, gross indecency with children, robbery, kidnapping, aggravated burglary, or arson.

Concerning the question of whether other European countries provide for the conditional discharge of similar patients or have legislation for equivalent coercive powers aimed at identified offender patient populations, information was sought from six countries. Norway, Germany, Sweden, France, and Finland have such legislation, while Denmark does not. In France the legislation is reportedly used very rarely. In Finland the conditions attached to release can be enforced for only 6 months.

COMMUNITY TREATMENT ORDER (CTO)

The debate concerning CTO in England and Wales has a history reaching back to certain legal decisions made in 1985. These essentially took away from psychiatrists the power they had hitherto exercised to release civil patients from hospital under a "long leash" and coerce them into accepting treatment and supervision in the community under the threat of recall to hospital—a situation somewhat similar to that outlined above under the Restriction Order.

A CTO would apply to patients with severe mental illness who required, among other things, treatment with antipsychotic medication and were in the community, having been either discharged from, or not admitted to, hospital. Such an order might oblige patients to, for instance, reside in a particular place or attend a treatment centre or accept treatment with medication. One of the key issues is whether it could or should carry the power to impose treatment with medication involuntarily and, if so, whether this should happen in the patient's home or at a hospital or clinic.

Recent English legislation (1995) has made provision for a so-called "supervised discharge," which carries with it the power to convey a patient from A to B—for example, from his or her home to a clinic. It does not, however, provide any power to impose treatment against the patient's wishes and has been criticized as being a fudge. The take-up rate has remained low. A survey done 6 months after the law came into effect showed that of 115 eligible consultant psychiatrists only 15 had implemented supervised discharge, and each of these had only one patient placed under an order (Mohan, Thompson, & Mullee, 1998). It remains to be seen how popular and effective this particular piece of legislation will be in England and Wales (Pinfold, Bindman, Freidli, Beck, & Thornicroft, 1999).

One of the objections to a CTO with power to coerce patients in the community to accept treatment against their will has been that it would be in breach of Article 5(e) of the European Convention on Human Rights (ECHR). Article 5 states: "No one shall be deprived of his liberty save in the following cases and in accordance with a procedure prescribed by law...(e) the lawful detention of persons with unsound mind." This was elaborated upon in the well-known case of *Winterwerp v. the Netherlands* (1979), as follows: (1) true mental disorder must be established by objective medical expertise, (2) the mental disorder must be of a kind or degree which warrants compulsory confinement, and (3) continued detention should be determined on the persistence of the disorder.

It can readily be seen that this is really to do with confinement or detention rather than treatment, but it is relevant if compulsory admission to hospital as a sanction against failure to take the required treatment in the community is being considered.

However, authoritative legal opinion in England disagrees on whether a CTO would really be in breach of Article 5(e). The answer to this question is obviously important in relation to the future of this sort of legislation in Europe as a whole.

In Australia and New Zealand, CTOs with heavy coercive power are widespread: the 1993 South Australian Mental Health Act, for example, refers to the issuing of (Community) Treatment Orders after a patient has been received into guardianship (conservatorship). The statute empowers medical practitioners, assisted if necessary by police and/or ambulance officers, to physically impose treatment with medication on an unwilling patient subject to such an order, at a medical clinic or even in his or her own home (South Australian Mental Health Act, 1993). The notion of patients being physically forced to receive a depot injection of antipsychotic medication in their own home is widely felt to be unacceptable in England, and it appears that even if the law is changed such powers will not be introduced.

Supporters of CTOs argue that they would help with the management of patients who are difficult to engage, non-compliant, lacking in insight, and liable to repeated relapse and (therefore) re-admission to hospital. It may be that such patients are more likely to be young and male and to show comorbid substance misuse and therefore be at relatively higher risk of showing criminal and violent behaviour. An extended debate about CTOs in England has rehearsed the pros and cons over a number of years, but it would be beyond the scope of this chapter to discuss them further here. It is, however, relevant to consider other European countries to see whether any have legislation providing equivalents of the CTOs already described for Australasia, or of involuntary outpatient commitment (IOC) as found in the US.

Of six European countries surveyed (Denmark, France, Germany, Norway, the UK, and Sweden), none, with the possible exception of Norway, provided legal powers to force medication on civil patients in the community. France, Norway, and Sweden provided powers to force medication on such patients provided they were taken (but not necessarily admitted) to hospital. All six countries except Denmark provided powers to convey such patients from one place to another.

Administrative and Organizational Aspects

The real difficulty here lies in making valid and sufficiently detailed comparisons between one place and another. This is a serious problem for researchers, managers, administrators, and clinicians interested in comparing, for example, different European countries. An illustrative example is the first European attempt to replicate the

Madison PACT study (Stein & Test, 1980), carried out in London and first reported in 1992 (Muijen, Marks, Connolly, Audini, & McNamee, 1992). How are the substantial outcome differences to be explained? Was the London implementation of the PACT model incomplete or flawed in some way, or was it that the control services in London already contained more effective PACT components than the ordinary services in Madison, so the comparison between PACT and control services in London showed fewer differences? It is impossible to be sure from the published data.

The task of steering a course between providing general descriptions referring to excessively large areas on the one hand and data from a specific service, from which it is difficult to extrapolate, on the other is a daunting one. It would be unhelpful, for instance, to provide a wealth of detail about the National Health Service (NHS) in the UK and its current round of reforms—the sectorization and organization of general and specialist (e.g., forensic) psychiatric services, the important role of primary care, and so on—to those who are unfamiliar with it.

In an attempt to provide a general framework that might be applied across time and space, Tansella and Thornicroft (1998) have proposed a matrix model, which is represented in a simplified form in Table 1.

Reference is made to a geographical dimension operating at three levels—country, local (catchment) area, and the individual patient—and also to a temporal dimension subdivisible into input, process, and outcome phases. "Input" refers essentially to the resources put into a mental health care system, "process" to those activities which take place to deliver mental health services, and "outcome" to changes in functioning, morbidity, and mortality, both at the level of the individual patient and at the level of population.

Table 1. Matrix model

Geographical	Temporal dimensions					
	(A)	Input phase	(B)	Process phase	(C)	Outcome phase
(1) Country/ region level	1A	Mental health law	1B	Performance indicator (e.g., compulsory treatment rates)	1C	Suicide rates
(2) Local level (catchment area)	2A	Population needs assessment	2B	Patterns of service use	2C	Decrease of local stigma
(3) Patient level	3A	Individual needs assessment	3B	Quality of treatments	3C	Symptom reduction

Source: Tansella and Thornicroft (1998)

Inter-country comparisons are particularly difficult to make in relation to process, where, even at the highest level of aggregation, no common currency exists to define and measure variables.

Tansella and Thornicroft (1998) point out that their matrix applies particularly to mental health systems which are mainly state-funded and provided within a mental health framework. This of course applies to most European countries, as most have an administrative infrastructure which organizes health, social services, and other public services for defined geographical areas.

In attempting to use this matrix with reference to the UK, some particular administrative and organizational features are worthy of mention, though it remains difficult to avoid descending into excessive detail. Such features include the chronic under-funding of the NHS, the important role of primary care—general or family practitioners—in providing mental health care in the first instance, and the sectorization of psychiatric services so that in many settings inpatient and outpatient psychiatric care are provided by the same catchment area teams, though the extent to which those teams are based primarily in hospitals as opposed to the community varies. This integration of inpatient and outpatient care stands in contrast to the situation in some other European countries.

There is also in England an administrative separation of health and social care from the top down, with separate departments of health and social services.

Having a direct bearing on the treatment of patients in the community in England are two administrative measures: first, and most important, the care programme approach (CPA); and second, supervision registers. CPA, really case management by another name, was introduced in 1990 throughout England by the Department of Health (Department of Health, 1990). Confusingly, social services were obliged to introduce SSCM—social services "care management"—at about the same time.

CARE PROGRAMME APPROACH (CPA)

The basic principles of the CPA are those of case management, and they can be summarized as follows: systematic assessment of client need, development of a care plan, identification of a care worker, and regular review of the patient's progress. The implementation of CPA in England has been slow, uneven, and controversial. In 1997, 7 years after it had been introduced, one prominent editorialist said of CPA that "only when it is clear what it is can it be properly researched" (Burns, 1997). The Cochrane Collaboration reviewers mentioned above have essentially called for it to be scrapped and have concluded that it is questionable whether there is a case for further research on existing case management approaches. It has taken years, but it is now widely used throughout NHS psychiatric services, even if there is continued tinkering at the edges.

The Cochrane reviewers have been criticized in their turn by Brugha and Glover (1998), who state that as case management is a process or protocol its effectiveness needs to be judged in terms of desired changes in systems and processes, rather than simply on relative health gain, even if the latter is a desired outcome. In other words, they appear to be saying that it is a mistake to try and treat case management or CPA as one would a single specifiable treatment and therefore to focus exclusively on RCTs, as the Cochrane reviewers have attempted to do.

SUPERVISION REGISTER

The supervision register is an administrative measure introduced in England and Wales in 1994 (NHS Management Executive, 1994). The register was largely a response to growing media and public concern about homicides by the mentally ill, and it obliged psychiatric hospitals to establish registers identifying patients with severe mental illness who might be at significant risk of harming others, of suicide, or of severe self-neglect. The fact of a patient's inclusion on the register is supposed to be communicated to all local agencies that may come into contact with the patient, thereby enhancing clinical risk assessment and management by helping to make it less likely that patients will fall through the "net" of care. There were no legislative changes made to complement the register and no allocation of extra resources to help with its implementation. It was viewed with suspicion by the Royal College of Psychiatrists and with outright hostility by many individual mental health practitioners and organizations representing the interests of mental health consumers.

A survey done at the end of its first year of operation showed that 119 (32%) of 367 consultant psychiatrists surveyed had no patients on the register. The remaining 248 consultants had 1,151 patients registered with a mean of 4.6 patients per consultant and a range of one to 30 entries (Vaughan, 1996).

In a 1998 follow-up survey, 19 consultant psychiatrists and 28 keyworkers—mostly Community Psychiatric Nurses—were interviewed (Vaughan, 1998). Each consultant had between two and six patients on the register. Only four of the consultants and nine (one third) of the keyworkers were positive about the register, and most remained antagonistic, regarding it as a political ploy with adverse civil liberties implications. It seems likely that most professionals remain indifferent or hostile to the register, regarding it as a clinically unhelpful measure imposed centrally to satisfy bureaucratic and political needs with the result that keyworkers "on the ground" are placed at greater risk of being scapegoated if anything goes wrong.

OTHER ADMINISTRATIVE ISSUES

Among the most recent round of reforms and administrative changes, NICE, the newly established National Institute for Clinical Excellence, is worth mentioning. This centre has the task of establishing standard "best practice" guidelines and protocols for the treatment of all diseases, including mental disorders, and will act as a kind of national standard-bearer. However, concerns have been expressed about the possible resource implications of its recommendations.

There are a number of topics not mentioned at all in this section because of space constraints and because of their questionable relevance to the subject of violence or crime prevention. Examples include mandatory homicide inquiries, crisis intervention services, and partial hospitalization.

Conclusion

To sum up, with regard to the UK and the rest of Europe:
1. There is a good deal of evidence that ACT and ICM can effectively achieve the following: reduced time in hospital and improved housing stability, especially among patients who are high service users; some effect on reducing symptom level and intensity; and improvement in overall quality of life, with reduction or withdrawal of services producing a deterioration.

2. There is little evidence for a positive effect of either ACT or ICM on social functioning, vocational functioning, arrests, or time spent in jail. As far as the research on community treatment done to date is concerned, the latter two outcome indices appear to be the most relevant for evaluating violent or criminal behaviour. The modest amount of evidence that has emerged arises mostly from uncontrolled studies of specialized forensic community programmes devised to treat established offenders.

3. There appears to be almost no empirical evidence relating to direct measurement of violence, equivalent to that, for example, carried out in the MacArthur Foundation study (Steadman et al., 1998), that any community treatment programmes can reduce or prevent violence.

Researchers in this whole area of community treatment have clearly been unwilling or unable to focus on the area of violent and criminal behaviour in their subject groups: they simply have not done so.

This is in striking contrast to other sectors of society, including politicians and the media, which seem to have become increasingly intolerant of and preoccupied with the perceived threat of violence posed by the mentally ill in the community, leading to a widespread perception that "care in the community" has failed, certainly in the UK. If serious violence is to be the measure, it is difficult to sustain the conclusion that it has failed. As Gunn and Taylor (1999) have recently shown, the rate of homicides committed by those with serious mental illness in England and Wales has decreased slightly over the years—rather than increased—while at the same time, as in other European countries, the number of psychiatric beds has been dramatically reduced, from 151,000 in 1954 to 40,000 in 1992 (Davidge et al., 1994).

This long view seems lost on the general public. A sufficiently historical perspective might lead to appreciation of the fact that a person living in Oxford today is 80 times less likely to be murdered than, for example, in 1340. Records show that in England even during the late 19th century—the 1870s—there were 98,000 assaults per year, compared to a rate of just 16,500 in 1975 (Stanko, 1998).

In considering possible future developments it is relevant to note that Steadman et al. (1998) have observed that discharged hospital patients do not form a homogeneous group in relation to violence in the community, so "community patients" subject to the kind of treatment programmes discussed in this chapter may be even less homogeneous. Even within the overall group suffering from serious mental illness, given the group's modestly overall increased risk of violence there are higher risk subgroups, particularly those with comorbid substance misuse (Scott et al., 1998).

Despite the lack of convincing empirical evidence about the kind of programmes that would help reduce violence and crime, there are a number of pointers towards the configuration of the ideal programme. Such a programme might have the following features:

- ACT or ICM with small case loads of not more than 15 patients per worker
- psychiatrist presence within the team
- support from a sufficient number and range of inpatient beds, including secure beds, to avoid having workers dissipate their energies in arranging or monitoring inpatient care (when necessary) for their clients in out-of-catchment-area sites.

- avoidance of an organizational split between mental illness and alcohol/substance misuse, thereby retaining a capacity to deal with dual-diagnosis patients
- the taking seriously of early intervention
- a country/regional context of legislative power to coerce defaulters or the non-compliant into treatment without necessarily re-admitting them to hospital
- proper provision of accommodation in the public, private, or voluntary sectors to house the mentally ill, maybe including specialist hostels with specialist staffing
- services organized to facilitate separate and specialized provision for forensic patients while at the same time promoting maximal integration/reintregation of forensic patients into general services as early as is appropriate.

The widespread provision of such services has profound resource implications, and it is clear that deployment of sufficient resources to care for the deinstitutionalized in the community has probably never occurred anywhere in a comprehensive, widespread way. The challenge for the future, then, may be seen as twofold: first, to carry out research that will support or refute the claim that a service with the kinds of features outlined above really does reduce violent or criminal behaviour without reinstitutionalizing patients en masse; and second, assuming that such resource-intensive, costly programmes are not going to be provided for the "ordinary" seriously mentally ill, the challenge is to find and then implement means of identifying and selecting out high-risk subgroups, so that appropriately intensive, resource-rich programmes can be effectively targeted on them.

References

Aberg-Wistedt, A., Cressell, T., Lidberg, Y., Liljenberg, B., & Osby, U. (1995). Two-year outcome of team-based intensive case management for patients with schizophrenia. *Psychiatric Services, 46,* 1263–1266.

Audini, B., Marks, I.M., Lawrence, R.E., Connolly, J., & Watts, V. (1994). Home-based versus out-patient/in-patient care for people with serious mental illness: Phase II of a controlled study. *British Journal of Psychiatry, 165,* 204–210.

Bailey, J., & McCulloch, M. (1992). Patterns of reconviction in patients discharged directly to the community from a special hospital: Implications for aftercare. *Journal of Forensic Psychiatry, 3,* 445–461.

Bond, G.R., Miller, L.D., Krumwied, R.D., & Ward, R.S. (1988). Assertive case management in three CMHCs: A controlled study. *Hospital and Community Psychiatry, 39,* 411–418.

Bond, G.R., Witheridge, T.F., Dincin, J., Wasmer, D., Webb, J., & De Graaf-Kaser, R. (1990). Assertive community treatment for frequent users of psychiatric hospitals in a large city: A controlled study. *American Journal of Community Psychology, 18,* 856–891.

Brugha, T., & Glover, G. (1998). Process and health outcomes: Need for clarity in systematic reviews of case management for severe mental disorders. *Health Trends, 30,* 76–79.

Buchanan, A. (1998). Criminal conviction after discharge from special (high security) hospital: Incidence in the first ten years. *British Journal of Psychiatry, 172,* 472–476.

Burns, T. (1997). Case management, care management and care programming. *British Journal of Psychiatry, 170,* 393–395.

Burns, T., Beadsmoore, A., Bhat, A.V., & Oliver, A. (1993). A controlled trial of home-based acute psychiatric services. I: Clinical and social outcome. *British Journal of Psychiatry, 163,* 49–54.

Burns, T., Raftery, J., Beadsmoore, A., McGuigan, S., & Dickson, M. (1993). A controlled trial of home-based acute psychiatric services. II: Treatment patterns and costs. *British Journal of Psychiatry, 163,* 55–61.

Bush, C.T., Langford, M.W., Rosen, P., & Gott, W. (1990). Operation outreach: Intensive case management for severely psychiatrically disabled adults. *Hospital and Community Psychiatry, 41,* 647–649.

Chandler, D., Meisel, J., McGowen, M., Mintz J., & Madison, K. (1996). Client outcomes in two model capitated integrated service agencies. *Psychiatric Services, 47,* 175–180.

Cohen, L.J., Test, M.A., & Brown, R.L. (1991). Suicide and schizophrenia: Data from a prospective community treatment study. *American Journal of Psychiatry, 147,* 602–607.

Conway, M. (1995). Care-management for mental illness. *Lancet, 345,* 926–927.

Creed, F., Burns, T., Butler, T., Byford, S., Murray, R., Thompson, S., & Tyrer, P. (1999). Comparison of intensive and standard case management for patients with psychosis; rationale of the trial; UK 700 group. *British Journal of Psychiatry, 174,* 74–78.

Davidge, M., et al. (1994, March). *Survey of English mental illness hospitals March 1994: Monitoring the closure of the water tower, prepared for the mental health task force.* University of Birmingham, UK.

De Cangas, J.P.C. (1994). Le "case management" affirmatif : Une evaluation complète d'un programme du genre en milieu hospitalier. *Santé mentale au Québec, 19,* 75–92.

Degen, K., Cole, N., Tamaye, L., & Dzerovych, G. (1990). Intensive case management for the seriously mentally ill. *Administration and Policy in Mental Health, 17,* 265–269.

Dent, S. (1997). The Home Office Mental Health Unit and its approach to the assessment and management of risk. *International Review of Psychiatry, 9,* 265–271.

Department of Health. (1990). *Caring for people: The care programme approach for people with a mental illness referred to the specialist psychiatric services* [HC (90) 23]. London: Author.

Essock, S.M., & Kontos, N. (1995). Implementing assertive community treatment teams. *Psychiatric Services, 46,* 679–683.

Ford, R., Beadsmoore, A., Ryan, P., Repper, J., Craig, T., & Muijen, M. (1995). Providing the safety net: Case management for people with a serious mental illness. *Journal of Mental Health, 4,* 91–97.

Ford, R., Rafferty, J., Ryan, P., Beadsmoore, A., Craig, T., & Muijen, M. (1997). Intensive case management for people with serious mental illness – site 2: Cost-effectiveness. *Journal of Mental Health, 6,* 191–199.

Ford, R., Ryan, P., Beadsmoore, A., Craig, T., & Muijen M. (1997). Intensive case management for people with serious mental illness – site 2: Clinical and social outcome. *Journal of Mental Health, 6,* 181–190.

Gunn, J., & Taylor, P.J. (1999). Homicides by people with mental illness: Myth and reality. *British Journal of Psychiatry, 174,* 9–14.

Hedderman, C. (1995). The supervision of restricted patients in the community. *Research Findings, 19,* 1–4 (Home Office Research and Statistics Department).

Herinckx, H.A., Kinney, R.F., Clarke, G.N., & Paulson, R.I. (1997). Assertive community treatment versus usual care in engaging and retaining clients with severe mental illness. *Psychiatric Services, 48,* 1297–1306.

Kuhlman, T.L. (1992). Unavoidable tragedies in Madison, Wisconsin: A third view. *Hospital and Community Psychiatry, 43,* 72–73.

Lafave, H.G., deSouza, H.R., & Gerber, G.J. (1996). Assertive community treatment of severe mental illness: A Canadian experience. *Psychiatric Services, 47,* 757–759.

Lear, G. (1993). Managing care at home. *Nursing Times, 89*(5), 26–27.

Lehman, A.G., Dixon, L.B., Kernan, E., & Deforge, B. (1995). *Assertive treatment for the homeless mentally ill.* Paper presented at the 148th annual meeting of the American Psychiatric Association, Miami, FL, USA.

Marshall, M., Gray, A., Lockwood, A., & Green, R. (1999). Case management for people with severe mental disorders (Cochrane Review). In *The Cochrane Library, Issue 1.* Oxford: Update Software.

Marshall, M., & Lockwood, A. (1999). Assertive community treatment for people with severe mental disorders (Cochrane Review). In *The Cochrane Library, Issue 2.* Oxford: Update Software.

Marshall, M., Lockwood, A., & Gath, D. (1995). Social services case-management for long-term mental disorders: A randomised controlled trial. *Lancet, 345,* 409–412.

Marx, A., Stein, L., & Test, M. (1973). Extra-hospital management of severe mental illness. *Archives of General Psychiatry, 29,* 505–511.

Marx, I.M., Connelly, J., Muijen, M., Audini, B., McNamee, G., & Lawrence, R.B. (1994). Home-based versus hospital-based care for people with serious mental illnesses. *British Journal of Psychiatry, 165,* 179–194.

McCrone, P., Beecham, J., & Knapp, M. (1994). Community Psychiatric Nurse Teams: Cost-effectiveness of intensive support versus generic care. *British Journal of Psychiatry, 165,* 218–221.

McGrew, J.H., Bond, G.R., Dietzen, L., & Salyers, M.P. (1994). Measuring the fidelity of implementation of a mental health program model. *Journal of Consulting and Clinical Psychology, 62,* 670–678.

Merson, S., Tyrer, P., Onyett, S., Lack, S., Birkett, P., Lynch, S., & Johnson, T. (1992). Early intervention in psychiatric emergencies: A controlled clinical trial. *Lancet, 339,* 1311–1314.

Mohan, D., Thompson, C., & Mullee M.A. (1998). Preliminary evaluation of supervised discharge order in the south and west region. *Psychiatric Bulletin, 22,* 421–423.

Morse, G.A., Calsyn, R.J., Allen, G., Tempelhoff, B., & Smith, R. (1992). Experimental comparison of the effects of three treatment programs for homeless mentally ill people. *Hospital and Community Psychiatry, 3,* 1005–1010.

Morse, G.A., Calsyn, R.J., Klinkenberg, W.D., Trusty, M.L., Gerber, F., Smith, R., Templehoff, B., & Ahmad, L. (1997). An experimental comparison of three types of case management for homeless mentally ill persons. *Psychiatric Services, 48,* 497–503.

Mueser, K., Bond, G., Drake, R., & Resnick, S. (1998). Models of community care for severe mental illness: A review of research on case management. *Schizophrenia Bulletin, 24*(1), 37–74.

Muijen, M., Cooney, M., Strathdee, G., Bell, R., & Hudson, A. (1994). Community Psychiatric Nurse Teams: Intensive support versus generic care. *British Journal of Psychiatry, 165,* 211–217.

Muijen, M., Marks, I., Connolly, J., Audini, B., & McNamee, G. (1992). The daily living programme: Preliminary comparisons of community versus hospital based treatment for the seriously mentally ill facing emergency admission. *British Journal of Psychiatry, 160,* 379–384.

NHS Management Executive. (1994). *Introduction of Supervision Registers for mentally ill people from 1 April 1994.* HSG [Health Service Guideline], 94, 5.

Pinfold, V., Bindman J., Freidli, K., Beck, A., & Thornicroft, J. (1999). Supervised discharge orders in England: Compulsory care in the community. *Psychiatric Bulletin, 23,* 199–203.

Quinlivan, R., Hough, R., Crowell, A., Beach, C., Hofstetter, R., & Kenworthy, K. (1995). Service utilization and costs of care for severely mentally ill clients in an intensive case management program. *Psychiatric Services, 46,* 365–371.

Richardson, G., Chiswick, D., & Nutting, I. (1997). *Report of the Inquiry into the Treatment and Care of Darren Carr.* Commissioned by the Berkshire Health Authority, Oxfordshire Health Authority, Berkshire County Council, and Oxfordshire County Council.

Rosenheck, R., Neale, M., Leaf, P., Milstein, R., & Frisman, L. (1995). Multisite experimental cost study of intensive psychiatric community care. *Schizophrenia Bulletin, 21,* 129–140.

Rosenheck, R., Neale, M.S., & Gallup, P. (1993). Community-oriented mental health care: Assessing diversity in clinical practice. *Psychosocial Rehabilitation Journal, 16,* 39–50.

Rossler, W., Loffler, W., Fatkenheuer, B., & Riecher-Rossler, A. (1992). Does case management reduce the re-hospitalisation rate? *Acta Psychiatrica Scandinavica, 86,* 445–449.

Scott, H., Johnson, S., Menezes, P., Thornicroft, G., Marshall, J., Bindman, J., Bebbington, P., & Kuypers, P. (1998). Substance misuse and risk of aggression and offending among the severely mentally ill. *British Journal of Psychiatry, 172,* 345–350.

Solomon, P., & Draine, J. (1995). The efficacy of a consumer case management team: Two year outcomes of a randomised trial. *Journal of Mental Health Administration, 22,* 126–134.

Solomon, P., Draine, J., & Meyerson, A. (1994). Jail recidivism and receipt of community mental health services. *Hospital and Community Psychiatry, 45,* 793–797.

South Australian Mental Health Act (1993), Part 5 Section 23 (5)–(8).

Stanko, E.O. (1998). *Taking stock: What do we know about violence?* Economic and Social Research Council Programme. Middlesex, UK: Brunel University.

Steadman, H.J., Mulvey, E.P., Monahan, J.M., Clark Robbins, P., Appelbaum, P.S., Grisso, T., Roth, L.H., & Silver, E. (1998). Violence by people discharged from acute psychiatric inpatient facilities and by others in the same neighbourhoods. *Archives of General Psychiatry, 55,* 393–401.

Stein, L.I., & Test, M.A. (1980). Alternative to mental hospital treatment. 1: Conceptual model, treatment progress, and clinical evaluation. *Archives of General Psychiatry 37,* 392–397.

Swartz, M.S., Burns, B.J., Hiday, V.A., George, L.K., Swanson, J., & Wagner, H.R. (1995). New directions in research on involuntary outpatient commitment. *Psychiatric Services, 46,* 381–385.

Tansella, M., & Thornicroft, G. (1998). A conceptual framework for mental health services: The matrix model. *Psychological Medicine, 28,* 503–508.

Test, M.A., Knoedler, W.H., Allness, D.J., Burke, S.S., Brown, R.L., & Wallisch, L.S. (1991). Long-term community care through an assertive continuous treatment team. In C.A. Tamminga & S.C. Schulz (Eds.), *Advances in neuropsychiatry and psychopharmacology. Vol. 1: Schizophrenia Research* (pp. 239–246). New York: Raven Press.

Tyrer, P., Coid, J., Simmonds, S., Joseph, P., & Marriott, S. (1999). Community mental health teams for people with severe mental illnesses and disordered personality (Cochrane Review). In *The Cochrane Library, Issue 2.* Oxford: Update Software.

Tyrer, P., Evans, K., Ghandi, N., Lamont, O., Harrison-Reed, P., & Johnson, T. (1998). Randomised controlled trial of two models of care for discharged psychiatric patients. *British Medical Journal, 316,* 106–109.

Tyrer, P., Merson, S., Onyett, S., & Johnson, T. (1994). The effect of personality disorder on clinical outcome, social networks and adjustment: A controlled clinical trial of psychiatric emergencies. *Psychological Medicine, 24,* 731–740.

Tyrer, P., Morgan, J., Van Horn, E., Jayakody, M., Evans, K., Brummell, R., White, T., Baldwin, D., Harrison-Read, P., & Johnson, T. (1995). A randomised controlled study of close monitoring of vulnerable psychiatric patients. *Lancet, 345,* 756–759.

Vaughan, P.J. (1996). The supervision register: One year on. *Psychiatric Bulletin, 20,* 143–145.

Vaughan, P.J. (1998). Supervision register in practice. *Psychiatric Bulletin, 22,* 412–415.

Wilson, D., Tien, G., & Eaves, D. (1995). Increasing the community tenure of mentally disordered offenders: An assertive case management program. *International Journal of Law and Psychiatry, 18,* 61–69.

Winterwerp v. the Netherlands. (1979). European Court of Human Rights, series A, 33, 24 October.

Wolff, N., Helminiak, T.W., Morse, G.A., Calsyn, R.J., Klinkenberg, W.D., & Trusty, M.L. (1997). Cost-effectiveness evaluation of three approaches to case management for homeless mentally ill clients. *American Journal of Psychiatry, 154,* 341–348.

Robert Ferris is Consultant Forensic Psychiatrist and Clinical Director, Department of Forensic Psychiatry, Oxford Clinic, Oxford, UK.

Author's Note

Comments or queries may be directed to Robert Ferris, Department of Forensic Psychiatry, Oxford Clinic, Littlemore Mental Health Centre, Littlemore, Oxford, Oxon OX4 4XN, UK. Telephone: 44 1865 223 118. Fax: 44 1865 223 348. E-mail: <Rob.Ferris@oxmhc-tr.anglox.nhs.uk>.

TREATMENT OF MENTALLY ILL OFFENDERS IN THE COMMUNITY

A Clinical Perspective

PETER GOTTLIEB
ASMUS FINZEN

Treatment Instead of Punishment

Marcus Aurelius, a Roman emperor in the second century AD, has often been cited for the following comment on a case of matricide on which he was consulted by a local governor:

> If you have clearly ascertained that Aelius Priscus is in such a state of insanity that he is permanently out of his mind and so entirely incapable of reasoning, and no suspicion is left that he was simulating insanity when he killed his mother, you need not concern yourself with the question how he should be punished, as his insanity itself is punishment enough. At the same time he should be kept in chains; this need not be done by way of punishment so much as for his own protection and the security of his neighbours. (Spruit, 1998)

And right up to the present, the concept of Not Guilty by Reason of Insanity has remained more or less intact.

Mental Hospitals

Ironically, it was not until after "the liberation" of the mentally ill around the year 1800 by Pinel that mental hospitals began to be built in the Western world, and locking up—institutionalization—became the solution for society as well as for the patients. Thus the discipline of psychiatry was, from the beginning, closely connected with a custodial setting. The building of hospitals in the old style and in isolated rural, often very beautiful, surroundings ended by and large at the turn of the 20th century. However, at the end of the 20th century the thinking of psychiatry is still centred around the old mental hospital. This is illustrated when we speak of intramural versus extramural services, about inpatients and outpatients—as if psychiatry necessarily has to relate to a hospital surrounded by walls.

S. Hodgins (ed.), Violence among the Mentally Ill, 409–416.
© 2000 *Kluwer Academic Publishers. Printed in the Netherlands.*

Psychiatry in the Community

It is only quite recently that psychiatric services have been established in the community. After the Second World War, new, efficient drugs and financial wealth previously unseen in the Western world, as well as the extension of liberties and human rights to the mentally ill, gave policy-makers the virtually inalterable idea of closing down the old institutions. "La libertà è therapeutica," declared the Italian Franco Basaglia (Finzen, 1980), and the idea spread throughout the Western world.

Mentally Ill Patients and Criminality

During the era of institutionalization, prevention of criminality and violence among the mentally ill was not a great problem. In 1936 an internationally respected authority on psychiatry, the Danish professor August Wimmer, published a textbook for medical students (Wimmer, 1936). The book comprised some 500 pages and covered every known aspect of psychiatry. Not surprisingly, the description of schizophrenia took up almost one fifth of the book. Neuroleptics had not yet been discovered and the subject of treatment required only a single page, half of which was concerned with castration, abortion, and sterilization. On the subject of criminality among schizophrenic patients, a few lines were sufficient to cover the issue:

> Some cases exhibit more antisocial or criminal behaviour, especially in the initial phases—that is, before the patient is subject to internment in a mental hospital. However, it must be stated that, overall, schizophrenic patients rarely commit offences, particularly serious crimes.

As further illustration, a footnote added:

> In 1,577 consecutive court-ordered psychiatric evaluations, only 40 cases of schizophrenia were found.

Deinstitutionalization and Criminality

Since the introduction of deinstitutionalization, however, violence and criminality among the mentally ill have become major problems. This is not surprising when one considers that mental illness is accompanied by a variety of social handicaps. Many discharged patients will, understandably, have so much difficulty in procuring food, clothing, housing, and employment, in trying to structure their day, and in coping with alcohol and drugs that criminality may seem unavoidable.

Kramp and Gabrielsen (1994) found that the number of mentally ill patients sentenced to treatment for criminal behaviour in Denmark had increased by a constant 7% annually for 2 decades. Five years later, the same annual 7% figure is still valid. Not surprisingly, most criminal patients in Denmark suffer from schizophrenia, and—as opposed to findings for the United States and Canada (Steadman et al., 1998)—only very few belong to the affective spectrum.

A person with schizophrenia poses nine times the risk of committing a violent crime compared to a person without schizophrenia. That is the odds ratio found by Peter Kramp in a cross-sectional study of psychiatric and criminal files in Denmark. Hodgins, Mednick, Brennan, Schulsinger, and Engberg (1996) found corresponding elevated risks using Danish birth-cohort data in longitudinal studies.

Thus the decrease in the number of psychiatric beds has been followed by an increase in the risk of violent crime among mental patients. Kramp is currently in the final stage of data collection—county by county—in order to determine whether there is a close and direct connection between the two variables (Kramp & Gabrielsen, personal communication, 1999).

Outpatient Services

The quantity and quality of psychiatric services vary considerably from region to region. For example, two neighbouring areas, the canton of Basel in Switzerland and the region of Lörrach in Germany, are, psychiatrically, two different worlds. The Swiss region, with a population of 200,000, has 300 psychiatric beds, 150 practising psychiatrists, and 120 therapeutic psychologists. An outpatient unit employs 15 psychiatrists as well as other mental health professionals. Forensic patients are offered inpatient as well as outpatient services. There are halfway houses and sheltered institutions. The German region of Lörrach, just across the border, has 250,000 inhabitants but just five to six practising psychiatrists and one small outpatient clinic. The nearest mental hospital is 60 miles away. There are no specific forensic psychiatric services.

Similar differences may be found elsewhere. These appear to stem mainly from long-established local tradition. Another possible source of difference is the variation in opinion on the boundary between "mad" and "bad," which is always difficult to discern precisely. Thus, while the concept of "psychosis" is basically the same the world over, opinions can be nuanced and can vary a great deal on how broadly the definition of "mentally ill" should be understood.

Even when the boundary is undisputed, it may be subject to change over time—for example, after legislation has been amended (Grant, 1997). The elevated risk of violent behaviour by mentally ill persons seems to have increased in the decades since the introduction of deinstitutionalization, as a reflection of increasingly liberal ideas about patients' rights to autonomy in matters of treatment and care. For example, a comparison of Häfner and Böker's (1982) results with those of Lindqvist and Allebeck (1990) and those of Hodgins et al. (1996) shows that the more recent the study the greater the risk of violence among the mentally ill.

It may be that countries or cultures which regard the idea of personal freedom with the greatest respect tend to hold their citizens more personally responsible than more so-called socially oriented countries. Thus some persons who would be labelled mad in Central Europe or Scandinavia would, in the Anglo-American sphere, be held fully responsible—that is, labelled bad. The mentally ill patients in Sweden cited by Belfrage (1991), for example, seem to differ from those in the US cited by Wiederanders, Bromley, and Choate (1997).

One consequence of the above differences is that outpatient treatment programmes and their outcomes can be compared from one place to another and from one time to another only with great caution.

Another consequence of moving the treatment of forensic psychiatric patients to the outside—following the current trend in general psychiatry—is reduced capacity for managing the more severely personality disturbed among the mentally ill, many of whom will end up in prison because they are "untreatable" as outpatients and thus pose a risk to public safety.

The authors of this chapter believe that the literature, allowing for the above-mentioned differences in culture and scientific methodology, is in accord with common sense—that is, the best outpatient treatment depends on the availability of:

* the best inpatient treatment before discharge (Bar El et al., 1998)
* the best protection against alcohol and drug abuse and the best programmes to ensure compliance with medication therapy (Swartz et al., 1998)
* the best resources for housing, employment, and daily life within a flexible and stable social network (Wilson, Tien, & Eaves, 1995)
* the best staff training and supervision (Lamb, Weinberger, & Gross, 1988)
* the best collaboration among members of an interdisciplinary team of social, legal, and health professionals (Greenberg, 1998; Mendelson, 1992) and between general and forensic psychiatry (Nedopil & Banzer, 1996)
* the most vigorous reaching out to patients (Müller-Isberner, 1996).

In essence, outpatient programmes should be as flexible as possible in order to be able to assess and meet the special needs of each individual patient.

The Current Situation in Copenhagen

In recent decades the trend is to rely more and more on outpatient services, not only in general psychiatry but in forensic psychiatry as well. This trend has been obvious in many countries, including Denmark:

* While previously sentencing to inpatient treatment was the rule, in recent years the courts have been sentencing more and more mentally ill offenders to outpatient treatment. Although such sentencing allows for the possibility for their admission to hospital, the reality is that, overall, more and more forensic patients are being treated in outpatient settings.
* Psychiatric centres in the community are gradually becoming attuned to also receiving offender patients, even though these patients may be potentially violent and substance abusing.
* A new kind of facility for the homeless is appearing—a small unit in a social or pedagogical setting. The primary criterion for admission is that the person be both mentally ill *and* difficult to "integrate." The three most recently established communities of this kind in Copenhagen each house between five and 12 residents, nearly all of whom are mentally ill offenders.
* Nursing homes have increasingly been opening their doors to forensic patients. They have found that a sentence of treatment may function as a kind of safe-

guard, in that when a forensic patient causes trouble in the nursing home the sentence will be used to have him or her admitted to a psychiatric hospital.

- Mental health agencies and social services seem to be gradually realizing that cooperation is not only necessary but mutually beneficial, and potentially beneficial for the patient.

Data on forensic outpatients are currently being collected by Peter Gottlieb in an attempt to evaluate the change from inpatient to outpatient setting in the realm of forensic psychiatry. The data thus far collected appear to imply that mentally ill offenders treated in the community are at high risk of dying from drug overdose. At the moment, analysis of the data on criminal recidivism and relapse of mental illness is still in its initial phase.

Implications

When general psychiatry moves from intramural to extramural services the risk of criminality must be expected to increase, and when treatment of mentally ill offenders increasingly takes place in outpatient settings the risk of relapse and more criminality may again increase. The above-mentioned factors still seem to be the best explanation for the 3-decade-long and ongoing rise in the number of mentally ill offenders in Denmark. It might therefore be expected that more and more patients will eventually be assessed as beyond therapeutic reach and—in the interests of public safety—sent to prison instead of a psychiatric clinic.

Those who offer programmes for incarcerated criminal offenders are already establishing programmes for mentally ill patients. When asked if this is not a task for the mental health system, they respond by referring to "the real world," where mentally ill patients are, in ever-increasing numbers, trans-institutionalized from the health system to the mercy of the prison system (Porporino, 1999). This development has taken place not only in the US (Torrey, 1995) and Canada. According to recent publications (e.g., Birmingham, 1999), the trend can be found in the United Kingdom as well. Its spread to still other countries is demonstrated by, for example, the comment that the lack of outpatient facilities for mentally ill offenders in Austria has meant that general psychiatry increasingly regards treatment for these patients to be less a mental health responsibility and more a legal one (Knecht, Schanda, Berner, Morawitz, & Haubenstock, 1996).

A clinical approach is highly relevant. The now well-documented connection between violence and severe mental illness (see, e.g., Monahan et al., 1984; Steadman et al., 1998) implies that psychiatric intervention as soon as the illness breaks out is in the best interest of all parties, and also will serve as a kind of primary prevention of violence. To treat means not only to address symptoms of imminent danger like imperative commanding voices or delusional ideas of being persecuted and thus having to defend oneself; to offer treatment is to recognize the whole mentally ill person —to fulfil not only medication needs but also social needs in the broadest possible sense. In the psychiatry of today, most patients are treated in an outpatient setting, where the possibilities for legal coercion are limited. Thus, crucial to the success of treatment is the establishment of a therapeutic alliance between staff and patient.

If violence has already occurred, what is called for is secondary prevention—prevention against relapse. The ingredients are basically the same—that is, therapeutic means adjusted to the needs of the individual. However, in these cases there is an awareness that because violence has occurred once there is considerable risk that it will occur again. This is acknowledged in many pieces of legislation concerning outpatient treatment as well. Thus, different coercive options may be used when they cannot be avoided. The use of coercion can take many forms—from the subtle verbal hint to the patient to the open use of police force. Since rarely is violence effectively prevented by more violence, it could be argued again—and perhaps even more so than in the case of non-forensic patients—that the quality of the patient-staff alliance is of fundamental importance as a predictor of therapeutic success or failure.

Conclusion

A professional clinical alliance with the patient is characterized by keeping an objective overview of the situation while at the same time being subjectively "with" the patient in the situation. Thus if we are to improve our knowledge and skills in the best interests of our patients and of society, we need empirical quantitative as well as psychodynamic qualitative research on how to deinstitutionalize forensic psychiatry.

References

Bar El, Y.C., Durst, R., Rabinowitz, J., Kalian, M., Teitelbaum, T., & Shlafman, M. (1998). Implementation of order of compulsory ambulatory treatment in Jerusalem. *International Journal of Law and Psychiatry, 21,* 65–71.

Belfrage, H. (1991). The crime preventive effect of psychiatric treatment on mentally disordered offenders in Sweden. *International Journal of Law and Psychiatry, 14,* 237–243.

Birmingham, L. (1999). Between prison and the community: The "revolving door psychiatric patient" of the nineties. *British Journal of Psychiatry, 174,* 378–379.

Finzen, A. (1980). La libertà è therapeutica—zum Tode von Franco Basaglia. *Psychiatrische Praxis, 7,* 207–209.

Grant, I. (1997). Canada's new mental disorder disposition provisions: A case study of the British Columbia Criminal Code Review Board. *International Journal of Law and Psychiatry, 20,* 419–443.

Greenberg, D.M. (1998). Forensic psychiatric services. *Current Opinion in Psychiatry, 11,* 679–682.

Häfner, H., & Böker, W. (1982). *Crimes of violence by mentally abnormal offenders.* Cambridge: Cambridge University Press.

Hodgins, S., Mednick, S.A., Brennan, P., Schulsinger, F., & Engberg, M. (1996). Mental disorder and crime. *Archives of General Psychiatry, 53,* 489–496.

Knecht, G., Schanda, H., Berner, W., Morawitz, I., & Haubenstock, E. (1996). Out-patient treatment of mentally disordered offenders in Austria. *International Journal of Law and Psychiatry, 19,* 87–91.

Kramp, P., & Gabrielsen, G. (1994). Tilsynsklienter idømt psykiatriske særforanstaltninger. *Nordisk Tidsskrift for Kriminalvidenskab, 81,* 375–384.

Lamb, H.R., Weinberger, L.E., & Gross, B.H. (1988). Court-mandated community out-patient treatment for persons found Not Guilty by Reason of Insanity. *American Journal of Psychiatry, 145,* 450–456.

Lindqvist, P., & Allebeck, P. (1990). Schizophrenia and crime: A longitudinal follow-up of 644 schizophrenics in Stockholm. *British Journal of Psychiatry, 157,* 345–350.

Mendelson, E.F. (1992). A survey of practice at a regional forensic service: What do forensic psychiatrists do? Part 2: Treatment, court reports and outcome. *British Journal of Psychiatry, 160,* 773–776.

Monahan J. (1984). The prediction of violent behavior: Toward a second generation of theory and policy. *American Journal of Psychiatry, 144*(1), 10–15.

Müller-Isberner, R.J. (1996). Forensic psychiatric aftercare following hospital order treatment. *International Journal of Law and Psychiatry, 19,* 81–86.

Nedopil, N., & Banzer, K. (1996). Out-patient treatment of forensic patients in Germany: Current structure and future development. *International Journal of Law and Psychiatry, 19,* 75–79.

Porporino, F. (1999, May). Oral presentation at meeting of NATO Advanced Study Institute, The Prevention of Criminality and Violence by the Mentally Ill, Tuscany, Italy.

Spruit J.E. (1998). The penal conceptions of the Emperor Marcus Aurelius in respect of lunatics. *International Journal of Law and Psychiatry, 21,* 315–333.

Steadman, H.J., Mulvey, E.P., Monahan, J., Robbins, P.C., Appelbaum, P.S., Grisso, T., Roth, L.H., & Silver, E. (1998). Violence by people discharged from acute psychiatric inpatient facilities and by others in the same neighbourhoods. *Archives of General Psychiatry, 55,* 393–401.

Swartz, M.S., Swanson, J.W., Hiday, V.A., Borum, R., Wagner, H.R., & Burns, B.J. (1998). Violence and severe mental illness: The effects of substance abuse and non-adherence to medication. *American Journal of Psychiatry, 155,* 226–231.

Torrey, E. (1995). Jails and prisons—America's new mental hospitals. *American Journal Public Health, 85,* 1611–1613.

Wiederanders, M.R., Bromley, D.L., & Choate, P.A. (1997). Forensic conditional release programs and outcomes in three states. *International Journal of Law and Psychiatry, 20,* 249–257.

Wilson, D., Tien, G., & Eaves, E. (1995). Increasing the community tenure of mentally disordered offenders: An assertive case management program. *International Journal of Law and Psychiatry, 18,* 61–69.

Wimmer, A. (1936). *Speciel klinisk psykiatri for studerende og læger.* Copenhagen: Ejnar Munksgaard.

Peter Gottlieb is associated with St. Hans Hospital, Roskilde, Denmark. Asmus Finzen is associated with Psychiatrische Universitätsklinik Basel, Basel, Switzerland.

Authors' Note

Comments or queries may be directed to Peter Gottlieb, St. Hans Hospital, Retspsykiatrisk afd. R, DK-4000 Roskilde, Denmark. Telephone: 45 46 33 46 06. Fax: 45 46 33 43 54. E-mail: <peter.gottlieb@shh.hosp.dk>.